THE SCIENCE AND ROMANCE OF SELECTED HERBS

USED IN MEDICINE
AND
RELIGIOUS CEREMONY

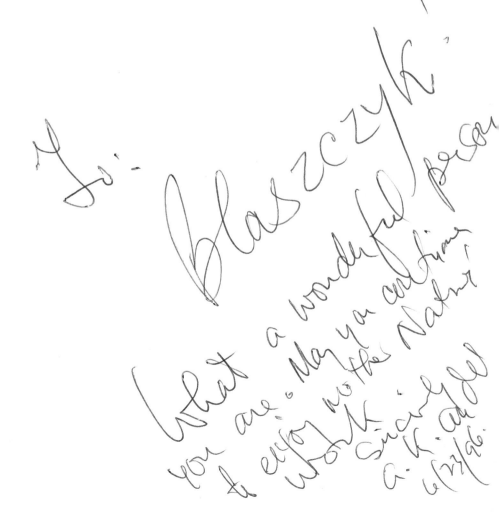

ABOUT THE AUTHOR

Anthony K. Andoh was born in Kumasi, Ghana, West Africa where his botanical training began at a young age; first, by his father's side, Joseph Andoh, a Kew-trained forest botanist, then later spending four years in Herbarium of the Forestry Department with another Kew-ite, botanist and taxonomist, Mr. Albert A. Enti, Fellow of the Linnean Society (London).

Thereafter he pioneered the developments of the first botanical garden at the University of Science and Technology in Kumasi. This project enabled him to investigate and experiment with the flora of the tropical and subtropical ecosystems around the world during his first four year tenure.

Andoh's success as a horticulturist and taxonomist earned him a four-year scholarship to the Royal Botanic Gardens at Kew in England. After completing his training at Kew, he worked as a government horticulturist in Zambia. During this time he took extensive field trips throughout the environs of Central and southern Africa.

Andoh came to America in the 1970's for further education in business administration, labor relations and arbitration and agricultural education. He has utilized all this training as a successful businessman in San Francisco, California where he grows rare and exotic plants along with important medicinal and spiritual plants.

He is the Director of the North Scale Institute, the education and research group dedicated to the preservation of ethnobotany and traditional medicine. The NSI has sponsored research into the medicinal and spiritual practices of indigenous cultures on a world-wide basis, and has published many books and articles on these subjects. Andoh was elected a fellow of the Linnean Society of London in 1988.

At the request of the Ghana Embassy in Washington, D.C. in 1988, Andoh began to work with the traditional doctors and herbalists of his native land of Ghana. As a member branch of the International Organization of Traditional and Medical Practitioners and Researchers headquartered in Zimbabwe, Ghana's traditional doctors were determined to raise the status and respectability of their healing art within their own nation and throughout the world. Andoh has been instrumental in bringing to the attention of the world the important work and the contributions to modern medicine of Africa's traditional healers.

As the North American representative of the IOTMPR, Andoh has also pioneered a quarterly journal on behalf of this Pan-African group of healers. *SANKOFA JOURNAL* is the authentic voice of the traditional healers of Africa. *SANKOFA* has given a voice to a people whose voice had never been heard; it will keep the entire world informed of the important developments in medicine and healing emanating from the continent of Africa.

THE SCIENCE AND ROMANCE OF SELECTED HERBS USED IN MEDICINE AND RELIGIOUS CEREMONY

by

Anthony K. Andoh

Director, The North Scale Institute
Education & Research Group,
San Francisco, CA 94116

Library of Congress Catalog in Publication Data

Andoh, Anthony K.
Library of Congress Catalog Card Number: 86-61735

First Printing, 1987
Second Printing, 1991

ISBN 0-916299-01-5   (CLOTH)
ISBN 0-916299-24-4   (PAPER)

II

Dedication

*This book is herewith dedicated to the great
assistance given by my Spirit Guide and in
fond memory of
JOSEPH EMMANUEL ANDOH*

TABLE OF CONTENTS

TABLE OF CONTENTS

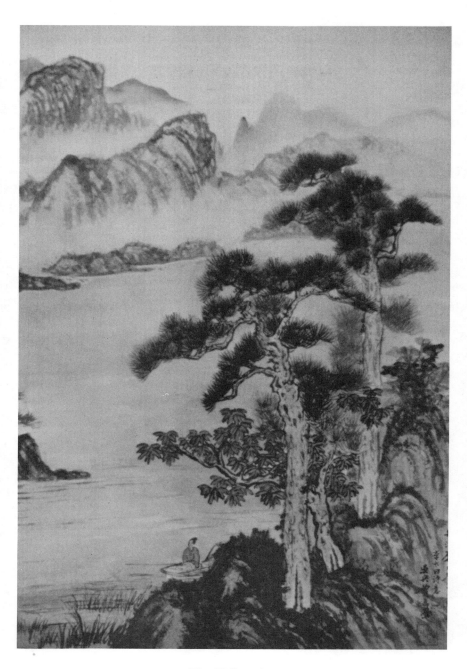

The Philosopher
Painting by Andrew Tseng, C.A., O.M.D.

FOREWORD

It is a great honor to be asked to comment on this very special botanical treatise done by Anthony Andoh, Ph.D., Agricultural Education.

Dr. Andoh has accomplished a feat worthy of the greatest botanist's life's work. He has painstakingly labored to scientifically and correctly classify some of the world's plants which are held in highest esteem, either for their medicinal value or for their religious and spiritual significance. In so doing, he has managed to demonstrate that legend and lore, as well as medicinal practices and herbal usage of traditional doctors, can be scientifically supported.

Traditional medicine on all continents and from all cultures seem to have a common beginning. Perhaps this knowledge of the healing wonders of the plant world is available to all persons through some source which we do not as yet understand.

Dr. Andoh has been pursuing the task of collecting data for this book for some eleven years and his meticulous work will, I am sure, be greatly appreciated by anyone interested in plants and especially students of ethnobotany. He deserves our gratitude for his perseverance and achievement.

This book is special in that it gives scientific data in an interesting, entertaining and intriguing manner. It opens the door for other scientists to take a more open-minded and investigative look at the healing practices of traditional cultures.

Further investigation must come soon, so as to preserve this ancient knowledge -- before it has been swept away and discarded, along with the trees and forests, by the new technology.

Andrew E. Tseng, C.A., O.M.D.
Professor of Traditional Oriental Medicine
San Francisco College of Acupuncture
San Francisco, California

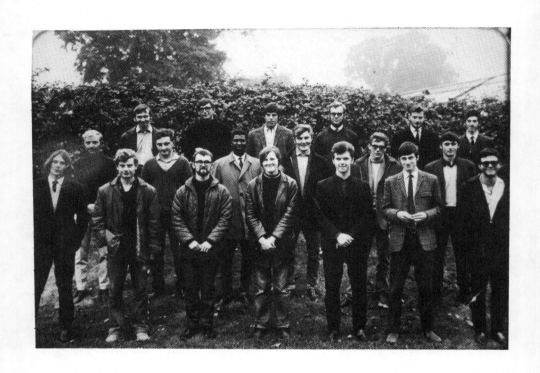

Anthony Andoh with classmates
Kew Gardens, England, 1969

ACKNOWLEDGEMENTS

I am greatly indebted to a number of people who have aided me in my botanical studies over the years. Special mention might be made particularly of the last five years which I spent in Southern Florida in preparation of this treatise. It is simply impossible to name and record my gratitude and appreciation to all those persons who assisted me in getting about the often difficult terrains and into the back countries in pursuit of the study of plant life in their natural habitats.

First, I wish to express my sincere gratitude to Mr. Albert A. Enti, formerly the Curator of the Herbarium, Department of Botany, University of Ghana, who sparked my interest in plant sciences at a very early age. My thanks go also to Mr. Gavin R. Paul, former Curator of the Botanic Gardens, University of Science and Technology, at Kumasi, Ghana, who right at the outset, introduced me to the diverse and complex lives of plants on a world-wide basis; I shall always feel indebted to him for his friendship and encouragement.

Special gratitude is extended to Mr. F.N. Hepper, Botanist in charge of West African Section, The Herbarium, Royal Botanic Gardens, Kew, England, for his friendship during my student years at Kew; Mr. Clarence Thompson of Warren County, North Carolina, U.S.A., an authority on the Tascorora Indians, who exposed me to the various medical and spiritual uses of the flora in that part of the world.

Among others, I am grateful to Dr. Paul G. Orth, soil chemist, University of Florida, Homestead, who made it possible for me to work at the Research Center in his department. His friendship, patience and understanding was beyond description. I also wish to thank Dr. Andrew Duncan, Horticulturist and Director of the Center where much of the manuscript preparation work was done, and also for the use of the library and much incidental assistance; Dr. Carl Campbell assisted me with plant identification of a number of the local species; Dr. Ken L. Pohrenezy, with whom I had the pleasure of undertaking research in *"Integrated Pest Management"*. Sincere thanks are due, also, to Dr. Jorge Parrado, formerly of the University of Havana, Cuba and currently an agricultural research officer at the Center. He assisted with nomenclatural classification and translation of Spanish vernacular names; and Dr. Malcolm Manners with whom I spent many happy hours botanizing at the Research Center Arboretum.

I am especially indebted to my companion on many field trips, Mr. David L. Williams, Sr., of the United States Air Force Base in Homestead. To the many Santeros of the chiefly Hispanic-owned Botanicas whom I came in contact with during this study, I owe a special gratitude. Special mention is made of Mr. A. Adriano, Santero and owner of Oricha Botanica in San Francisco, CA; Mr. Orelio Martinez, Santero and owner of La Caridad de las Mercedes Botanica; and Mr. Jorge Fonseca, Santero and owner of Tamiami Botanica, both at Miami, Florida. They not only brought me up to date on the significant role of the uses of local flora, including their geographical limits, but they did expose me to the spiritual uses of many plant species I encountered during the study.

For confirmation of some taxonomical names of local species in Collier and Monroe Counties, I wish to thank Mr. George N. Avery, of Dade County Chapter of the Native Plant Society of Florida. A very special gratitude is due to Ms. Nella R. Thomas, Librarian, Florida International University, Miami, for her innumerable hours of assistance in bringing current botanical literatures to my attention, and also for her assistance on local botanical expeditions. To Mrs. Janet Avery of Sweetwaters, Florida, whose interest in the local flora encouraged me to continue the research. To Mrs. Lizzie Dawkins, an adherent of the Santeria religion and a resident of Florida City, who urged me to write a simplified version of this treatise to aid the lay person. To Dr. Julia F. Morton, Director of the Morton Collectenea, Botany Department, University of Miami, who kindly gave me an authoritative book, *"Checklist of Native and Naturalized Trees of the United States"*, to aid me in my work. Dr. Frank Almeda, Chairman of the Botany Department, California Academy of Sciences at San Francisco, and Mr. Walden R. Valen, Director of Strybing Arboretum, San Francisco, are thanked for their assistance and encouragement and for making it possible for me to complete the nomenclatural classification of the treatise including botanical determinations and comparative studies of herbarium specimens as well as living plant collections.

Many thanks to Mr. Philip Mills, Chairman, Business Administration Department, Miami-Dade Community College; Dr. Zola Sullivan of Florida International University, for her undying faith in my efforts. Special thanks go to Adebowale Epega, American-born Babalawo and practitioner of the Yoruba religion, who provided the links between the traditional theology of *"Ifa"* and the contemporary practice of *"Santeria"*.

A very special gratitude goes to Dr. Andrew E. Tseng, Doctor of Oriental Medicine and Professor at the San Franciso College of Acupuncture, who not only provided information on traditional uses of herbs in China, but whose great artistic talent and sensitivity enhances the cover and pages of this book. His artistic expression of the natural landscape gives a universal feeling of oneness of mankind. Ms. Charlene Lynell Mattox, Chairman of the Board, Lynell 's Cosmetics, Ltd., is thanked for her understanding and appreciation of aesthetic beauty. She commissioned me to design and implement a major landscape scheme at her mansion in Burlingame, California.

I wish to thank my California mentors in the nursery and landscape business. First, Mr. Jim Wilson, proprietor of *"Peters & Wilson Nursery"* in Millbrae, California, who exposed me to the lucrative opportunities in the nursery business in California, the tastes and needs of the people. His 50 years of business in Northern California has made him a giant and authority on consumer needs. Thanks to Mr. Albert Wilson, author of gardening books and television personality, who gave me secret *"tips"* on conducting a proper landscape consulting business in California.

Many thanks to Louis and Sylvia Rosenberg, proprietors of the *"Sunset Garden Supply"* nursery in San Francisco; they gave me my first opportunity to see how the nursery business is managed in California.

God, himself, must have sent Mrs. Ada Williams to my aid. She is a San Francisco community *"pillar"* who saw my humble beginnings in the nursery and landscape business in San Francisco; she gave me the use of her vacant commercial property so that I could expand and grow and offer a unique garden center and *"plant clinic"* to the public.

There are no words to express my appreciation of those who are so very close to me, whose faith in me, dedication and unwavering belief in my abilities has brought me to this point. My deep appreciation goes to my father, the late Joseph Emmanual Andoh, formerly of the Forest Herbarium, Ghana Forestry Department, who encouraged and supported my interest in Botany by taking me on botanical expeditions from the age of seven. His spirit has continued to roam the forests and jungles of the world with me even today, showing me the way to the location of specimens I am seeking. To my mother Agnes Kate Andoh, who encouraged and supported my studies, through great hardships, after my father's death. She has earned a special place in God's Book reserved for Naturalists. Finally, I must thank Kali Sichen-Andoh, professional colleague, collaborator in botanical research and landscape development, trail buddy, companion, critic, editor, nurturer and wife for her unwavering understanding, support and efforts in bringing this work to completion.

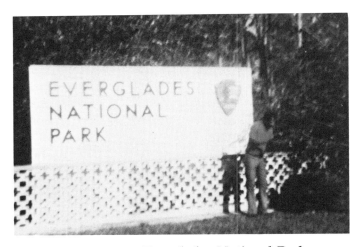

Entrance to Everglades National Park, Florida, 1981

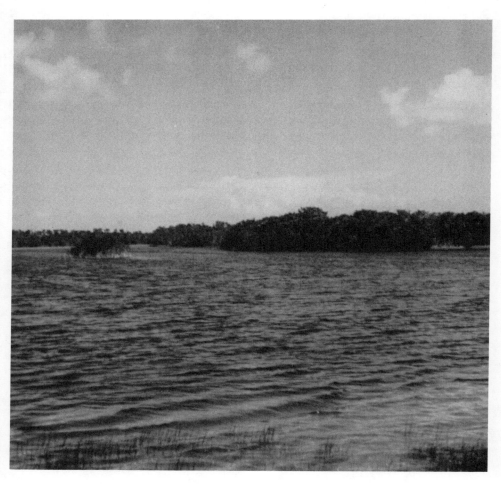

Sunset in the Everglades

PREFACE

Over the past nine years, I have been involved in ethno-botanical studies in search of the secrets of the natural steroid producing plants which are so much in demand by modern medicine. (Steroids -- a group of compounds containing four carbon rings interlocked to form hydrogenated cyclopentophenanthrene-ring system; it includes many hormones, cardiac glycones, bile acids and sterols.) These steroids have shown to be the salvation and life-sustaining force in so many diseases and bodily dysfunctions. Many plants are known to yield these steroids, the most important ones being some members of the families **Dioscoreaceae** and **Solanaceae**. Additionally, many kinds of aloes, yuccas, cassava and other less suspecting plants are known to contain a certain amount of these important compounds.

A considerable amount of time has been devoted to studying the ecological limits and intra-specific variations in these two families. As far back as 1973, I was afforded the opportunity to undertake botanical expeditions in Southern Africa to some of the less spoiled eco-systems where I encountered a number of these steroid-producing species. Extensive field work was undertaken in the vicinity of the River Zambezi eco-system in South-Central Africa between latitudes 15° to 25° South of the Equator, with a varying altitude from sea level to 3,000 meters. This area, encompassing the vast veldt, is botanically rich and contains a substantial number of these medicinally valuable plants. The vast sub-continent has been amply and correctly described as a botanist's paradise because of the profusion of diverse species of the flora and fauna, due to varying climatic and other edaphic conditions. One of the interesting plants I encountered being used by the inhabitants for kidney problems was **Dioscorea bulbifera** L., commonly called *"kiya"* in Chianga districts as well as parts of Sabi valley. Medicinal use of this plant is interesting from the standpoint of the *"Doctrine of Signatures"* as the stems bare aerial, kidney-shaped brown tubers; these are also edible.

I proceeded to undertake these botanical expeditions in the Western Hemisphere, beginning in Northern California, U.S.A. During the course of the study of native flora of the Pacific Coast, a number of the **Solanaceous** plants were found to flourish in this eco-system. Among them, **Solanum xanti** Gray, commonly known as violet nightshade, which is gregarious in southern California and up in the Sierra Mountains environs.

My movement proceeded toward the Southeastern Seaboard of the United States, concentrating in the Blue Ridge Mountain area, the highest mountain range in Eastern U.S.A., which is known to have the richest varieties of wild growing plants. Botanically speaking, this area is one of the most interesting sections of the continental U.S.A., there being more species per square foot than in almost all of the United States except perhaps in the Florida Everglades environs. This lavish collection of species, many of which are endemic to the area, is attributed to the variable topography and wide range of edaphic factors, including the prevailing climatic conditions. In traveling through the state of North Carolina, one can encounter plant growth which can be condusive to eco-systems as far south as the sub-tropical climes of 20° latitude, as well as plant communities one would normally associate with the temperate zones and colder climates of the far north. A great deal of America's crude drugs are produced from the area embracing the Blue Ridge Mountains. My private collection of botanical specimens, samples of which will be at the Smithsonian Institute and other herbaria, attest to the habitat, occurence and variation as well as their geographical distribution.

Continuing my expeditions to the sub-tropical Florida, I undertook extensive botanical surveys. I wish to quote my field notes of July 4, 1981, taken at Cape Sabel, a flat landmass area, being the southernmost point of the continental United States, and located at the periphery of the Everglades National Park, one of the most unique eco-systems in the world.

"Today is America's Independence Day, a general public holiday in the nation. It is celebrated just in the same spirit and exuberance which commonly characterizes the celebrations of similar historical significance around the world. On this particular day, I saw a film at the Park's auditorium on the state and philosophy of the National Park. One salient point that I learned from this film was that the eco-system of the Everglades Park ought to be viewed and treated as one entity rather than a series of unrelated components. A cardinal theme and perhaps the most basic message of the film was the fact that all living things, in some manner, are related to each other."

"This fact, while mainly important as a physical principle, carries implications even of a spiritual nature, for at this level of evolutionary dynamism something very remarkable and funda-mental is at stake -- the very existence of the local species as a link in the order of Nature."

"Today has been very wet, raining almost incessantly through-out the day, allowing me just enough time to roam about in this heaven. Finding myself in this environment made it one of the soothing and serenely happiest moments of my life. It reminded me of the Biblical "Garden of Eden", a concept which I believe was used and associated with the beginning of the creation of mankind; and for a very good and valid reason at that! I can vouch that association and proper appreciation with Nature in its true and authentic form, soothes the nerves. One cannot fail to come to grips with Life itself, especially when viewed from a close perspective of this profusion of diversified life forms. It clearly shows the eco-system as being a series of interrelated niches, all in harmony with each other and whose total sum equals the environment. Conversely, it could be viewed as a natural community in action, developing and restructuring its own environment and continuously altering it until the plants and animals that started there can no longer inhabit the area and must give way to others better adapted to live in the newly created environs. An orderly progression of such changes occur until, at last, a condition of balance or 'climax' is attained and the cycle begins anew."

"One cannot harm or endanger one species without threatening the life-line of a totally different species. In short, it can be seen as a perpetual chain that must be maintained at all times, if any semblance of equilibrium of life is to be sustained. Although the balance of nature is a complex business and often enough seems unattainable, I hold the view which is shared by many naturalists and aptly expounded by the late Aldo Leopold, the eminent ecologist who said that "Unless one approached conservation with an ethical as well as an economic perspective, the problem has not been adequately defined."

"From my own point of view, a lot of work remains to be done in this area in the form of educating the public. A concerted effort by the Federal Government and whole-heartedly supported by the individual states, with the full cooperation of the various business conglomerates must be undertaken. This action not only calls for the highest order of patriotism to conserve the natural endowments, it assures the individual a sense of preserving their own identity as well as their natural heritage. We have not inherited the earth from our parents, we have only borrowed it from our children."

"This is something we cannot fail to do in our time; long-term advantages far outweigh any other considerations if only we will compare and contrast the merits or benefits to be derived from undertaking these steps toward conservation. For example, if an oil company even dared to undertake prospecting for oil in these sacred grounds, I dread that day for the flora and fauna, many of which are now categorized as an endangered species. I do hope that the American people are not blinded by greed and short-sightedness. I do hope that my fears will fall on infertile ground."

"As I trekked the various areas of the Reserve, I encountered an area set aside and designated as a Mahogany Hammock. I found the vegetation here to be drastically different from the rest of the eco-system. It is essentially made up of a very few sparsely distributed species which consists mainly of pines, palmetto palms and mahogany trees, these being the dominant species of this area. The land is still completely flat with only a few clumps of species dotted here and there in the landscape. Most of the young mahogany trees in this area have a heavy infestation of bacterial gall attack. The symptom is similar to the attack on **Khaya senegalensis,** a true mahogany of the savannah scrub forest of Ghana and most of the tropical African eco-system. I had a strong feeling that I was back home in Ghana because of the similarity of the vegetation and climate, and I wondered if, at some time in antiquity, these land masses were joined together."

16

"This is the largest and finest mahogany hammock and contains the largest mahogany tree in the U.S.A. It is also the finest example of a tropical lowland forest in the Everglades. This hammock developed on an elevated island of the Miami oolite. Surrounding water excluded fire and allowed tropical forest rather than pine wood to flourish here. As noted from a guide post, Mahogany Hammock lies close to a transition zone where fresh and salt water begin to merge. Between here and Flamingo, another section of the Park, the water becomes increasingly saline as it flows toward Florida Bay. This sharply influences the landscape and the character of the vegetation changes completely. Rare Paurotis Palm grows well here in the transitional zone on salt fringes, though they are also found in fresh water."

Cape Sabel, Florida
July 4, 1981

While in the Everglades and its environs, I encountered and studied from a taxonomical standpoint no less than 50 species of members of **Dioscoreaceae** and **Solanaceae**. A number of these were introduced but have since naturalized in the Florida Basin. I also observed the cultural practices of a number of these plants. One in particular was **Solanum quitoensis** from Ecuador, seeds of which were furnished to me by Dr. Malcolm Manners of Florida Southern College, when he was working on his doctorial dissertation at the University of Florida Agricultural and Education Center in Homestead. It was while I was working at this Research Station that I undertook the germination tests of this species, the findings of which will be published along with cortisone and other steroid producing plants in a subsequent publication.

April 3, 1983
San Francisco, CA

INTRODUCTION

Our forefathers were true naturalists. They lived close to the earth and the elements of their environment, and they were meticulously observant of the cycles of birth, growth and decay of the ambient vegetation. Because they understood the interdependence between man, the surrounding flora and fauna and the seasonal changes, they were able to group herbs into categories which these ancient peoples claimed were governed by certain natural phenomena, including spiritual and planetary forces.

In the human cultures of antiquity, the reverence for plants has always formed the link between the physical and the spiritual worlds. Our ancestors intuitively understood the Biblical verse, *"To everything there is a season, and a time to every purpose under the heaven..."* (Eccl. 3:1).

Should you decide to delve into the numerous claims of these ancients, rest assured that you are in good company. Hippocrates, known as the father of Western medicine[1] believed that all physicians should be trained to understand the relationship between the physical and spiritual sciences so that the phenomena of natural affinities could be utilized for the betterment of mankind.

In conformity with this thought, Franz Anton Mesmer, M.D. (1734-1815) the father of modern hypnosis, wrote for his doctoral dissertation entitled **Physical-Medical Treatise on the Influence of the Planets** that *"... My purpose is solely to demonstrate that the celestial bodies act on the earth, ... that all things which are here act upon these celestial bodies in turn ... and that all parts are changing."* Furthermore, he stated, *"The dominant role of the planets was revealed in agriculture, navigation and medicine, more than any other disciplines."* Mesmer further denounced the trend of the medical profession of his era, whereby it was confined to the auspices of a few aristocrats. He stated, *"I have too much respect for Nature to be able to convince myself that the individual preservation of Man has been left to the mere chance of discovery and to the vague observations that have been made in the course of a number of centuries, finally becoming the domain of a few (medical researchers)."* In continuation, he stated also that, *"The further we advance in our knowledge of the mechanism and the economy of the animal body, the more we are compelled to admit our inadequacy."*

In contemporary psychology, we encounter Carl Gustav Jung (1875-1961), who utilized the concept of "archetypes" in explaining human behavior, his concept being based on ancient symbolism and mythology, which owe their birth to the mother science of cosmobiology.

---

[1] Scholars familiar with ancient medicine have generally always held the view that the foundations of true medicine really began with the Egyptians and *not* the Greeks. Most medical authorities are in agreement that the Egyptians had far more *"excellent physicians"* than the Greeks ever did. (*Theories and Philosophies of Medicine*; Institute of History of Medicine and Medical Research, Delhi, India, 1962; p. 15). And some American doctors and Egyptologists seem to feel that the *real* Father of Medicine should have been an ancient Egyptian priest-physician named Imhotep, who initiated an important medical society around 2750 B.C., and not Hippocrates, as is now the case. (John R. Green, M.D., *Medical History for Students*; Springfield, Ill.; pp. 15 - 17). It is generally recognized by now that the Greeks borrowed most if not all of their medical ideas from the Egyptians.

In the final analysis, the survival of man directly or indirectly, depends on the plants around him, for his food, medicine, clothing, shelter and spiritual nourishment.

Since time immemorial, the ancient people have always used plants as a guide to the perpetuation of their species and for their philosophical and spiritual development. Knowledge of the environment has always correlated with the level of civilization. Thus, we find scattered throughout literature of the ancients, how the total sum of the eco-system of any given civilization was preserved and held in awe as a monument to the benevolence of Nature.

Because of the importance with which the ancients attached to the natural world, and again on their pointed observation of the growth, behavior and usage patterns of certain plants, some selected plants gained a place of worship and high esteem within the society. Consequently, the worship of certain trees, shrubs, herbs and grasses, supposed to possess spirits, has at all times been practiced throughout the world. These practices still remain a part of all societal and religious activities, from the so-called *"primitives"* of the darkest Amazon and the Congo to the modern temples and cathedrals of Europe, including the Vatican.

In the Old World, especially Africa and India, there abound numerous such plants which are regarded as objects of veneration or esteemed as emblems of some special virtue. Thus, the myrrh, belonging to the family **Burseraceae,** genus **Commiphora,** with approximately 160 species, all of which, with the exception of perhaps a dozen, occur in Africa, was so highly regarded that it was one of the three gifts from the Wise Men to the Baby Jesus at the event of the Savior's birth.

Other plants are said to be possesed of a soul or the spirits of ancestors. An example here is the *"up-side-down"* tree -- the Baobab tree, known botanically as **Adansonia digitata,** endemic to the dry veldt of Africa. This particular tree has many uses also. The leaves, pulp, seeds and oil extract are edible, the shells are used as containers, the bark is used for making ropes and baskets, the roots, bark and leaves are used as medicine. It should be borne in mind that not all sacred trees possess great utility. Some are used to erect shrines (the Cedars of Lebanon) for offering of prayers, while others such as the Bo-tree of India (**Ficus religiosa**) is used as a canopy under which devotees sit to pray and meditate for enlightenment; Gautama Buddha himself received his calling while meditating under a Bo-tree.

Much of today's modern advancements and discoveries in science and technology is simply a *"re-discovery"* of ancient Egyptian knowledge and wisdom. In Adele G. Dawson's excellent book, *"Health, Happiness, and the Pursuit of Herbs",* she correctly alludes to the fact that much of the new information in pharmacology is simply an application of the profundity of the ancient civilizations. An example here is how *". . . the ancient Egyptians' use of the cabbage seeds to prevent intoxication. Today, cabbage juice is being used to treat alcoholism."* Garlic was so highly valued as a natural cure-all that *". . . fifteen pounds of it was the going rate for an able-bodied slave."*

In pursuit of advanced scientific investigation, I had the opportunity to live and work in Miami, Florida, dwelling among a large population of people of Hispanic descent from the Caribbean Basin and South America. One of the customs and belief systems which captured my attention and imagination was their practice of the

Santeria religion. Many of the rites of this religion so reminded me of religious rites of many of the West African cultures, that I was compelled to delve into the background and historical significance of the religion, especially from the point of view of the herbal preparations used in the rites.

The Santeria religion had its beginning with the arrival of the African slave trade in the New World. It has been suggested that, on the esoteric level, the sole purpose of the slave trade was to assure the preservation and propagation of the ancient Yoruba religion. As it is well documented in contemporary literature, the principles of the basic African religions correlate precisely with the ancient Egyptian Theology. Christianity was established as the state religion by Roman Emperors, Theodosius and Justinian, for the purpose of suppressing the practice of the Egyptian Theology in Rome, which at that time, was the religion of Isis. Remnants of the Isis religion still remain in the Roman Catholic Church as the *"Black Madonna"*, Isis with her son, Horus. The Romans actually adopted the Egyptian Theology from the Greeks who called it the Egyptian Hoi Aiguptoi which meant Black people.

The movement of missionaries into the heartland of Africa over the past four centuries had also as its prime objective, the suppression and obliteration of the African Theology which was quickly dubbed Paganism. Migene Gonzales-Wippler in *"Santeria"* (1975), states: *"Many advocates of the sect believe that Santeria is one of the new religions of the Aquarian Age. They believe also that the migration of the Africans to the New World was pre-ordained by spiritual forces in order to ensure a widespread belief in the 'Orishas' (African deities)."* She further asserts that *"some people go so far as to say that the entire slave trade was conceived as a means to ascertain that the African cults would find roots in the Americas, and from there, spread to the rest of the world."* If all these beliefs hold any truth, it is ironic that Santeria has actually taken the face of the very religion, Catholicism, which had intended to destroy its origin in the ancient Egyptian Theology.

It is well to remember at this time that Santeria is essentially a fusion between the Yoruba Pantheon and the Roman Catholic faith. The Yoruba is a nation with an ancient civilization which is located in Nigeria, West Africa. The necessity for the amalgamation of these two faiths was because the captive Africans were not allowed to practice their native ceremonies in the New World, so they had to hide behind the Catholic deities, this being the religion of the Spanish colonialists. Originally, the practices of the Santeria was confined to the Africans, but in time it has emerged as the dominant spiritual practice of the majority of the people of the Caribbean Basin and the South American mainland, crossing all socio-economic barriers and emerging in the governmental circles and the secular orders. It has become so acceptable from its inception as a practice of a *"bush people"*, that it now holds its own in the sophisticated places of Miami, New York, San Francisco, Los Angeles and throughout the metropolis of the New World wherever Hispanics are located. The conservative estimation of the number of followers now exceeds 100 million people. These followers hail from all classes and educational backgrounds, many of whom have turned to the Santeria after prayer and confession in contemporary church did not work to bring about desired results.

There is a striking similarity between the African Pantheon and the Greek mythology, with the Africans identifying God as the Universe, and everything in the universe being a manifestation of this One Supreme Being. Both the Greeks and the African have identified these manifestations of God in the personification of certain deities, who possessed distinct powers and virtues. In recent history, the fathers of these *"Greek Philosophies"* being Plato, Pythagorus, Socrates, Aristotle, Hippocrates, and Theophrastus have been revealed as students of the initiated Priests of ancient Egypt. Therefore, the doctrine of the *"One God"*, along with the philosophies which these Greek scholars were purported to have authored, indisputably have their origin on the continent of Africa.

The subject of the true origin of civilization and the knowledge of the ancients being preserved until modern times by the people of West Africa is treated extensively and in a most scholarly manner by Robert K. G. Temple in his invaluable book *"THE SIRIUS MYSTERY"*. In this treatise he presents the folklore and mythology of the Dogan people of Mali, West Africa. It appears that these people have preserved astronomical information which would have been much too far advanced for our modern astronomers even 50 years ago. Mr. Temple proves through innumerable references to ancient writings that the religion, mythology and philosophical beliefs of the Dogan people have a direct link to ancient Egypt. The Dogans live close to the site of the now destroyed University of Timbuctoo (Timbuktu) where many European scholars studied during the Middle Ages. Of the ancient Greeks and their myths he states . . .

"Perhaps some of the true meaning of the myths is now becoming evident. The ancient peoples were not concealing information from us out of spite. Their purpose in disguising their secrets was to see that those secrets could survive. In fact, so successful were the ancient Egyptians in accomplishing their purpose that the Greeks often preserve earlier Egyptian secrets in total ignorance of their true meaning, retaining only through an innate conservatism certain peculiar archaic details which we now find to be so important. Not only are the stories mythical and symbolical in that they are not meant to be taken at face value, but they even involve 'characters' and 'events' which have a strictly numerical significance . . . It is, admittedly, difficult for those of us who have been brought up in our strictly literal civilization, where there is no such thing as hidden meaning and everything is on the surface, to think in such a way as to understand the ancient myths. It was, after all, only a century ago that supposedly intelligent people were maintaining that the Earth was created in 4004 B.C., on the basis of what the Bible was reputed to have said! And it is only half a century ago that the courts of Tennessee in the famous Scopes trial decided that the theory of evolution was not only unholy but illegal and could not be taught in the schools. We mistakenly assume that because we have superlative technology and science we must also be extremely civilized and come from a subtle background of sophisticated thinkers. But this is all a base illusion."

Temple continues that . . . *"we are on a low rung of the ladder of evolutionary intelligence, and in many ways (such as ethics and aspirations to excellence) we have gone backward since those early mutants in our paltry intellectual history on this planet, Confucius, Socrates, the Buddha, and the others of whom every reader may substitute his own favourites."* Temple makes further reference to the herb *"saffron"* (**Crocus sativus**) by relating the myth of *"Argonautica"*, Jason and the

Golden Fleece. The fact that the true saffron has been confused with *"meadow saffron"* (**Colchicum**) until recent botanical history. Saffron has been used as a gout medicine since ancient Egypt and still remains one of the only medicines effective against the dread disease of gout.

The Yoruba people hailed from West Africa, along the bulge of the River Niger, and have a long and colorful history of being a well advanced civilization dating back as far as 3,000 years when they were producing exquisite works of art in bronze, gold, silver, ivory and other precious metals and stones. They had a series of Kingdoms, the Kingdom of Benin being one of their most advanced periods, flourishing from the 12th century A.D. to the late 1800's. The Africans had an intricate and intimate knowledge of their physical environment as well as a great wisdom of the entire universe in the form of astronomy -- knowledge which is just beginning to surface in modern astronomy with the advent of modern technology. Their medicine and social order were well advanced. The power within the society was held by the Oba (King) who was, at that time, also a priest in the religion. The Yoruba Kingdom began to disintergrate with the coming of the English and the ensuing deportation of the Africans to the Americas.

One of the ancient occult sciences of Egypt which forms a part of the present Santeria religious practice, has been the custom of the indigenous people of Western and Central Africa from time immemorial. What is now practiced by the Santeria of the Americas is known amongst the Yoruba people as *"Ifa"*. *"Ifa"* is the ancient art/science of divination. *"Ifa"* can be compared to the *"I Ching"* of ancient Chinese philosophy, and is a proven method of divination and prediction. According to the eminent African scholar, Professor J. A. Aboyomi Cole, in his treatise of *"Astrological Geomancy in Africa"* (1898). *"So ancient is the history of its (Ifa) introduction into the West (Africa) from the East (Egypt), it is to this day preserved in this fable:*

> *"In those early days of the world's history, when the gods associated with men and rendered them valiant help in all their struggles for existence, sacrifices were offered unto them. At these offerings they became so delighted that they came down from heaven in such great numbers that it was not possible to obtain sufficient meat to distribute amongst them."*
>
> *"Having cultivated the taste for flesh, and the worshippers not being able to supply all they demanded, the gods were therefore obliged to resort to various pursuits so that they might obtain food."*
>
> *"Ifa, the God of Divination, took to fishing.*
>
> *"On a certain day Ifa returned from the sea hungry and exhausted, having caught no fish, he thereupon consulted the god Elegba what to do.*
>
> *"Elegba, in reply, said that there was near the forest a farm belonging to Orunga, the son of the goddess Yemaja. It was planted by Odudua, the wife of Obatala (Heaven). It bore only sixteen nuts, and if Ifa can succeed to obtain the sixteen palm nuts from*

Orunga -- who now owns the lands -- he would, with them, teach him the art of Divination, by which food will be secured for the gods without resorting to labour; for everyone wishing to consult the Oracles will pay a goat, and knowing the anxiety of mankind to pry into the future, he was sure that the gods would thereby have more flesh than they would need, stipulating at the same time that first choice of all such offerings should be his."

"Ifa at once proceeded to the farm of Orunga. He bargained for the sixteen palm nuts, promising in return for them to teach Orunga how to forecast the future, assuring him that by this knowledge he will become very rich, and at the same time be of great service to mankind."

"Orunga went and consulted his wife, Orisabi, who agreed that they would part with the palm nuts, if by so doing they would become both rich and useful. Both of them set out to get the nuts, which they collected by the aid of monkeys."

"All sixteen in number, were wrapped in a bundle of clothes, and Orisabi tied the bundle on her back in the manner in which babes are generally carried, and she with her husband took them to Ifa."

"Ifa received and took them to Elegba, who taught him, as he promised, the art of divination; Ifa in turn taught it to Orunga, who thus became the first Baba-alawo (i.e., Father of Mysteries)."

Santeria received its name from the Spanish word, *Santo*, which means Saint, and connotes the worship of saints. The aim and purpose of the Santeria priests/priestesses includes the intervention into the life processes of their adherents. They do this by the use of offerings and sacrifices to these *"saints"*. This is coupled with the application of the will power to bring about a particular desire. This custom is similar to the belief system as practiced by the *"New Thought"* movement where the power of positive thinking, using prayer along with the application of a positive will power is stressed. Methods employed by the priests and priestesses are through the use of chants, medicinals, herbs, oils, incenses, candles, animal parts, dance, music, prayer and sacrifice. Although some priests engage in evil practices, most practitioners are dedicated to the spiritual enlightenment and enrichment of their adherents.

When the Africans found themselves in the New World, they had no choice other than to continue to practice what they knew to be effective medicine, as little concern was given for the physical and spiritual well being of the slaves. When illness befell these Africans, little sympathy was offered them by the masters, and often they were not given the benefit of a European doctor's care. Therefore, they collected herbs from their environment which resembled the medical preparations used in their native land. This gave rise to a greater exploitation of the *"Doctrine of Signatures"* aspect of traditional medicine, this concept still being widely used today.

This *"Doctrine of Signatures"* , according to Nicholas Culpepper during the mid-1600's, was developed by the ancients because they related the image of a plant with its metabolic action within the human body. Culpepper's view was that *". . .by the icon or image of every herb, man first found out their virtues."*

Some contemporary botanists, however, scorn this ancient *"unscientific"* belief as a superstition. It has been proposed that perhaps it was through this approach, nonetheless, which determined that an herb resembling a human organ will aid the healing of that same organ, that the first investigators actually were able to classify medicinals according to their mode of action. Even though man as a species is inquisitive by nature, he would never be so naive as to experiment too extensively with his life using unfamiliar plants. Therefore, it seems most appropriate that our first knowledge of the properties of plants was derived, in most part, from the *"Doctrine of Signatures"*.

Another important *'signature'* which pointed to the healing properties of herbs is the eco-niche within which a plant grows which tells the curative properties of the plant. For example, the willow tree which grows in damp places has been used in the treatment of rheumatism, a condition which results from exposure to cold and dampness affecting the body. One of the major progenitors of aspirin, salicylic acid, is related to the compound glucoside salacin, which is found in the bark of the willow. Aspirin is still most commonly used for treatment of the pain of rheumatism. The root plant ginsing, **Panax qinquefolia**, resembles the human form and is said to prolong life by benefiting the spleen. The traditional Chinese medicine considers the spleen as one of the most important organs in the body as it controls the blood.

Essentially, African and Santeria ceremonies revolved around the use of plant materials as a medium to employ the planetary forces and the gods to aid them in their worldly and spiritual endeavors. Customarily, one-hundred and one plants are required as part of the traditional ingredients known as the *"OMIERO"*, which is used in the initiation ceremony of the priests and priestesses of the religion. But this number has decreased owing to the unavailability of plants in this eco-system.

The *"OMIERO"*, the sacred elixer, is prepared with twenty-one crushed herbs mixed with either of the following, depending on the *"Orisha"* (African deity) for which the elixer is being prepared; sea water, river water, holy water, rum, honey, manteca de corojo, cocoa butter, cascarilla, pepper or kola nuts. Often some blood of an animal is added to the elixer. The resulting liquid has a very offensive smell caused by the herbs and the rapidly decomposing blood of the sacrificed animals. Nevertheless, the Santeros claim it has great medicinal properties, and everyone present at the ceremony eagerly drinks a few mouthfuls of the *'Omiero'* for good luck and better health. Also, beads and talismans which are to be worn by the initiates are soaked in the *'Omiero'* to increase their powers.

Because the religion was imported from West Africa, all of the plant materials were not readily available in the New World. Substitution for many of the ingredients became an absolute necessity for those plants which could not be obtained locally. As a result of the movement of people in the Caribbean Basin and the South American mainland, many of the practicing Santeros have erroneously been using wrong plants to prepare the sacred elixer *"Omiero"*. Even though the plant usage has sometimes been in error, this has not negated the value and spiritual significance of the *"Omiero"*, as the power of belief in the sacred elixer out-weighs the disadvantage of ignorance of botany

The purpose of this book is intended to fill a gap in botanical literature, a gap which becomes more noticeable as the interest and importance of knowledge of the medicinal practices of the traditional healers and doctors of Africa, commonly known as *"witch doctors"*, gains more recognition in the forefront of ethno-botany and traditional medicine. Indeed, this book has been written for scientists as well as laymen. It is a summary account of established knowledge and current research concerning the modern practitioners of an ancient tradition.

During the investigative studies for this work, one of the cardinal points which continually surfaced was the commonality of the spiritual principles which hold true between the African belief systems, Qabalistic, Greek and Egyptian philosophies and their deities. The spiritual and mental significance, mythological background and meanings/relationship to the cosmic forces, all seem to bare the same affinity. The old adage, *"We are the microcosm of the macrocosm"*, suggests that everything which exists in the universe also exists in the human body. This supports the fact of the interrelationship of all things, both physical and spiritual. This appears to extend beyond the racial, religious and cultural boundaries and alludes to a common origin of all knowledge and all life.

I have spent considerable time on the comparison of the *"Ifa"* to the *"Santeria"* Pantheon. As mentioned previously, *"Santeria"* is a fusion between *"Ifa"* and the Roman Catholic faith. It appears that there are discrepancies between the two Pantheons, perhaps as a result of the fusion as well as the fact of the oral tradition being passed down in another language, from the Yoruba and other West African dialects, to Spanish and Portuguese. These discrepancies were confirmed by Adebowali Epega, an *"Ifa"* Babalawo in Oakland, California as well as Ifayemi Eleburuibon, the Chief Priest and Babalawo of The Ancient Philosophy International House of Culture, Oshogbo, Nigeria. He has traveled throughout North and South America to attend and address conferences on *"Ifa"* and *"Santeria"*.

Even though the deities or *"Orishas"* are inconsistent between these two religions, there appears to be no desire on the part of the *"Santeria"* priests to change. We must remember that belief and faith in one's belief hold power over and above language barriers; therefore, though the *"Orishas"* may differ somewhat, the results are comparable.

This prevalence of herbal curative knowledge from cross-cultural origins has demonstrated the principle of *"signatures"* as being a basis for herbal medicine globally. Plant species which grow thoughout the world also appear to possess the same or similar healing properties, and are used in the treatment of the same type of physical dysfunctions,. regardless of the continent on which it is found. This fact suggests that, either there is a common origin of medical knowledge or that the principle of the Universal Mind, or the Race Consciousness, pervades all mankind, and that all truth is available to everyone who is open to receive it. This fact should certainly be applied to the healers, shamen, witch doctors and spiritual leaders, as they are the ones who prepare themselves spiritually to be receptive to this Universal Wisdom.

For these reasons above stated, I have included the *"romance"* of the named *"herbs"* as it appears in the lore of five continents, Africa, Asia (China, Middle East, India), Europe, North and South America, including the Caribbean whenever the information is at my disposal. To erase error insofar as the science of these spiritual/medicinals is concerned, I have gone to great lengths to systematically classify the plants and to give as much scientific data as is available for me to disseminate at this time.

In addition to the *"Twenty-one"* herbs of the *"Omiero"*, the sacred elixer of the initiated religious leaders of Santeria, I have also included additional plants which are known throughout the world for their religious, medicinal and spiritual significance. I earnestly hope that this work serves as a guide to assist serious students, botanists, pharmacists, chemists, and practitioners to identify the plants as they grow in their natural habitat, and that this work will serve as a guideline for further research and investigation into this most worthy scientific discipline.

It may seem at times that the information contained in the lore, legend and romance is superfluous. This information has been included, not because it is always true, but because such records should be included in the hope that this information will be sifted and checked by scientific experiments. Wherever possible, the results of such experiments already made have been recorded.

This books lists 446 species in 75 families of plants, occuring around the world, under their standard scientific binomials. 65 are illustrated or have photographs depicting important salient points pertaining to the species.

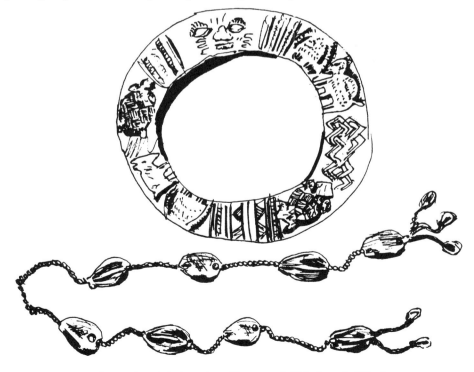

Yoruba "Ifa" Divination Tray and Diviner's Chain

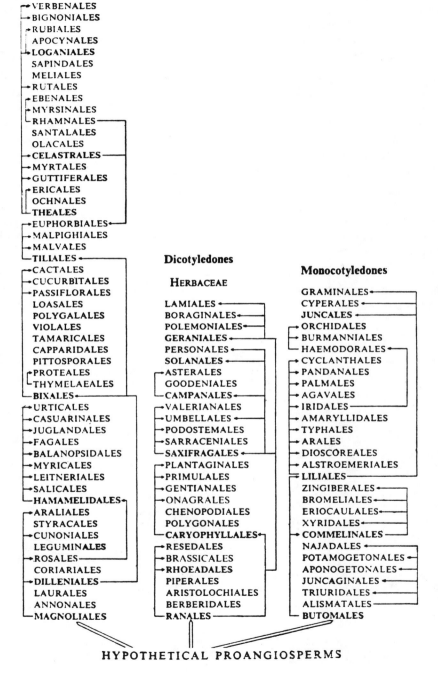

The range and order of natural groupings of families of plants
[After Hutchinson, 1973]

THE FORMAT OF THE BOOK

BOTANICAL NOMENCLATURE

The plants treated in this book are arranged in the following order. First, the *"TWENTY-ONE HERBS"* used in the Santeria religious ceremony have been arranged alphabetically according to the generic names. The remaining spiritual and medicinal plants are arranged according to THE KEYS TO THE FAMILIES OF FLOWERING PLANTS based on ENGLER'S CLASSIFICATION as given in "DIE NATURLICHEN PFLANZENFAMILIEN" and revised in his syllabus, Edition Seven.

I follow many giants in the field of taxonomy in supporting this system, which to many, may appear to be revolutionary. Understanding human nature and the reluctance to change, especially in these well established scientific fields, I look to the future generations of botanists who have opened their consciousness to the inter-relatedness of plants to their environment, not just to the microscopic determinations, in classifying plants. Throughout this work, I have on numerous occasions cited differences in plant species which could possibly be a result of edaphic factors. The old maxim, *"When in Rome, do as the Romans"*, also applies to the plant world as all living things must adapt to new environments, thereby subjecting themselves to change. I do hope that the mainstream of the Botanical Brotherhood will not judge me too harshly.

I leave with these two thoughts, first in reference to cytology, then to the hierarchical world of science and religion:

> *"When we probe the mystery of the cell*
> *We find even more mystery.*
> *When we probe the mystery of the Human Spirit*
> *We find Answers."*
>
> *Kali Sichen-Andoh*

and from the late Professor J. A. Aboyomi Cole

> *". . . And he who would employ the higher faculties of the Soul*
> *and thereby enter into the Sacred Temple of Knowledge,*
> *must be prepared to be regarded in the scientific world*
> *as a Maniac, and in the religious world as an Infidel."*

TAXONOMY

In its basic definition, taxonomy may be viewed as the study of the principles and practices involved in the orderly classification of both living and nonliving objects into appropriate categories on the basis of relationships among them. It should be pointed out that there are only two basic functions possible in the universe. These are analysis and synthesis; it is simply to divide and to unite. Thus, if anything is to be altered, some unit must be added to it or subtracted from it. This regularity forms the basis of all scientific work. Therefore, the scientist's first thought is to classify and measure his specimens. He deduces that *"this nightshade leaf resembles that nightshade leaf; this nightshade leaf is unlike this wormwood leaf."* The Scientific Method is understood and appreciated only when this concept is grasped.

The term taxonomy has come to be much more associated with the principles of biological classification since it was first introduced by the Swedish born French Botanist, A.P. de Candolle (1778-1841) in his *"Theorie elementaire de la botanique"* published in 1813. It is in this biological sense that *"THE SCIENCE AND ROMANCE OF SELECTED HERBS USED IN MEDICINE AND RELIGIOUS CEREMONY"* is concerned.

It may suffice here to mention that due to the era in which de Candolle lived, an era of rapid scientific development, he chose to concern himself with classifying the various methods and systems of classification. He postulated on the following two basic approaches for which he is remembered:

(1) Empirical Classifications: an arbitrary approach to naming objects, using as an example the alphabetical classification of initial letters as a standard norm.
(2) Rational Classifications: stressing the factual aspects of the objects classified. These were further sub-divided into three distinct groups, namely:
   (a) Practical Classifications: the value of the plants to us as a human species.
   (b) Artificial Classification: emperically devised approach to aid in the recognition and identification of unascertained plants.
   (c) Natural Classification: delineation of the factual natural affinities between plants.

DeCandolle felt that *"rational"* classifications were the only ones meriting serious scientific attention, and of these he favored artificial classifications in which, according to Hutchinson, 1973, it was shown that the relationships of plants were best ascertained by the comparative study of the structures and development of their organs (morphology) and not by their functions (physiology). This system of classification had many similarities and resembled the *"keys"* contained in contemporary botanical flora. Prior to the publication of de Candolle's *"Theorie elementaire"*, Lamarch in 1778 published his *"Flora Francaise"* of artificial classification on a large scale of what came to be known as a dichotomous key.

Just before the publication of *"Theorie elementaire"* a number of systems using all modes of morphological characters of the entire plant parts as a starting point in their classification, i.e., artificial groupings, had in fact, been broached.

It is interesting to note here that the most popular of these diverse systems was the so called *"sexual system"* which was proposed by the father of modern botany, the most lauded naturalist of all time, Carolus Linnaeus. Linnaeus was born in Sweden in 1707, the son of a Lutheran pastor, was educated at Upsala University, Sweden, in Medicine and eventually became professor of Medicine and Botany at Upsala. Linnaeus stressed the inflorescent nature of a plant as a primary basis of classification emphasizing their reproductive organs. He recognized twenty-four classes, determined mainly by the number, or some obvious character, of the stamens. The classes are sub-divided into orders according to the number of the styles. The simplicity and convenience of this novel system led to its universal adoption, and it held the field superseded by the more natural arrangement of Jussieu, and later of de Candolle.

The spectacular success of the sexual system lies in its own strength. This sexual system received an instant and overwhelming acceptance by the scientific community; its main strength lies in the ease of application and readiness of comprehension. It cannot, of course, be denied that the great personality of its author has a lot to do with its immediate wide acceptance. Although Linnaeus was a botanist, he extended his system of nomenclature to include animals and adopted as its basic unit the species, which were after the manner which had already been regularized by the French botanist Joseph de Tournefor. To Linnaeus as to many of his predecessors, genera appeared as a *"natural"* unit, comparable in this respect with the species of which they were composed of in the sexual system, the genera were grouped simply by reference to a few flora characters. In 1738, he published an account of sixty-five natural families, and a few years later he produced a *"Fragmenta Methodi Naturalis"*, a unique and unparalleled scientific work of its day which is known as the *"Natural Systems"*.

It can be said that Linnaeus brought orderliness to classification by instituting what became known as the binomial system of nomenclature. He believed quite early in his career, that the ideal classification would be one which gave full expression to this natural affinity.

In this system, he used two names (binomial) or words derived from Latin or Greek. This method of naming many organisms avoided the confusion in identifying particular plants and animals often called different names by different people. In the binomial system the first name of an organism is called the genus (plural - genera); the second name is called the species (plural species). The genus name is written with a capital letter and the species name is written with a small letter. The generic name of the common black nightshade is **Solanum**; the species name is **Solanum nigrum**, with **nigrum** being the specific epithet. With this system of naming living things, the scientific name of a particular organism is used and recognized by scientists and technical officers of any nationality, regardless of the language with which they are familiar. To the extent that this system, or approach is important and of absolute necessity would be appreciated when attempts are made to identify and classify at least the plants named in this book.

For a long time, people used simple descriptive words in naming plants or animals. We still do so today, but with the knowledge that each organism also has a scientific name. Names such as *"bloodroot"* give an immediate and unforgetable mental picture of a particular organism. However, the use of these names may lead to false notions. The red juice of the blood root plant is not blood. A catfish is not a fish with cat-like structures and functions. To add to this type of confusion, one region of a country may call a plant by one name, another region may give the same plant a different name. Scientific names prevent such confusion.

Linnaeus realized the weaknesses in using common names for both plant and animal classification, and Aristotle, who has been credited with being the first in Western science to devise a system of classification for living things, was grossly in error in his method of classification. It is interesting to note that in classifying plants Aristotle used the divisions -- trees, shrubs, and herbs. This seems fair enough but he grouped such diverse plants as moss and clover together as herbs because they grow close to the ground. Actually, clover is a flowering plant and moss is not. Also, an apple tree is grouped with a pine tree only because both are trees, with no consideration taken of the difference between them. Aristotle was completely unaware of the fact that a single plant family, such as the rose family, has representatives of all three groups of plants -- shrubs, trees and herbs. Included in this family are the rose, hawthorn, raspberry, and spirea, which are shrubs; the cherry, apple and pear, which are trees; and the strawberry, which is an herb. Where as these plants appear to be very different from one another, they are very much alike in their flower structure and in their methods of reproduction. As new varieties of organisms were discovered, Aristotle's method of classifying plants and animals became more confusing and more difficult to use.

Today we know that the possession of similar flowers is a more reliable guide to relationship than stems because flower structure is a stable characteristic. That is, stems may differ in size in response to environmental variations in light, temperature, soil, water and minerals. However, the form of flowers seldom changes in response to these environmental variations.

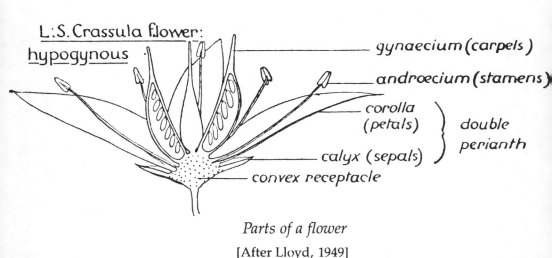

Parts of a flower

[After Lloyd, 1949]

THE SPECIES CONCEPT

When we speak about different kinds of living things, whether extinct or existing, we really mean different species of living things. Thus, a species is a taxonomic category subordinate to a genus and superior to a subspecies or variety, composed of individual specimens possessing common characteristics distinguishing them from other categories of individual specimen of the same taxonomic level. John Lindley in his *"Introduction to Botany, 1832"* wrote: *"A species is an assemblage of individuals agreeing with each other in all essential characters of vegetative and fructification capable of reproducing by seed without change, breeding freely together and producing perfect seeds from which progeny can be reared. Such are the true limits of a species . . ."* The idea of the interfertility between members of the same species and, by implication, sterility between members of different species, gives these definitions a strikingly modern ring.

In Linnaeus's system the species formed the basic units; downwards they were divided, if necessary, into varieties, whilst upwards they were grouped into genera, genera into orders and orders into classes.

Thus far, the species then is the basic unit, or building block, upon which the classification of living things is constructed. Following are the levels of division of classificaton:

Taxonomic Unit	Characters its members have in Common	Taxonomic Category	Rank
Primula vulgaris	18. Flowers pale yellow 17. Flowering stem very short or absent 16. Corolla-lobes flat 15. Flower-stalks with shaggy hairs	Species	Low ↑
Primula	14. Leaves all at the stem base 13. Corolla-tubes long 12. Fruits many-seeded	Genus	
Primuleae	11. Ovary superior 10. Fruit opening by longitudinal splits 9. Corolla-lobes not overlapping in bud 8. Roots fibrous	Tribe	
Primulaceae	7. Plants herbaceous 6. Flowers without bracteoles 5. Fruit a capsule 4. Ovary of 5 united carpels	Family	
Primulales	3. Flower-parts in fives 2. Ovary unilocular 1. Placentation free-central	Order	↓ High

TAXONOMIC HIERARCHY

Taxonomic Categories:

FAMILY
LABIATAE

RANKS

GENUS
Ocimum

SPECIES
Ocimum basilicum

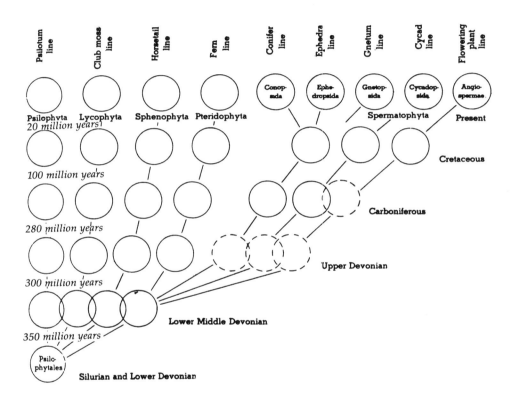

Evolutionary development of plants through geologic time.

THE PRINCIPLES OF MODERN TAXONOMY

Plant taxonomy, otherwise known as systematic botany, like any other branch of science, has its own principles or basis upon which it operates. The most important basis of classifying living things into related groups includes the following: The pattern of structure and function, the manner of development, similarities in the molecules making up the deoxyribonucleic acid (DNA) of cells, and adaptations the organisms possess that help them to survive. Essentially then, plant taxomony is concerned with the identification, classification and naming of plants.

DEFINING SPECIES

Species are distinct from one another in recognizable and subtle ways. Variation between species are discontinuous, i.e., they are not connected with one another by intermediate forms. Within species variation between individuals occur. This variation may not be uniformly distributed, but may give rise to local intra-specific populations that are recognizably distinct and are known as races. Finally, individuals of a species are interfertile with one another, but do not interbreed with individuals of other species. In other words, between species there exists barriers which prevent interbreeding. These barriers are genetically controlled and result in the reproductive separation or isolation of species from one another. If we summarize these features even more precisely we arrive at a definition of a species more or less as follows:

"A species is a series of intergrading and interfertile populations, recognizably distinct from other such series, and separated from other such series by genetically controlled barriers preventing interbreeding. Different species, therefore, are different such series. Hence: Specific name = generic name + specific epithet. This constitutes the binomial nomenclature or otherwise the binomial system as initiated by Linnaeus (1707 - 78).

THE SCIENTIFIC NAMING OF PLANTS

Nomenclature is the system of naming in the field of plant taxonomy or systematic botany. It is distinct from identification which leads up to classification; it is only there that naming becomes imperative. The purpose of a name is to act as an easy means of reference; in other words, to aid in communication. The naming of plants facilitates easy reference and further aids communications. Naming

- avoids descriptive phrases every time we need to refer to plants
- therefore stands for the object itself
- must be completely unambiguous
- avoids the breakdown in communication

The various common or vernacular names of plants often mislead and are not suitable for scientific purposes. For these reasons, it is imperative that scientific plant nomenclature adhere to one set of rules that would transcend all national boundaries. In order to achieve this, a set of rules known as the International Code of Botanical Nomenclature (ICBN) have been drawn which gives a guideline to the formulation and usage of all scientific plant names except those of cultivars which are governed by a separate code, the International Code of Nomenclature for Cultivated Plants (ICNCP).

One of the basic fundamental provisions of the International Code of Botanical Nomenclature is that scientific plant names must be in Latin. This provision at once overcomes the difficulty of the multiplicity of different languages while making common and vernacular names so unsatisfactory as a means of world-wide communication. Latin has been chosen as a language for two main reasons. First, it was in the past for a long time the common language of learned men of Europe, where the science of modern botany originated and first developed. Secondly, being a dead language, it avoids any element of national bias, and therefore any possible national jealousy which might have arisen had a modern language been chosen. It is no longer spoken as a native tongue by any people and its use avoids any such possibilities.

CITATION OF AUTHORITIES

Botanical names are written down followed by the name of a person (usually abbreviated); e.g., **Solanum nigrum** L. This is the authority citation and the person is said to be the author of the name concerned. Thus, Linnaeus is the author of the name **Solanum nigrum** L. The author of a name is the person who first published that name. His name is not a part of the botanical name but is often added for the purpose of precision. The author of a name may also be referred to as the authority for that name.

SYNONYMS AND SYNONYMY

Two or more names that are considered to apply to the same taxon are known as synonyms; i.e., synonyms are different names for the same plant. Thus we encounter **Eriosema andohii** Milne-Redhead with synonym **Eriosema cajanoides** Hook.f. partly.

Double citation indicates that there has been either a change in taxonomic position or a change in taxonomic rank. An example of a change in taxonomic rank is afforded by **Populus canescens** (Aiton) Smith. In 1789 Aiton described a new variety of the species **Populus alba,** for which he validly published the name **Populus alba var. canescens** Aiton. In 1804, Smith showed this to be a distinct species and raised Aiton's variety to specific rank, validly publishing for it the name **Populus canescens** (Aiton) Smith.

COMMON / VERNACULAR NAMES

The local common and vernacular names used in this publication as with all popular and folk names, must always be regarded critically and not as embodying complete accuracy. The reason for this is simple; the same name may be used for two or more botanically distinct plants; and conversely, the same plant may be known by two or more distinct popular names. When used with caution, however, popular names can often lead to correct identifications. One should always verify these identifications through botanical literature or through a herbarium.

CENTERS OF DIVERSITY

The Centers of Diversity is taken as the origin and distribution of a particular species. I have chosen this approach to indicate the geographical and ecological ranges within which the named species occur. This is not to say that locations named are the only places where the species occur, but that these are the genetical centers, the boundaries of the gene pools. According to deCandolle, 1882; ". . . *the region where a species is abundant is not necessarily its center of origin.*" Also, Vavilov, 1927, theorized conclusively that a center of origin was characterized by dominant alleles while towards the periphery of the center, the frequency of recessive alleles increased and the diversity decreased. The cause was an inbreeding and geographical isolation (drift). Vavilov further discovered "parallelism" which was especially clear for plants which belong to the same general group (annuals, herbaceous) and which are characterized by the same areas of distribution and have followed geographically the same route in their evolution. One point in Vavilov's theory is that a primary center is marked by a high frequency of dominant alleles.

GEOGRAPHICAL DISTRIBUTION

The present distribution of plants over the earth's surface also provides evidence supporting the evolutionary view. One example only can be mentioned here — the flora of the Galapagos Islands, 500 miles off the coast of South America. These islands are of volcanic origin and were formed in relatively recent geological times. Darwin found that of the 175 species of flowering plants occurring on the islands, 100 were not known elsewhere in the world. Some of these latter species, known as *"endemic species"*, belonged to genera which were also peculiar to these particular islands.

It seems clear that the species from the mainland which colonized the islands became so modified during the succeeding period that, by the time Darwin examined them, they had in fact evolved into new species. In some examples, the modifications had been so profound that they could not even be placed in the same genus as their relatives on the mainland.

Isolation by geographical barriers such as seas (as in the case of islands just considered) or mountain ranges often leads to the development of new species. This result is due to the fact that favorable variations arising after isolation will have a better chance of persisting than if free inter-crossing with the parent species were possible.

Genotype

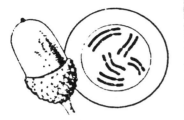

The genetic information stored in the chromosomes of the individual

Environment

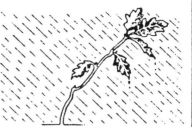

The sum total of the conditions affecting the individual throughout its lifetime

Phenotype

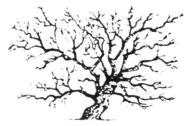

The physical structure and physiological make-up of the individual

Genotype + Environment = Phenotype

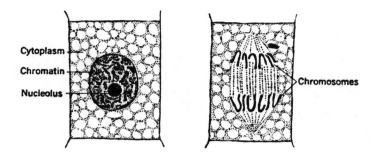

Cells of onion root tip

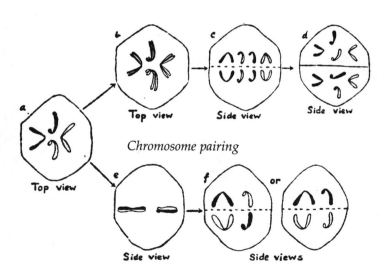

Chromosome pairing

Body cell divisions

Somatic chromosome number and genome constitutions are presented for each plant where this information is available. Most of the chromosome numbers are derived from Zeven et al (1975). In recent years, taxonomists have employed the shapes, numbers and form of chromosomes as an aid in identification and classification. Where the chromosome numbers could not be traced, a space has been left and hopefully these will be filled when scientific investigators have had the opportunity to work on them. Corrections, criticisms and any other related data on chromosome numbers would be highly appreciated. These should be sent to: The Editor, The North Scale Institute Publishing, Educational and Research Group, P.O. Box 27555, San Francisco, CA 94127.

Some groups of plants are relatively simple to identify, classify and provide with names, as for example, the Sugar Maple, Red Maple, Mountain Maple and Stripped Maple; each one is distinct in leaf, twigs and bark. But there are groups of plants which are extremely difficult, if not impossible, to identify and name using the conventional morphological characteristics. Any one who has grown mints will know and appreciate the difficulty gardeners and botanists alike have in classifying and ascribing names to these interesting and aromatically useful plants. Within the last three decades or so, the science of botany has provided a new tool to unravel the discreet relationships certain groups of plants have with one another which have baffled plant systematics for quite some time. This new scientific tool in taxonomy is cytology, the study of cells and their origin, including their structure and functions with particular emphasis on the chromosomes which have become important to taxonomy in two ways. First, because the chromosome numbers, sets and shapes often have taxonomic value in the same way as any other morphological character, and second, in a rather fundamental role, the link the organism has with its hereditary maternal past.

Thinly sliced root tips are usually treated in these taxonomic studies when chromosome numbers or hereditary units are observed. The information as to the chromosome numbers, sets and shapes often are very helpful. Examination of chromosome complements is now a routine operation in critical taxomonography in such plant groups as **Mentha** spp.; **Mentha rotundifolia** and **Mentha longifolia**, each of which has two sets of twelve chromosomes. Other species and varieties have four sets, as for instance, **Mentha spicata.** The stage at which the chromosome set is seen at its best is at the metaphase of mitotic division.

For taxonomic studies, it is customary to prepare sections of root-tips, young leaves or other meristematic tissues in which rapid cell division is in progress to obtain nuclei in this state, and to use differential staining techniques to make the chromosomes visible for microscopic study. The appearance of the chromosomes at mitotic metaphase is known as the karyotype.

Based on Heslop-Harrison, 1953, *"in referring to chromosome numbers in polyploid series, a conventional reference system is adopted. The base number of the series is symbolized as "X", so the lowest member of the series would have a* somatic number of "2X", a tetraploid, "4X", a hexaploid "6X", and so on. However, in the chromosome number of an individual plant, whether it is in a polyploid series or not the gametic number is symbolized as "N", and the "diploid" (somatic) number as 2n, even though it may be polyploid with the reference to the base number "X" if the plant happens to belong in a polyploid series.

It seems probable that the only variations which can be passed on to the offspring are those which are related to the actual mechanism of heredity.

In Mendel's experiments with peas bearing different types of seeds, it was seen that in the F_2 generation there appeared seed types differing from base of the parents (round, green seeds, for example). This example indicates the result of associating genes already in existence in various recombinations. This phenomenon of recombination is, in fact, one of the commonest sources of variation. It always occurs when sexual reproduction is followed by meiosis. This latter process, too, is always associated with crossing-over and, as we have seen, this leads to new combinations of characters.

BOTANY

Plants depend directly on the physical and chemical conditions of their environment, which are included in the science such as geology, meteorology and soil science. The study of botany is also intimately related to the applied sciences of forestry and agriculture. Furthermore, the fact that all animals depend upon a food chain which contains plant products as its fundamental link renders the study of vegetation a basic necessity in relation to all questions affecting animal nutrition.

Green plants, by the miracle of photosynthesis, capture a tiny fraction of the Sun's awesome physical energy and convert it into enough chemical energy to support all life on this planet. Without green plants, all living things would perish, and the Earth would revert to its original barren state. Mankind survives on the Earth only because green plants grow here. Indeed, "all flesh is grass". (Isaiah 40:6).

The relationship between man and plants has been very close throughout the development of human cultures. To quote from Professor Richard Evans Schultes, Director and Curator of Economic Botany, Botanical Museum of Harvard University:

"Through most of man's history, botany and medicine were, for all
practical purposes, synonymous fields of knowledge, and the
shaman, or witch-doctor — usually an accomplished botanist —
represents probably the oldest professional man in the evolution of
human culture."

It is generally believed in the scientific world that the Plant Kingdom consists of no less than 500,000 species. This figure, though incomplete, because of our lack of knowledge of the entire plant world, still represents a bewildering array of complex organisms, each of which is a different chemical factory. Of these plant species, only a fraction of a percentage plays any part in our economic lives, and hardly more than a thousand have any financial significance in international markets. But most astonishing, only 15 species of plants and nine species of animals provide almost all the food for the world's population (Janick et al., 1974; Ehrlic & Ehrlic, 1970). The

15 staple food plants are: rice, wheat, maize, barley, sorghum, sugar cane, sugar beet, potato, sweet potato, cassava, bean, peanut, soybean, coconut, and banana, the forage grasses and legumes, the fiber and forest plants. The nine principal domestic animals are cattle, swine, sheep, goats, water buffaloes, chickens, ducks, geese and turkeys.

No distinction between pure and applied science can be drawn in the case of biological studies, since a sound knowledge of taxonomy, morphology, histology, physiology, ecology, genetics and kindred subjects is directly relevant to all practical questions.

THE CHANGING ENVIRONMENT

Under natural conditions, the forms of plant and animal life which survive in a particular region represent a kind of *"balance of Nature"* in which constructive and destructive factors are in general equilibrium. The balance involves both the vitality of organisms and their surroundings.

In a mechanical sense, the balance of nature is not a simple balance, but a complex system of levers and links all balanced with each other, so that extra weight placed on any part of the system may cause the whole to change its equilibrium.

In the case of wild plants, it is largely a matter of chance whether the seeds or spores reach a suitable habitat, that is, a situation favoring their germination and healthy development. If they do reach a favorable habitat, they will establish themselves; otherwise they will perish or develop feebly. With cultivated plants it is different, for cultivation means that the plant is assured of a suitable habitat; then, once developed, the conditions are kept suitable, artificially by man so far as he is able. For example, soils are manured, they are ploughed, hoed and harrowed, and water is supplied when there is insufficient rain. It is not easy to supply suitable temperatures and light intensities outside, but this can be done in the greenhouse; and even soil temperatures are controlled in some cases by heating the soil by electricity or steam pipes. Light intensity, too, is not easy to control, though in the case of some valuable plants this is done by a system of artificial electric lighting to raise the intensity or the use of green glass to lower it. In controlling conditions, man has been able to make plants grow in situations which otherwise would be unsuitable for them.

In nature, there is a vast range of habitats, varying in the condition of the soil and climatic conditions. Each habitat tends to have its own distinctive vegetation, or plant community, consisting of species which, in the course of evolution, have become adapted to the particular habitat conditions. The study of this relationship between plants and their environment is called *"Ecology"*.

42

WHAT IS A HERB?

The standard definition is a plant whose part above ground does not become woody, that dies down every year, and is valued for its medicinal properties, flavor or scent. A spice, on the other hand, is defined as a pungent or aromatic plant used as a seasoning or preservative.

For the purpose of this book, I define a herb as a plant, woody or otherwise, that may or may not die down every year and is used for food and medicine, drink, flavoring, preservative or scent. This is a somewhat more inclusive definition, which allows us to include as herbs such medicinally valuable woody plants as myrrh, wintergreen, sage, and even Eucalyptus trees.

Readers are strongly warned against attempting to carry out cures mentioned in this book, as distressing results may occur. It is surely unnecessary to point out how easily a plant's identity may be confused, e.g. a poisonous plant may be gathered by mistake. Also, when so little is known about doses and so few facts are given here about dosage, the obvious danger here also should be evident to readers.

GLOSSARY

The glossary contained in the book is designed to assist the lay person and students alike in understanding some of the scientific information included. The purpose is to direct these persons who are interested in seeking out the medicinals, so that they may make correct identifications. It is also designed to assist the scientist who may not be familiar with the lore or mythology which is alluded to, and to direct his thought in the integration and the assimilation of this spiritual knowledge.

There are two separate glossaries, one devoted to medical terminology and the other to botanical science.

SUGGESTIONS FOR PRACTICAL WORK

Any serious study of taxonomy includes both theoretical and practical aspects. Taxonomy, like gardening, is essentially a down-to-earth activity. Theorizing on plant classification falls short of actual hands-on and eyes-on observation and focus. This book gives only the bare fundamentals of the theories of plant classification. The seemingly superflous bibliographical list of this work includes some excellent books on General Botany. For the serious student, this list should be consulted for further insights into plant taxonomy.

I must highly recommend these resource books in particular: *"The Families of Flowering Plants"*, J. Hutchinson, (1973); *"The Flowering Plants of Jamaica"*, C.D. Adams, (1972); *"Atlas of Medicinal Plants of Middle America"*, Julia F. Morton, (1981); *"New Concepts in Flowering Plant Taxonomy"*, J. Heslop-Harrison, (1953); *"An Introduction to Plant Taxonomy"*, C. Jeffrey (1968); *"Woody Plants of Ghana"*, F. R. Irvine, (1961); *"Diccionario Botanico de Nombre Vulgares de la Espanola"*, A.H. Liogier, (1974); *"Plants of the World"*, H.C.D. deWit, (1966); *"Flowering Plants and Ferns"*, J.C. Willis, (1966); *"A Dictionary of the Indigenous Plants of Yoruba-land"*, Royal Botanic Gardens, Kew, (1891). I used the foregoing resources extensively for this work, and I humbly pay tribute to these giants in the field of Plant Sciences.

The greatest tribute, however, must be paid to my Alma Mater, the Royal Botanic Gardens, Kew in England. Throughout my travels around the world, in meeting distinguished plant scientists, I realize that my education and training at Kew has prepared me to meet all these great scholars on equal footing. I now pray that Kew will be proud of this modest contribution to the field of plant sciences.

In spite of all the assistance and help that I received in the preparation of this treatise, any factual error or otherwise should rest solely on me and no one else.

For purposes of general familiarity with plant classification, the majority of the time should be devoted to the study of living specimens. Students should first acquaint themselves with the terminology of botanical description and the pertinent features of the most important families of flowering plants. To this end, I have included a limited section on botanical illustrations (pages 242-280) and a glossary of taxonomic terms (pages 281-288). Most cities and universities feature botanical gardens where a wide variety of plant specimens can be found growing; for the most part, they have been classified by family, genus and species, and when applicable, by cultivar. The observation of these specimens through their seasonal changes will give you a working knowledge of the basics of plant taxonomy.

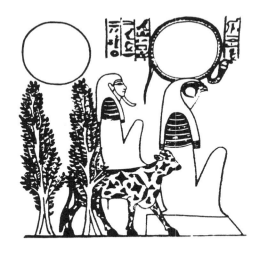

Balance of Nature—Ancient Egyptian

depiction of Nitrogen Cycle

ADDENDA

LEGUMINOSAE — Legume family

Since the times of Linnaeus some two centuries ago, there has been a trend toward breaking larger families of plants into smaller genera representative of fewer species. This trend tends to fluctuate, and appears to follow popular fashions, oscillating as the field of botany is further sub-divided into more confining specialties. The fact that there are still inconsistencies 200 years after the binomial theorem was generally accepted, suggests that this concept of smaller genera is less satisfactory as the recognition of differing groups varies.

Very few groups treated in this book are affected by this anomaly; the **Leguminosae** family being one where the greatest anomolies and inconsistencies arise. For instance, the distinguishing factors which characterize the *"unacceptable"* small genera within the **Cassia** complex are easier to discern than the characters which distinguish *"acceptable"* genera in the sub-family of **Leguminosae, Mimosaceae.** The factors which segregate **Caesalpiniaceae** as genera from **Mimosaceae** are not as clear cut. In the subfamily **Caesalpiniaceae**, genera can be based on the many different kinds of flowers, whereas in the **Mimosaceae**, the burden of genus definition is carried by the fruits and foliage, as the flowers are quite uniform.

The family **Leguminosae** is the third largest and most economically important family of all the flowering plants. This family contains 13,000 or more species, smaller only than the **Asteraceae (Compositae)** and **Orchidaceae,** but much more widespread than these groups and more cosmopolitan. The family **Leguminosae** has been subdivided into three subfamilies, the **Mimosoideae** with small actinomorphic flowers in dense inflorescens, and the **Caesalpinioideae** and **Papilionatae,** both with zygomorphic flowers. It has been the desire of some taxonomists to treat the subfamilies as full families and to raise the **Leguminosae** to the rank of the order **Fabales.**

Although this split would give the family **Mimosoideae** approximately 1500 species and **Caesalpiniaceae** about 2000 species, the **Papilionaceae** would still remain the third largest family of the plant kingdom. The one common characteristic of all **Leguminosae** is that the fruits are all formed from a single carpel, splitting along the dorsal and ventral sutures, and usually containing a row of seeds borne on the inner side of the ventral suture as in all pea pods. Another distinguishing factor is that the **Mimosoideae** and **Caesalpiniodeae** are mostly tropical whereas **Papilionoideae** species are both tropical and temperate plants.

PRACTICAL WORK SHEET FOR PLANT STUDY I

Botanical Name	**Family**
Common/Vernacular Name	**Chromosome Number**
Habitat	

Description	**Roots:**
	Stem:
	Leaves:
	Stipules:
Uses	**Inflorescence:**
	Flowers:
Lore, Legend & Romance	**Perianth:**
	Calyx: No. Sepals:
	Corolla:
	Form:
Gynoecium ( ) Female	**No. Petals:**
Androecium ( ) Male	

Student: **Coll. #:**   **Date:**

The Tree of Life

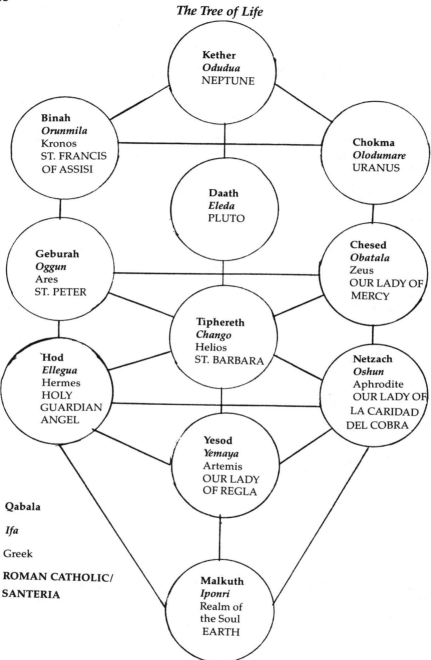

The TREE OF LIFE, stated simply, is a guide to the path one should take to reach one's fullest potential in spiritual development, thereby becoming the "Immortal Man." The above illustration reflects the Pantheons of the Jewish Qabala, the Santeria Pantheon along with their Catholic counterparts and the Greek Pantheon. This "Tree" represents the "Grand Man of the Universe" and expresses the descent of man from the Throne of God, as spirit, falling into matter to live bound by the body on Earth. This symbolic "Tree" teaches man how to climb back to the Throne of God through the unfolding of his consciousness.

THE TWENTY-ONE HERBS
of the
"Omiera"
The Sacred Elixir

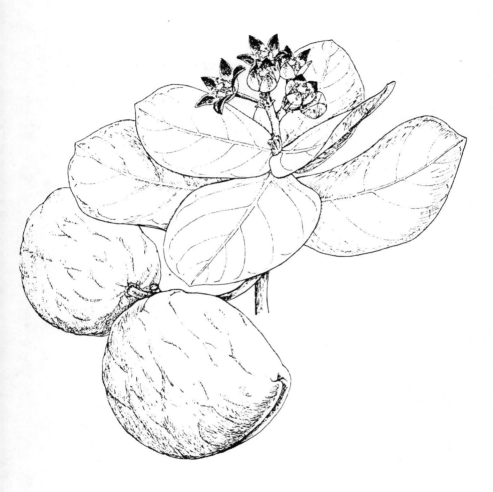

Calotropis procera

CALOTROPIS PROCERA (Ait.) Ait. f   Asclepiadaceae

Syn. Asclepias procera Ait.   **Milkweed family**

Centers of Diversity: Arid regions of Tropical Asia and Africa. Senegambia to Uganda, Egypt, Saudi Arabia and India. Introduced and naturalized elsewhere in the warmer parts of the globe.

Common/Vernacular Names: *English:* Sodom apple, Swallow wort, Dead Sea apple, Aurecula tree, Dumb cotton; *Spanish:* Algodon, Algodon de seda; *Africa:* Gbo-loba (Ghana), Bomu-bomu (Nigeria), Mpamba mwitu (Swahili)

Somatic Chromosome Numbers and Genome Constitution: 2n=(20), 22, (24)

Description: A shrub to small tree, gregarious in disused areas in South Florida and the West Indies, attaining 4.6–6 m in height. It exudes a white, milky latex. Leaves opposite and subsessile, greyish-green or hoary white, 30 x 15 cm, oblong-ovate, cordate at base, shortly acuminate at tip. Flowers white outside, with purple-brown tips, pinkish within, May-Dec. Fruits with inflated follicles, sub-globose to obliquely ovoid up to about 10 cm long; pericarp thick and spongy, seeds numerous, with silky white pappi.

Lore, Legend and Romance: This is one of the *"Twenty-one"* plants forming a basic ingredient in the sacred elixir used in the Santeria religious ceremony. The plant is claimed by the Yoruba deity, Obatala, the father of the gods, whose counterpart is Our Lady of Mercy of the Catholic faith. Obatala is accorded the dominion over bronchitis, asthma, tumors and earaches. Obatala, as father of the gods, it equated with the Chesed, the plane of love and mercy of the Qabalistic Tree of Life, while he has Zeus, the Greek god as his counterpart and is ruled by the planet Jupiter.

In Northern Nigeria, the pithy stems and leaves are burned and the smoke inhaled by the Hausas for asthma and coughs; they may also smoke the leaves in a pipe, like tobacco, for the same ailments. The roots, soaked in the latex, are pulverized and prepared in the form of candles and burned, the smoke being inhaled in India by people with asthma and cough problems. The bitter acrid root-bark, which has a characteristic odor, is probably the most important part medicinally. It is emetic and has been used as an *"ipecacuanha"* substitute, as a bitter tonic, and in mild cases of dysentery.

The latex is used by the Fulanis to curdle milk and cheese. Macerated plant, along with salt, or lye from ashes, is used in dehairing hides. The floss is used as cotton in Sierra Leone and weaves into a strong cloth. The plant is used in Ghana as an enema. The roots are used by the Ewes for a disease called kuku. In Northern Nigeria the root is pounded and macerated in water in which corn has been soaked. After standing 1–2 days the liquid is drunk copiously to cause vomiting and diarrhea, which it is believed expels the *"spawn"* of syphilis.

The dried, pulverized root-bark is used in parts of West Africa added to soup as a stomachic and for colic, and is believed to encourage lactation in women. The rootbark is used on the Ivory Coast for leprosy, alone or with **Antiaris toxicaria** and **Cochlospermum tinctorium** A. Rich. The charred roots and root-bark, usually made into ointment, are applied to skin eruptions, syphilis, leprosy, foul ulcers and camel sores. The bark is used in Senegal as an aphrodisiac. On the Ivory Coast, the bark is used, powdered or in decoction, for drinks and medicinal baths. In Ghana, barren women are treated by local application of pulverized, fresh leaves with pepper, while for difficult labor, a leaf poultice is applied to the abdomen. The latex is used both in Northern Nigeria and Ghana for conjunctivitis. In Sudan and India the latex has been used for internal and external application in abortion and as an infanticide.

In Curacoa, West Indies, the fresh leaves, with the upper surface outward, are bound on the head to relieve headache; also bound on sprained or swollen feet or on the soles of the feet when a cold is coming on. In Barbados, the leaves or latex may be applied on rheumatic pains or swellings. The latex has been employed in Colombia as a diaphoretic, emetic, vermifuge and antisyphilitic; it also is inserted into painful tooth cavities. In India, the latex and root bark are administered in cases of syphilis, giving rise to the term *"vegetable mercury."*

The resin contains isovalerate acetate of d-lactuceryl, d-lactucerol, and fomiate of isolacturol. From a pharmadynamic point of view, the digitalis-like properties of calotropin compared with other cardiotonic substances, and the emeto-cathartic action of the resin and the caustic action of the latex, all justify the various therapeutic uses of this plant.

Besides resins and gutta-percha-like substances in the latex, the bitter principle mudarin or asclepin is also present. Mudarin is bitter and is emeto-cathartic while calotropin, which is a glycoside, is cardiotonic, capable of causing death by heart paralysis, though respiration may continue for some time.

The latex contains a proteolytic enzyme and, like all other parts of the plant, the cardiac calotropin, which acts on the heart like digitalis, has shown anti-tumor activity. The floral nectar is said to be toxic. The leaves are insecticidal. The latex is a skin irritant; it has been used in Africa as an arrow poison.

In South Florida, many of the Santeros use **Gossypium hirsutum var. punctatum** (Schumach.) J. B. Hutch, a variety of Short Stapel Cotton or Upland Cotton as it is called in the Anglophone areas of the Caribbean Basin, as **Calotropis procera.** The plant under discussion **G. hirsutum var. punctatum,** is called Algodon, the same vernacular name applied to **Calotropis procera,** particularly in Cuba and Venezuela. This may have accounted for their choice and use. It is to be noted that there are many plants of totally different affinity but all bearing the name Algodon. Thus, the following plants are similarly called Algodon: **Gossypium hirsutum** L; **Asclepias curassavica** L.; **Hibiscus brachypus** Urb.; **Gossypium barbadense** L.

Gossypium hirsutum var. punctatum is a herb to small shrub which is sparingly cultivated in Jamaica. Native of the coasts and islands of the Gulf of Mexico, Florida, Bahamas, Dominican Republic and Cayman Islands. In Senegal, **Calotropis procera** leaves and fruits are hanged over doorways of dwellings as a protection against witchcraft.

CANELLA WINTERANA (L.) Gaertn.   Canellaceae

Syn. Laurus winterana L.   **Canella family**

Centers of Diversity: Southern Florida, Cape Sabel and the Keys; Bahamas, West Indies; on the drier islands to Barbados, Cayman Island. Common in thickets and woodlands in arid areas. **Canella** as a genus has about seven species ranging from Southern Florida through the West Indies to Colombia. Naturalized in Brazil and cultivated in Venezuela.

Common/Vernacular Names: *English:* Jamaica Cinnamon, Canella, Wild cinnamon, White cinammon; *Spanish:* Canela, Canela blanca, Canela de la tierra, Tuerco, Paratudo; *Africa:* Agbababubu, Origbo (Nigeria)

Somatic Chromosome Number and Genome Constitution: 2n=42, 48.

Description: A small to medium-sized tree attaining 12.3 m in height, native of the Caribbean Basin and Tropical America, including Cape Sabel in Southern Florida. The orange-colored, deeply fissured bark is bitter and aromatic and is used to be exported to a limited extent, chiefly from the Bahamas, for medicinal purposes. Leaves alternate or in whorls at the tips of the twigs; leaflets obovate to oblanceolate, rounded at the tip, cuneate and decurrent on petiole at the base. Flowers hermaphrodite, actinomorphic, crimson marked yellowish at base within, anthers bright red; berry globular about 1 cm long, turning red, 1–4 seeds; seeds black. It is prepared in the form of long quills similar to cinnamon, and yield about 1% volatile oil containing l-d-pinene, engenol, cineole, caryophyllene, about 8% resin and 8% manitol.

Lore, Legend and Romance: This is one of the *"Twenty-one"* plants of the *"Omiero,"* the sacred elixir of the Santeria initiation. It is claimed by the Yoruba deity, Oshún, whose counterpart is La Caridad del Cobre of the Catholic faith. Oshún corresponds with Netzach of the Qabalistic Tree of Life, the emotional sensitivity plane, and is equated with the Greek goddess of love, Aphrodite. It is under the rulership of the planet Venus. Oshún is reputed to have dominion over intestinal trouble and love philters.

In the West Indies the bark is used as a condiment and the twigs are thrown in the water to stupefy fish in order that they may be easily caught. The powdered bark with aloes is commonly called *"heira picra"* or *"pulvis aloes et canellae,"* and is used as an emmenagogue. In Brazil the bitter bark decoction is taken as a febrifuge and is gargled to relieve soreness of the tonsils. Puerto Ricans take the bark infusion as a tonic. In Cuba, the bark is macerated in alcohol and then later used as a rub for rheumatic pains. The bark decoction is taken to relieve indigestion and fever in new mothers.

I suspect that **Canella winterana** was substituted for **Canarium schweinfurthii** Eng, a Tropical African species, which is known by the Yorubas as *"Agbababubu"* and *"Origbo."*

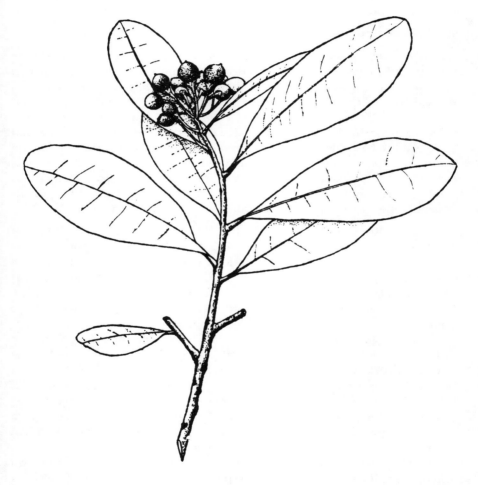

Canella winterana

CASSIA OCCIDENTALIS L.   Caesalpiniaceae (Fabaceae)

*Syn. **Ditremexa occidentalis** (L.) Britton & Rose*   **Pea family**

Centers of Diversity: Senegambia to Kenya, southwards to Cape Province, South Africa; Virginia to Indiana and south to Florida and Mexico; Caribbean Basin countries.

Common/Vernacular Names: *English:* Senna coffee, Florida coffee, Styptic weed, Wild coffee; *Spanish:* Yerba hedionda, Cafe negro, Brusca; *Africa:* Bazanfari, Rai-dore, Sanga-sang, Aborere, Kofi, Kere (Nigeria), Ananse-dua Ghana), Mrumbuzi (Swahili); *China:* Wan-chian-nan, Pi-hohono.

Somatic Chromosome Numbers and Genome Constitution: 2n=26

Description: A woody herb to sub-shrubby, sometimes with many stems radiating from the base and attaining one m in height. Leaves pinnate; leaflets 4–6 pairs or sometimes up to 8 pairs or more; ovate, lanceolate, acuminate, 10 x 4½ cm; closing at night and with a gland near the base of the petiole. Flowers nearly actinomorphic, yellow and showy. Fruits somewhat flattened to linear and abruptly beaked, measuring 15–20 cm in length, borne on woody peduncle; pods contain numerous broadly ovoid, small, dark olive seeds about 4 mm long. The plant is propagated from seed, preferring sandy loam and full sun to partial shade. Higher percentage of germination rate is obtained when seeds are placed in boiling water and left to set and cool in the water overnight.

Lore, Legend and Romance: This plant is one of the *"Twenty-one"* herbs of the *"Omiero,"* the sacred elixir used during the Santeria initiation ceremony. The herb is claimed by Elegguá, one of the most powerful deities of the religion, known as the messenger of the gods. He opens and closes all doors. His image is always kept on the floor, behind a door, as he protects the entrances to all the homes where he is kept. He is generally represented as a head made of clay or sandstone, with the eyes and the mouth formed with seashells.

All the importantYorubadeities that became part of the cult of Santeria were identified with Catholic images. Thus, Elegguá came to be associated with the Holy Guardian Angel and St. Anthony of the Catholic faith. An interesting and perhaps a remarkable resemblance exists between this deity and the Hod of the Qabalistic Tree of Life, this *"Tree"* having been described as one of the gifts of the New Age. Hod as a stage in the Tree of Life governs intellect and clarity in communications. Elegguá corresponds with the Greek god Hermes. Astrologically, the herb comes under the rulership of Mercury.

Cassias have had a remarkable and colorful history for a millenium. There is a recorded history of Cassia being one of the medicinal plants used in the ancient Babylon. The code of Hammurabi, the ruler of Babylon, engraved circa 2100 BC, mentioned the cassia plant as being among other medicinal species used in his day. These medicinal plants would later be used by the Semetic races who followed each other into the *"fertile valley."* The drug plants which Hippocrates used were few by comparison to the Indian and Egyptian practice; one of these, nevertheless, was Cassia.

Cassia as a name is an unfortunate one because of its application to totally different plants, different not only in structure, but also in their affinity. It has been suggested that there is more confusion of this genus than any other group of medicinal plants.

The Bible mentions qiddah (Exod:30:24 and Ezek:27:19) and qetzioth (Psalms:45:8). These two names are translated by botanical authorities as "*Cassia*." The word qinnamon which occurs in Exod. 30:23, Prov. 7:17 and Canticle 4:14 has very naturally been translated "*cinammon*." It is very doubtful indeed, in the minds of contemporary botanical authorities, if any of the above translations is correct. It has been suggested by many contemporary authorities that qinnamon, qiddah and qetzioth may very well be a species of **Cassia** but of different varieties, or that the passages refer to other aromatic products altogether, of which a number are mentioned elsewhere in the Bible. Examples are, Kashmir plant of the **Compositae** family, **Saussurea lappa** Clark, Orris root, botanically called **Iris germanica var. florentina.**

In the United States, the word "*cinammon*" is used identically with "*cassia.*" The cassia buds which are used medicinally, are the unripe fruits of **Cinnamomum cassia** and are imported from China. With slight exception, the Chinese make no distinction between the various species of Cassia; all the members are listed and treated as a source of drugs, especially for diseases of the eye. In Chinese herbal medicine, 3/10 of a pint of the juice of the seed forced into the nostril is considered to be an effective cure for epistaxis. **Cassia tora** L. is called "*Tsao-chueh-ming,*" yet the Pen ts'ao used the same vernacular name to ascribe to **Celosia argentea,** which incidentally, is also called "*the plant from Kunlun.*" The two plants, **Cassia tora** and **Celosia argentea** are used medicinally in the same way, their chief attributes being that of anti-scorbutic, anthelmintic, vulnerary and in the treatment of eye diseases.

All parts of **Cassia occidentalis** L. (seeds, roots, leaves) are used as a purgative, antiphlegmatic and antitoxic. The steeped root is used for gonorrhea and other hepatic troubles. The root infusion is used in Kenya for kidney dysfunction. The roasted and ground seeds which contain no caffein, are sometimes used in Cuba and elsewhere as a substitute for coffee. In Venezuela and Cuba, seeds are used for liver, stomach, asthma and malaria fever. A decoction is used as an application to sores, itch and inflammation of the rectum. Ointment from the leaves are used as dressing for sores by the southern Blacks of the United States. The roots are of value as a febrifuge either as an infusion or decoction. The root decoction with seeds are used for sore throat in Nigeria. The plant is used in Zambia for stomach aches and dysentery.

The seeds contain an oil, chrysarobin, 0.25% tannin. The root contains 0.3% methylanthraquinones. The leaves contain oxymethylanthraquinones. The leaves and flowers are used in Ghana as a vermifugal enema for both children and adults.

Raw seeds are toxic and roasting the seed destroys their purgative properties. As an edible herb, though not cultivated, the plant is used as food in Sri-Lanka. In West Africa, the leaves are used in the treatment of yellow fever and in the cure of skin diseases.

The plant is also used for colitis. In India, pulverized seed is taken orally in fever. It has been reported that its cultivation is supposed to be inimical to the root parasite, Striga, of cereal crop. The entire plant is used in Hawaii in the treatment of skin troubles such as ring-worm and similar skin diseases.

In Jamaica, the leaf decoction is given to children as an antidiuretic to overcome nocturnal incontinence; the decoction is drunk and applied externally to treat skin diseases. In El Salvador and Guatemala, the roots are said to be anti-spasmodic and the decoction is taken in cases of difficult menstruation, hysteria and rheumatism. In Trinidad, root decoctions or infusions are taken to alleviate inflammation of the womb and after childbirth.

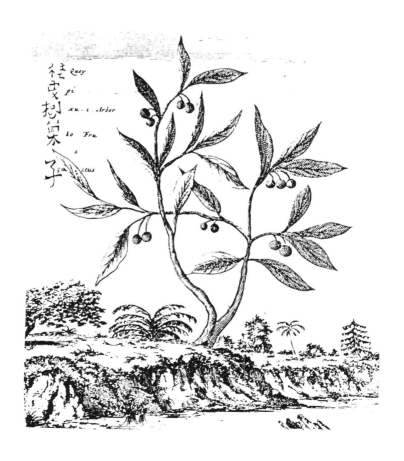

Cinnamomum cassia

Chinese illustration circa 17th century

CORCHORUS SILIQUOSUS L. — Tiliaceae

Linden Family

Centers of Diversity: Native to coastal thickets, especially on limestone, near seacoasts in Southern Texas, South Florida, the Bahamas, West Indies, Mexico, Central America and Isla Margarita off the coast of Venezuela.

Common/Vernacular Names: *English:* Broomweed, Slippery bur; *Spanish:* Malva té, Hierba té, Escova blanca

Somatic Chromosome Numbers and Genome Constitution: 2n=14

Description: An erect, bushy herb introduced into Florida as a fiber plant but now naturalized. The plant is woody at the base, taprooted, 50–120 cm high. Leaves ovate to lanceolate, acute or acuminate, glabrous or with a few hairs on veins beneath. Flowers solitary or two together, yellow tinged crimson. Gregarious on disused areas and thickets, mostly on oolitic (limestone) soils.

Lore, Legend and Romance: This is one of the *"Twenty-one"* plants used in the *"Omiero,"* the sacred elixir of the Santería religious initiation. The plant is claimed by the Yoruba deity Oshún, whose counterpart in the Catholic faith is La Caridad del Cobre. Oshún corresponds with Netzach, the plane of emotional sensitivity in relationships of the Qabalistic Tree of Life. She is also equated with Aphrodite, the Greek goddess of love; astrologically associated with the planet Venus. Oshún is credited with purification through spiritual bath.

The docoction of leafy twigs is taken as a treatment for venereal diseases in Yucatan. In Cuba it is a remedy for bladder troubles and also used for bathing the skin. Jamaicans have boiled the leafy twigs with leaves of **Piper umbellatum** and then taken the decoction, sweetened, as a remedy for colds and asthma.

It is postulated that the Africans who went to the New World had substituted **Corchorus siliquosus** L. for **Corchorus olitorius** L., commonly called Tossa Jute or Jew's Mallow, which they were familiar with in the Old World. DeWit confirms that **C. olitorius** comes from Africa.

Corchorus olitorius L. is commonly called Long-fruited Jute, Tossa Jute, Jew's Mallow, and in Ghana, it is known as Otoro. Its somatic chromosome number is 2n=14. Zeven, however, believes that the plant is native to South China and was probably taken to India/Pakistan. It is cultivated as a spinach in Ganges-Brahmaputra delta, where it may have run wild and escaped to the Middle East, Egypt, Sudan and Tropical Africa. It is a robust annual herb, 0.6–0.9 m high, usually woody towards the base with reddish stems. Leaves oblong-ovate, acute, truncated at the base. Flowers solitary or paired; sepals as long as or shorter than the petals, 7–8 mm long; seeds 1.5–2 mm long, rhomboidal. It is a mucilaginous pot herb much used in West Africa, and very popular in Sudan. The Zande (Sudan) and the Shuwa Arabs (N.E. Nigeria) sometimes dry and store the leaves, using potash later to break down fibers and shorten cooking time. It is used medicinally in Sudan.

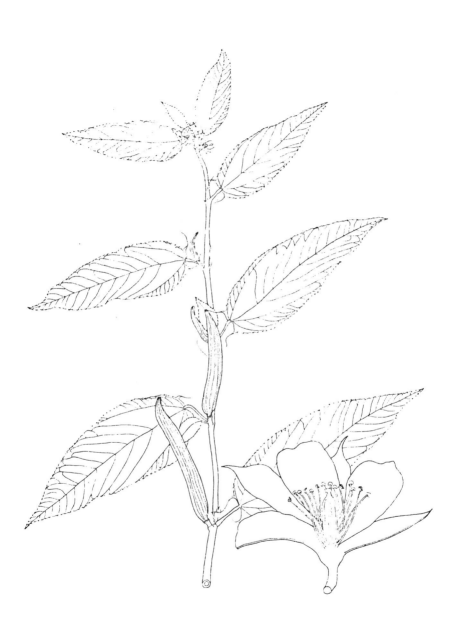

Corchorus olitorius

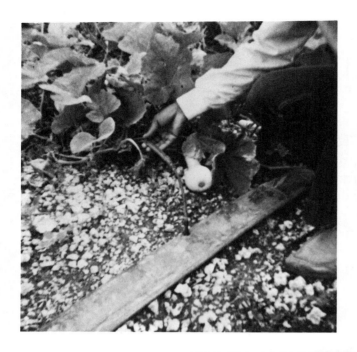

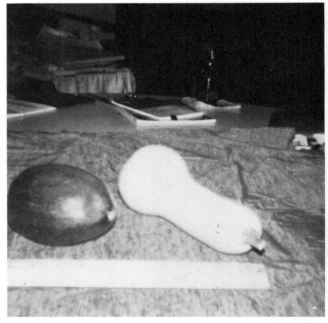

Cucurbita pepo—Golden Acorn Butternut variety. Univ. of Florida, Agricultural Research Center, Homestead, Florida. May, 1981.

CUCURBITA PEPO L.   Cucurbitaceae

Centers of Diversity: Native to Africa, but now cultivated and naturalized in South and Central America including the United States and the West Indies. It has been suggested that this species is a possible derivative of **Cucurbita lundelliana** Bailey, a wild gourd with somatic chromosome constituents of 2n=40, spreading into North Mexico and Southwestern United States. In Texas the related wild gourd, **Cucurbita texana** Gray is found. This species is either a weedy off-spring of **Cucurbita pepo** or may have been involved in the latter's formation. Whitaker and Cutler observed one seed, in a layer dated circa 8750 to 7840 BC, in a cave in Mexico. However, Mors and Rizzini (1966) confirmed its African origin in *"Useful Plants of Brazil."*

Common/Vernacular Names: *English:* Marrow, Pumpkin, Summer squash, Cold seed, Pompion; *Spanish:* Calabaza; *Africa:* Mboga (Swahili); *China:* Nan-kua, Nan-Kua-tz'u

Somatic Chromosome Numbers and Genome Constitution: 2n=(24,28), 40, (40-42, 44-46)

Description: An annual prostrating monoecious herb armed with tendrils whose dried oval, flat seed is used as a nutrient, and as an emollient, introduced into Europe in the sixteenth century. Edible fruits may weigh more than 45 kg. Flowers are yellow, campanulate, 5-lobed and up to 9 cm long.

Lore, Legend and Romance: This is one of the *"Twenty-one"* plants used in the elixir of the Santería religious ceremony. The plant is claimed by Oshún, the goddess of love and of gold, who is patron saint of the rivers. She corresponds with La Caridad del Cobre of the Catholic faith. Oshún is equated with Netzach of the Qabalistic Tree of Life, while it forms a natural affinity with the Greek goddess of love, Aphrodite. She comes under the rulership of the planet Venus and has dominion over burns, skin disease and whooping cough.

Many botanical writers are doubtful about Calabaza's true native home. It has been suggested that it is probably a native of Southwestern North America, for though no wild forms are known, related species abound in that region. The American Indians cultivated pumpkins in a number of forms long before the Europeans arrived. The Europeans took the plants back home, together with **Cucurbita mazima**, autumn and winter squash, whose edible fruits can be very heavy, and the mushy **Cucurbita moschata,** barbary squash.

The seeds, which furnish an essential oil, are also rich in methionine, an essential amino acid. These seeds have gained considerable reputation in the treatment of tape worms (taenia) by expelling them. The seeds are good in the treatment of scalding urine and affections of the urinary passages. The fruit is used for food, baked or boiled and made into pie. In Brazil, the seeds combined with coconut milk are employed in the treatment against tape worms, particularly in children.

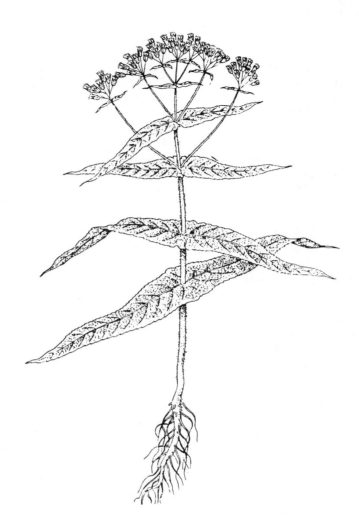

Eupatorium perfoliatum

The name squash is given in America to numerous varieties of gourds which bear variously-shaped fruits, ranging from ovoid to almost flat or shell-like forms. They are all extensively grown in the warmer parts of the United States where they are much appreciated as a vegetable. These varieties appear not to be suited to wet tropical climates. A variety, **C. pepo var. ovifera** (L.) Alef., is cultivated for its ornamental fruits.

It is interesting to note here that the staple food of the Native American diet was maize (corn) and pumpkin. Nutritional analysis shows corn to be deficient in methionine, an essential amino acid. At the same time, pumpkin seeds are shown to be exceptionally rich in methionine. The combination of the two vegetables makes a balanced, complete protein.

EUPATORIUM ODORATUM L.   Asteraceae (Compositae)

Syn. Osmia odorato (L.) Sch. Bip.   **Composite or Sunflower family**

Centers of Diversity: Southern Florida, Mexico to Paraguay, Caribbean Basin including Cuba; West Africa to Malaya; grows in proximity to rivers at medium elevation in almost all the Caribbean Basin countries and subtropical ecosystems; now a pan-tropical plant throughout the world.

Common/Vernacular Names: *English:* Bitter bush, Christmas bush, Jack-in-the-bush; *Spanish:* Rompe zaraguey, Alba haquilla, Hierba de chiva, Santa Maria; *China:* Tse-lan, Yeh-lan, Hsiang-Tse-lan

Somatic Chromosome Numbers and Genome Constitution: 2n=51

Description: A small shrub attaining 3.2 m or more in height; gregarious on disused oolitic soils. Leaves; truncate at base; Flowers white to light mauve, Nov.–April.

Lore, Legend and Romance: The plant is claimed by Changó. Changó's counterpart in the Catholic faith is the mystical St. Barbara. It corresponds with Tiphareth of the Qabalistic Tree of Life. Helios, the Greek god, corresponds with this deity. Astrologically, it comes under the rulership of the Sun. It is used to ward off evil influences by incorporating the leaves and flowers in the spiritual bath. The entire plant, including flowers, is used in the Santeria religious ceremony.

Medicinally, it is good for calming down nerves, especially for women. In Cuba, it is used for fever and skin diseases; the leaves and branches are used for rheumatism. In Brazil, it is used as diuretic, for diarrhea, intestinal colic and for the urinary system disorders.

According to the Pen ts'ao, the name *"tse-lan"* refers more to the genus **Eupatorium** rather than the species. The name of the genus **Eupatorium** is in honor of Mithridates Eupator, a king of Pontus about 120 BC, who supposedly discovered an antidote to poison among the species of the genus, **Eupatorium.** He was subsequently taken a captive by his enemies. He preferred death to captivity, and had one of his own men stab him to death for he had thoroughly fortified himself against poisoning. The genus includes over 400 species, quite a number of which are reputed to have medicinal virtues. Well over 80 species occur in the continental USA. Boneset and Joe-pye weed are among these species.

Boneset, with a botanical name of **Eupatorium perfoliatum** L., was never used as an antidote to poison, but it was a very popular antidote for colds and fever. The American Indians were the first to so use it. The Iroquois and the Mohegans used it for colds and fever, while the Menominees used it for fever.

It is reported as giving relief of stomach aches and general body pain. Until the advent of the publication of the *Materia Medica* of the United States, boneset was used by the Indians in intermittent fevers among other ailments. It was so much thoroughly used by them that the plant was associated with them and came to be known as Indian Sage. Through the 19th century, boneset continued to be held in high esteem for its healing powers, especially for fevers, particularly the variety called break-bone fevers. The name boneset is derived from the popular conception of the plant's efficacy in treating such cases. During the Civil War, boneset was recommended as a febrifuge medicine for Confederate troops. It is used in women's complaints of amenorrhea. It is most commonly used for grippe, laryngitis and as a decongestant.

In Barbados, Panama and Trinidad, the leaf decoction is a remedy for colds and coughs; in Jamaica and Cuba, for fever. Cubans also put it in baths to treat skin diseases. The root decoction is an emmenagogue. The plant is employed as a fish poison in India.

It is believed that the Santeros have used **Eupatorium odoratum** L. as a substitution for **Vernonia conferta** Benth. and **Vernonia amygdalina** Del. as these Yoruba species were not available in the New World. Another species of **Vernonia, V. biafrae** Oliv. & Hiern with Nigerian common names of *"Olubo,"* *"Ujuju"* and *"Ewuro"* is employed for the same purposes, the plant being used in Ghana for women's complaints.

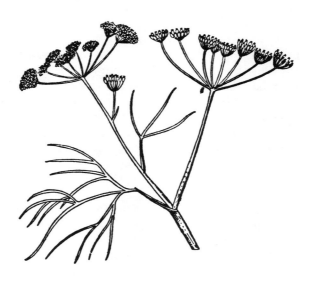

Foeniculum vulgare

FOENICULUM VULGARE Mill.   **Umbelliferae**

Syn. Foeniculum officinale Gaertn.   **Parsley or Carrot family**

Centers of Diversity: Indigenous to the Mediterranean countries. Cultivated there for a long time and has been introduced into many other temperate and subtropical regions of the world where it has naturalized in most regions.

Common/Vernacular Names: *English:* Fennel, Sweet fennel, Dill, Anise, Aniseed; *Spanish:* Anis, Hinojo; *China:* Shih-lo, Tzu-mo-lo, Hsiao-hui-shiang

Somatic Chromosome Numbers of Genome Constitution: 2n=22

Description: An erect biennial to perennial branched herb up to 2 m high with a white coating. Leaves finely divided into filiform segments, resembling feathers; peduncles 1.5–6.5 cm long. Flowers yellow, terminal in umbels with characteristic odor of licorice, bloom May–Sept. An almost obnoxious weed in disused places, especially Southern and Central California, where it is particularly abundant in coastal regions, occurring frequently on cliffs and sand dunes of the Pacific Coast. Cultivated for its blanched petioles in South France and Mediterranean region. **Foeniculum vulgare var. azoricum** (Mill.) Thell., Syn. **F. azoricum** Mill., *"Carosella"* or Italian fennel, originated in Italy.

Lore, Legend and Romance: The plant is one of the important ingredients of *"Omiero"* the sacred elixir used in the initiation ceremonies of the Santeria sect. The plant is claimed by the Yoruba deity, Oshún, who is generally credited with indigestion and hysteria. Oshún corresponds with Netzach, the emotional sensitivity plane of the Qabalistic Tree of Life. Her counterpart is Aphrodite, the Greek goddess of love. She comes under the rulership of Venus. Oshún further corresponds with La Caridad del Cobre of the Catholic faith. The plant is used to ward off evil spirits when carried on a person. When used as a *"tea"* it increases psychic ability.

    Ancient Egyptians, Hindus and Chinese used its seeds for spices. The Romans cultivated it for seeds and edible shoots. The fragrant fronds were made into garlands with which to crown victorious warriors. The name fennel is derived from the Latin foeniculum, supposed to be a variety of fragrant hay. Fennel was a symbol of success in ancient Greece and was called Marathon in reference to the famous battleground on which Greeks gained a victory over the Persians in 490 BC.

    In the words of the old master herbalist, Culpepper, those who are afflicted with obesity might take a consolation here. All parts of the fennel plant when used are in frequent demand as a condiment. The shoots of the young plant are considered to be carminative. The fruits are prescribed in fluxes, dyspepsia, colic, and other abdominal disorders.

    With carminative and purgative qualities, fennel expels wind, provokes urine, eases the pains of kidney stones and also helps to dissolve them. Fennel also can be a mother's friend, as the leaves and seeds boiled in barley water increase the yield of mothers milk and make it more wholesome. Fennel is the basis for the concoction called *"grip water"* used to correct flatulence in infants.

The fruits have been used as a carminative, stimulant, flavoring agent, galactogogue, aromatic, and stomachic and as a flavoring for other less pleasant medicines.

Fennel's principal constituents are anethol and fenchone, both volatile oils. In Southern Florida, there is a tendency of some of the Santeros to use **Pimpinella anisum** L., commonly called aniseed, as fennel. This is also a typical member of the plant family, **Umbelliferae.** Also used is **Anethum graveolens** L. commonly called dill and which yields an oil (Oleum anethi) which contains about 50% of carvone ($C_{10}H_{14}0$) and no anithole, and is often mistakenly used as fennel in South Florida.

INDIGOFERA SUFFRUTICOSA Mill. — Papilionaceae (Fabaceae)

Syn. Indigofera anil L. — **Pea Family**

Centers of Diversity: West Indies, Senegambia to Cameroon, and introduced into Central and Southern Africa and Madagascar. A native of tropical America, now a pan-tropical species.

Common/Vernacular Names: *English:* West Indian indigo, Guatemala indigo, Markham gunbo, Wild indigo; *Spanish:* Añil, Añil colorado, Azul de hojas, Plantanito de tinto; *China:* Lan-ts'ao, Lan-tien

Somatic Chromosome Numbers and Genome Constitution: $2n=12$

Description: A branched under-shrub up to 1.8 m high. Inflorescence brownish-hairy; pods reddish-brown, short with 5–8 seeds. A widely cultivated crop plant, especially in Southern and Central Africa and Tropical America. It forms a suitable perennial cover crop for coffee and for planting on contour ridges. Once much cultivated in the tropics for its dye. In the Caribbean Basin the plant is commonly encountered in rough pastures and disused lands. Flowers and fruit all the year.

Lore, Legend and Romance: This plant is claimed by Yemayá and Oshún. Yemayá corresponds withOurLady of Regla of the Catholic faith and is associated with Yesod of the Qabalistic Tree of Life. She also corresponds with the Greek goddess Artemis and astrologically under the rulership of the Moon. Oshún corresponds with La Caridad del Cobre, the patron saint of Cuba, and is associated with Netzach of the Qabalistic Tree of Life. The Greek goddess Aphrodite is Oshún's counterpart and she is astrologically associated with the planet Venus. Yemayá and Oshún are responsible for internal tumors and epilepsy.

The medicinal properties of indigo are said to be febrifuge, sudorific and antispasmodic. It is used as a diuretic. It is also used in herpes sores and in abortion. The plant causes diarrhea. It is used as a fish poison and insecticide. A number of **Indigofera** plants producing indigo are found in China, nearly all of which go by the common name of "Lan-ts'ao," the blue plant.

In West Africa, another plant belonging to the pea family is believed to be the original plant for which the **Indigofera suffruticosa** was substituted. The name for this plant is **Lonchocarpus cyanescens** (Schum. & Thonn.) Benth.

The common name for this plant is Yoruba indigo, or West African indigo. It is a shrub or weedy climber attaining 6 m in height. The flowers are reddish to bluish white, sweet scented and much frequented by insects. The flowers are in panicles, 30 cm long; pods flat, indehiscent, turning bluish-black on drying; May–June.

In West Africa, the ground roots are applied to sores. Women on the Ivory Coast drink the decoction of the roots and leafy stems after childbirth. The washed roots, boiled with other ingredients, are a cooling stomachic in Ghana. The roots are used in Sierra Leone for leprosy and cataract. The leaves are used as a poultice for ulcers of the foot and as a dressing for skin diseases.

The Indians in Panama drink the plant decoction as a blood purifier. The Mexican Indians take the plant decoction as a remedy for syphilis and they apply poultices to the heads of feverish infants. The physicians in Mexico declare that it is an effective antispasmodic and an effective treatment for epilepsy when 3-4 grams of the dried, powdered plant is taken daily. Experiments at the Medical University of Mexico have shown the physiological effects to be purgative by causing strong contractions of the lower bowel.

Some Santeros in Southern Florida and Cuba use **Indigofera lespedizioides** Kunth. as anil in the *"Omiero."* This is a perennial herb or undershrub 15–90 cm high. Leaflets 2–5 cm long, 4–10 mm broad, puberous on both surfaces. Flowers about 5 mm long, pink to reddish, July to Aug. Pods 1.5–3 cm long. Gregarious in pastures subject to periodic burning, and found most abundantly in Honduras and tropoical South America, Cuba and Dominican Republic.

INULA HELENIUM L.   Asteraceae (Compositae)

Syn. Helenium grandiflorum **Gilb.**   **Composite or Sunflower family**
Syn. Cornisaxtia helenium **Merat.**

Centers of Diversity: Central Asia; also wild westward to Central and Southern Europe. It is commonly grown in Europe, and has now made its home in temperate Asia, parts of India and is naturalized all over North America where it is encountered as a weed of roadsides and abandoned fields.

Common/Vernacular Names: *English:* Elecampane, Inula, Inul, Horseheal, Elfdock, Elfwort, Horse elder, Scabwort, Yellow starwort, Velvet dock, Wild sunflower; *Spanish:* Campana

Somatic Chromosome Numbers and Genome Constitution: $2n=20$

Description: A herbaceous plant, up to 1.2 m high occurring along roadsides and disused places, in damp pastures and in moist clay loamy fields along the Eastern Seaboard of the continental U.S.A. to the mountains of North Carolina. Flowers yellow and showy, terminal.

Lore, Legend and Romance: The plant is claimed by Obatalá, the father of the gods in the Yoruba region. His counterpart in the Catholic faith is Our Lady of Mercy. Obatalá is further equated with Chesed of the Qabalistic Tree of Life, the plane of love and mercy which is usually depicted as the archetypal persona of the laughing Buddha. Obatalá further corresponds with Zeus, the Greek god of joy, beneficence and expansion. Astrologically he is associated with the planet Jupiter.

Elecampane was a familiar plant to the Greeks and two legends link it to Helen, wife of Menelaus, who was believed to have had an armful of the plant when Paris abducted her to Phrygea. Another explanation of the name is that the best plants grew òn the island of Helena. Before Linnaeus, however, the plant was known as Inula campana, as it grew wild in Campania. Hippocrates, Dioscorides and Galen noted the beneficial effect of Elecampane on the uterus, the urinary passages and the respiratory apparatus, and it was subsequently discovered to act on the digestive organs. An ancient herbal summarizes its uses as follows: *"It will cause asthmatics to spit and soothe persons suffering from lung diseases. It is very useful in sicknesses of the stomach. It is also a laxative; it breaks up thickened matter and removes obstructions. For this reason it induces menstrual discharge and suppressed voidance."*

Julius Augustus was said to have eaten the root of elecampane every day to aid digestion and *"cause mirth."* In Anglo-Saxon medicine, elecampane was used in England before the Norman conquest. The Welsh physicians of the 13th century called it *"marchala."* Present day herbalists use the root of elecampane as a tonic for pulmonary complaints and for coughs.

The plant is widely used for weakness of the digestive organs, in dyspepsias, in tetter, itch, cutaneous diseases and as a stimulant. It produces confusion of the head, vertigo, burning of the eyeballs, dryness of the mouth and throat, and increases peristaltic action of the intestines. Its constituents are inulin, elecampane, camphor, helinin, alant-camphor, synanthrose, inulic acid, and resin. The dried rhizome was found to loosen mucous and causes patients to sweat profusely, thereby breaking fevers.

Two unrelated plants are sometimes used by the Santeros of South Florida either deliberately or erroneously as elecampane. The first of these plants is **Datura candida** (Pers.) Safford., Syn. **Bragmansia candida** Pers. It is called in the Anglophone Caribbean as Angel's trumpet. It is a small shrub to small tree up to 6 m in height, native to Peru, now naturalized in all warm countries. Flowers, campanulate, creamy-white, fading light pinkish-orange.

The other plant is **Trixis inula** Crantz., Syn. **Inula trixis radialis** Kuntze, and **Peridicium radiale** L., being described botanically as an illegitimate name. A herbaceous shrub with sub-erect, scrambling or climbing branches, pubescent at first, up to 2.5 m high. Leaves oblong-ovate, to elliptic lanceolate, obtuse or rounded at base, acute, mucronate, pubescent beneath. Flowers capitula, bright yellow, Nov.–June.

LACTUCA SATIVA L.   Asteraceae (Compositae)

Composite of Sunflower family

Centers of Diversity: Primary center is North Africa and the Middle East. The present marked variation of lettuce is probably a product of hybridization with **Lactuca seriola** L., but may have also been induced by some natural form of mutation. The first record of lettuce dates from 4500 B.C., a long-leaved form was depicted on the Egyptian tombs. Lettuce was grown by the ancient Greeks and Romans. The Moors developed many types. Lettuce reached China in the 7th century A.D. Lettuce is a compartively recent introduction into the tropics and no truly tropical races have been evolved.

Common/Vernacular Names: *English:* Lettuce, Garden lettuce, Sleepwort, Salad; *Spanish:* Lechuga, Alface comum, Alface cultiva; *China:* Wo-chu, Pai-chu, Shih-chu, Shen-ts'ai; *Africa:* Saladi (Swahili)

Somatic Chromosome Numbers and Genome Constitution: $2n = 18$

Description: An annual leafy herbaceous, caulescent plant preferring a rich, mellow, humus soil. The plant exudes a milky, bitter latex, which when dried is given the name lettuce opium, or *"lactucarium."* This substance is light green when fresh, but later turns brown and gives off a characteristic opium-like odor. The erect, glabrous herb has lower cauline leaves, coarsely toothed oblanceolate. Flowers light yellow, Dec.-Feb. Occasionally a weed of sandy or gravelly waste places.

Lore, Legend and Romance: The plant is claimed by Yemaya and Oshun. *"Lechuga"* is used to guard against evil. In the mysteries of Adonis the lettuce was considered a sacred plant. It is alluded to Emperor Diocletian, after his abdication, that a friend attempted to lure him back to the throne by promises of giving him the finest lettuce growing in his garden. It supposedly exerts a sedative action on the sexual drive. However, this must be only in the form of when taken as the extracted latex, as it has been said that hermits use the extraction to subdue the sex drive. It induces sleep.

Suetonius reports that a statue was raised to Musa, Physician to August, for having cured the emperor of a melancholy by making him eat lettuce. It was called the *"enuchs"* plant and was recommended that its juice tempers lust. It was said to increase milk production in wet nurses. It controls involuntary sexual excitation, spermatorrhea and is an anti-aphrodisiac. It is reported to be good for regulating bowels, for gastric spasms, palpitations, congestion of the liver and bronchitis, also for skin disorders when used for arthritis and gout and the flowers are prepared for a purgative. It is also used as a tonic in stomach and liver ailments. A syrup is prepared from the flowers as a laxative for children.

Many of the Santeros of Southern Florida erroneously use another Composite plant, **Lactuca intybacua** Jacq., commonly called *"Lechuga silvestre"* in the Spanish language and is called wild lettuce in Anglophone Carribean countries.

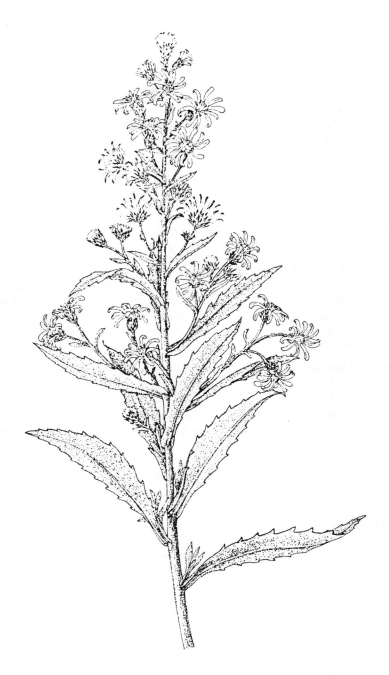

Inula spp.

LEPTOCHLOOPSIS VIRGATA (Poir.) Yates   Gramineae (Poaceae)

Syn. Uniola virgata (Poir.) Grieeb.   **Grass Family**

Centers of Diversity: Caribbean Basin. Grows wild in moist or dry pastures and waste places along roadsides from Mexico to Paraguay and the West Indies at low to medium elevation.

Common/Vernacular Names: *English:* Sea Oats; *Spanish:* Espartillo, Cola de buey, Palu-bia

Somatic Chromosome Numbers and Genome Constitution: 2n = 40

Description: An erect graceful perennial grass with small tufts of slender, smooth, wiry stems, up to 2 m. high. Leaves flattish, coarsely setulous. Flowers brown in color, Oct.–Jan., May–Aug.

Lore, Legend and Romance: This is one of the plants used in the preparation of the *"Omiero,"* the sacred elixer employed in the initiation of the Santeria ceremonies. The plant is claimed by Elegguá and Ochosi, the two Yoruba deities accredited with protection against evil spirits. Elegguá is synonymous with the Holy Guardian Angel of the Catholic faith while Ochosi corresponds with Saint Isidro. Elegguá is further equated with Hod of the Qabalistic Tree of Life, corresponding with Hermes, the Greek god of communication and comes under the rulership of Mercury.

In South Florida, many of the Santeros erroneously use another group of plants called **Sporobulus** spp. also a member of the grass family, **Gramineae,** as a substitute for **Leptochloopis virgata** (Poir.) Yates, the true *"Espartillo."* Three distinct species of **Sporobolus** occur in South Florida and all are commonly referred to as *"Dropseed."* These are: **Sporobolus domingensis** (Trin.) Kunth, with the Spanish name of *"Z'herbe a cotes,"* **Sporobolus virginicus** (L.) Kunth with the Spanish name of *"Chiendent,"* and **Sporobolus pyramidatus** (Dam.) Hitchc., also commonly called *"Chiendent."*

MELIA AZADERACH L.   Meliaceae

                                                       Mahogany family

Centers of Diversity: Indigenous to Iran, India and tropical Asia; now widespread throughout the tropics and sub-tropics including West Africa and Southern Europe. It also occurs in the Southern states of the United States of America and in the Caribbean Basin countries.

Common/Vernacular Names: *English:* China berry, Persian Lilac, West Indian Lilac, Bead tree, Pride of India, Hog bush, Bastard cedar, Tree of Paradise; *Spanish:* Paraiso, Lila, Pasilli, Arbol Santo; *Africa:* Nassara, Eke-oyinbo, Itchin-kurdi (Nigeria); *China:* Lien, K'n-lien, Sen-shu.

Somatic Chromosome Numbers and Genome Constitution: 2n = 28

Description: A small to medium-sized deciduous tree up to 15.2 m. high with slender straggling branches. Flowers purplish to pale lilac in large panicles, May–June. However, in the Caribbean Basin, the tree is known to flower and fruit throughout the year. Fruits a drupe, ellipsoid, about 1.5 cm long, ripening yellow. It contains five-sided, yellowish-brown stones. Seeds germinate freely near mature trees. Leaves, bipinnate, sometimes tripinnate; leaflets lanceolate, glabrous, 2–7 cm long giving a graceful, feather-shaped foliage.

Legend, Lore and Romance: This is one of the important ingredients of the *"Omiero,"* the sacred elixer of initiation ceremonies. The plant is claimed by Changó, the Yoruba deity who corresponds with Saint Barbara of the Catholic faith. In the Qabalah, Changó corresponds with Tiphereth. Tiphereth is the fifth stage of the Tree of Life; this signifies beauty and ethics in the psychological realm. Tiphereth is the heart of the whole tree and holds all the other spheres in their respective paths and in place. Changó also corresponds to the Greek god Helios and is astrologically associated with the Sun. (This is an interesting correspondence as both Tiphereth and the Sun hold the central place, or nucleus, in their fields of influence while everything revolves around them.) Changó is god of lightening and thunder in the Yoruba pantheon. He wards off evil spirits.

In Italy, the seeds are fashioned into rosaries, while in Southern Africa, where the plant is known as Cape Lilac, the seeds are worked into pretty necklaces. The plant is commonly cultivated in India, the scented flowers being esteemed for thanks offerings.

The active principle of this plant is the yellowish-white body soluble in alcohol and scarsely soluble in cold water, though it is more likely to be a substance still to be isolated which happens to be extracted with the resinous body. This explains the reason for the plant's use as a fish poison, for example, in China, by a water soluble substance, and why a water infusion is used as a vermifuge in India. This unknown substance is destroyed by boiling. An overdose of the extract produces symptoms like those of **Atropa belladonna** poisoning, and after stupor, death may follow. Recently, a toxic alkaloid, tazetine ($C_{18}H_{21}NO_5$) has been reported in the fruit and bark. The crushed, dried fruit has yielded azadirachtin, which is known to inhibit feeding of the desert locusts. The same property may be present in the leaves.

The tree exudes a clear, tasteless soluble latex which coagulates rapidly into gum which is used for colds, coughs and catarrhal fever, especially in India. The tree is used medicinally by Arabs and Iranians, the name azaderach suggesting poisonous properties, all portions being bitter and strongly purgative, antiseptic, germicidic, anthelmintic, vermifugic and insecticidal. The root bark is considered the best of anthelmintics, being especially used for roundworms. The leaf juice is used by Arabs and Iranians as a vermifuge, diuretic and emmenagogue.

Brushing the teeth with chewed twigs is common practice in India; this refreshes the mouth and arrests sore mouth, sore throat, gum and tooth troubles. The leaves and flowers are applied as a poultice, in India, to relieve nervous headaches. The root bark is used in North and South America as a cathartic and emetic.

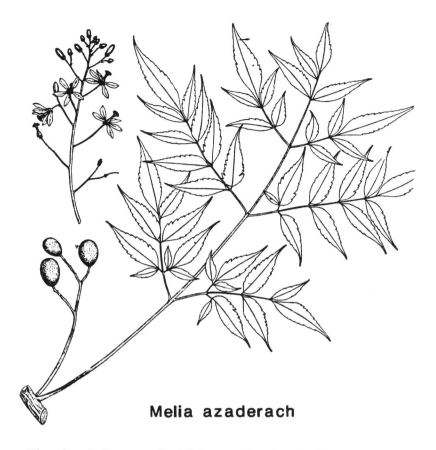

Melia azaderach

The plant belongs to the Mahogany family—**Meliaceae**, a relatively large and very homogenous family with very few species occurring outside the tropical rain forest. The family contains about 50 or more genera, and approximately 1400 species of hard wood trees and shrubs, often having scented wood, differing from **Rutales** in having their stamens fused into a tube. These Mahoganys have actinomorphic and mostly hermaphroditic flowers.

There appears to be widespread inconsistencies in the recognition and naming/classification of **Melia azaderach** L. from other **Melia** spp. in a number of botanical literatures. The problem is compounded by the plant's frequently changed scientific name, and further, many botanical authors erroneously misspelling and scientific name.

In China, no distinction is made between the **Melia azaderach** and **Melia toosendan** as far as medicinal properties and uses are concerned. However, the latter species, **M. toosendan** is usually preferred and considered the most chemically potent of the two species. In China, at the time of the Dragon Festival (fifth day of the fifth moon) bamboo sprouts and rice cakes are wrapped in **Melia azaderach** leaves, and tied with silk thread of five different colors. These parcels are then thrown into streams to propitiate the spirit of the water. This custom is similar to one of the religious rituals of the Santeria, which has its origin in Africa.

NASTURTIUM OFFICINALE R. Br.   Cruciferae (Brassicaceae)

Syn. Sisymbrium nasturtium aquaticum   **Mustard Family**
Syn. Rorippa nasturtium aquaticum (L.) Hayek.

Centers of Diversity: West Africa and South Europe; now cultivated and naturalized almost throughout the world.

Common/Vernacular Names: *English:* Water cress, Water cushie; *Spanish:* Berro, Berro cruz, Mastuerzo; *China:* Chin-lien-hua

Somatic Chromosome Numbers and Genome Constitution: 2n = 32 (48, 64)

Description: A low trailing perennial herb with soft stems and leaves; common in running waters throughout the world and sparingly naturalized in the United States. Flowers numerous, small and white; fruit, 15–18 mm long.

Lore, Legend and Romance: The plant is one of the ingredients of the sacred elixer used in the initiation ceremony of the Santeria religion . The species is claimed by the Yoruba deities, Yemayá and Oshún, who are generally reputed to have dominion over stomach irritations. Yemayá corresponds with Our Lady of Regla, and Oshún relates to La Caridad del Cobre. Yemayá is universally equated with Yesod, the plane of love and mercy of the Qabalistic Tree of Life, corresponding with Artemis, the Greek goddess and coming under the rulership of the Moon. Oshún, on the other hand, corresponds with Netzach, the emotional sensitivity plane of the Tree of Life, equating with the Greek goddess of love, Aphrodite, and having Venus as her ruling planet.

The pinatified pungent leaves are, in the young state, a favorite salad herb, containing some form of isothiocyanate, a characteristic compound of many members of the family **Cruciferae.** The fresh plant of this perennial herb is antiscorbutic and is used in the treatment of constipation.

The tips of the leafy stems are eaten as salad. It is also cooked as a vegetable. In New Zealand it is a serious river weed. The almost sterile hybrid plants (2n = 45) of watercress and its relative **Nasturium microphyllum** (Boenn.) Rchb. (2n = 64), are cultivated for salad (Purseglove, 1968). It is vegetatively cultivated, though it can be propogated from seeds as well.

The Salernitan school of medicine, the leading light of science in the Middle Ages, recommended rubbing the juice of watercress into the scalp to strengthen and thicken the hair, and one of the most common popular prescriptions for promoting hair growth is still to rub the scalp with lotion composed of a mixture of 100 grams of watercress juice with 100 grams of alcohol (90%) and 10 grams of geranium essence. The Salernitan doctors similarly advocated the use of watercress juice in the treatment of skin complaints, a treatment which has survived as a beauty treatment for freckles and clearing the complexion; (mix 60 g. of watercress juice with 30 g. of honey, strain through a cloth, dab on the face with a wad of cotton wool morning and evening.)

Hippocrates held it to be a stimulant and expectorant. Dioscorides believed it to be aphrodisiac. Ambrose Pare considered it the specific for scabies in children. Others have used it in the treatment of skin diseases, diabetes, scurvy and weak chest.

One can chew watercress to strengthen the gums and prevent them from bleeding; it is also effective against aphtha (ulcerations of the mouth). But one must be cautioned here as wild watercress may be contaminated by a deadly parasite, the liver fluke (found especially in the livers of sheep) present in animal droppings; it is consequently wiser to eat only watercress that has been grown in watercress beds.

There is more confusion over this plant among the various Santeros in South Florida. A number of plants are mistakenly used as watercress. The problem is compounded by the Spanish vernacular names of Berro or Berron or Bay-rum being ascribed to **Pimenta racemosa** (Mill.) J.W. Moore, as well as **Nasturtium officinale** R. Br.

In Venezuela, the juice extracted from the fresh plant has long been given as a remedy for tuberculosis; the leaves are applied as poultices on skin afflictions. The plant is rich in vitamins "A" and "E" and has a fair amount of vitamin "C". It yields 0.06% of a pungent volatile oil containing mainly phenylethyl isothiocynate. This is a well known herb and popular salad plant in Mexico, Central and South America. In Guatemala it is often cooked as a vegetable.

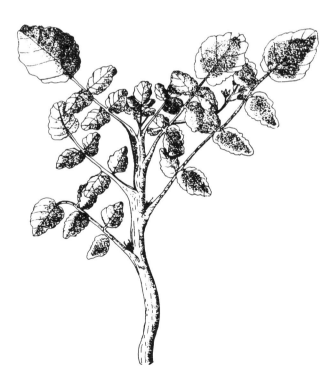

Nasturtium officinale

MENTHA AQUATICA L.   Labiatae

Syn. Mentha citrata Ehrh.   **Mint Family**

Centers of Diversity: Asia and North Africa, Southern Europe. Native to the Middle East but widespread across the globe because of their growth characteristics and the great esteem with which they are held by all who came in contact with them.

Common/Vernacular Names: *English:* Bergamot mint, Water mint, Orange mint, Citrus mint, Lemon mint; *Spanish:* Yerba buena; *Asia:* Podina (India); Bok-ho (China)

Somatic Chromosome Numbers and Genome Constitution: 2n = (36, 60), 96

Description: Rampantly spreading perennial inhabiting moist, rich soils of the world. Common in ditches and damp places. It is noted for its distinctive citrus-like fragrance. Its rounded, broad underside of the leaves often have a reddish hue and in the spring the entire plant is distinctly reddish-purple, hairy; stems square, leaves opposite. Flowers zygomorphic, pale mauve, July–Sept. Inflorescens of 2–3 whorls. It is a source of an essential oil. Its A^{aq} genome is partial homologous to the **Mentha x piperata.** This species is cultivated **Mentha citrata** in the United States for its lavender-like oil for perfumery (Todd & Murray, 1968).

Lore, Legend and Romance: The mint family, **Labiatae**, is a large one, having about 200 genera and 3200 species; this includes the thyme, sages, marjorams, basils, hyssop, horehound, rosemary, lavender and lemon balm. The true mint, however, are the members of the genus **Mentha**. The best known of the mints, are Spearmint and Peppermint, the two most common flavors of chewing gum. The mint family, **Labiatae**, are closely related to the Vervain family, **Verbenaceae.**

It is common knowledge in the taxonomical field that botanists often have difficulty classifying mint plants. This is due to the fact that there are so many variants among each species due to their mode of pollination. As a result of this, cuttings and root divisions are the best method of propagation to obtain desired plants which ultimately would be true to type.

Mentha aquatica L. is claimed by the Yoruba deita, Yemayá, with Our Lady of Regla of the Catholic faith as her counterpart. Yemayá corresponds with Yesod of the Qabalastic Tree of Life and equates with the Greek goddess Artemis, with the Moon as her astrological ruling planet. Yemayá has control over skin troubles. In the language of flowers, mint is *"Homeliness."* **Mentha aquatica** is used by the Santeria religion as one of the ingredients of the *"Omiero,"* the sacred elixer.

There are numerous references in the literature of all ages concerning the desirability of the mints in the Bible, the writings of the ancients, in Chaucer's writings and in Greek mythology.

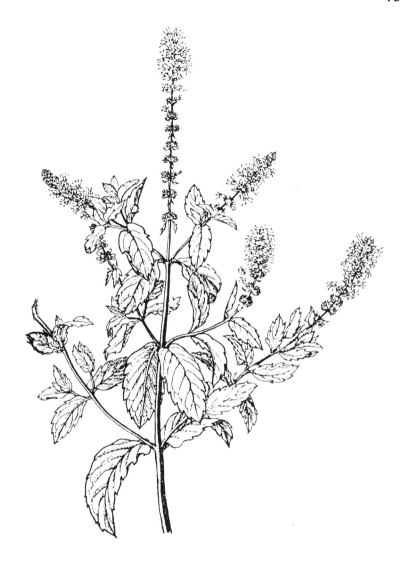

Mentha spicata

The genus, **Mentha**, was first connected with the mint plant by the Greek philosopher/scientist, Theophrastus more than 300 years before Christ. He based the connection on Greek mythology. Mintho, the story went, was a beautiful nymph who was loved by Pluto, god of the underworld. Persephone, who had been abducted by Pluto to reign with him over his domain, became jealous and changed Mintho into a fragrant and lowly plant which to this day waits at the shady edges of Pluto's dark world.

MYRIOPHYLLUM BRASILIENSE Camb.   Haloragidaceae

Syn. Myriophyllum proserpinacoides   **Water Milfoil family**

Centers of Diversity: South and Central America; cultivated in small hot house pools.

Common Vernacular Names: Parrot's feather; *Spanish:* Pluma de cotorra, Helecho que resucita; *China:* Shui-t'sao

Somatic Chromosome Numbers and Genome Constitution: $2n = 42$

Description: An Aquatic plant with attractive floating or submerged feathery whorled leaves borne on shoots that spring from rhizome-like creeping stems. The family has a close nomenclatural affinity with **Lentibulariaceae** containing the genus **Utricularia**, the bladder wort.

Lore, Legend and Romance: The plant being one of the *"Twenty-one"* herbs of the *"Omeiro,"* the sacred elixer of the Santeria initiation ceremony. It is claimed by Yemayá and Oshún, the Yoruba deities who are given dominion over evil spirits. Yemayá corresponds with Our Lady of Regla of the Catholic faith, while she is equated with Yesod of the Qabalistic Tree of Life, and Artemis the Greek goddess. Astrologically, Yemaya is associated with the Moon. Oshun, on the other hand, corresponds with La Caridad del Cobre of the Catholic faith, Netzach of the Qabalistic Tree of Life, Aphrodite the Greek godess of love, and is.ruled by the planet Venus.

In China, several halorageous and adaceous plants of which the genus **Myriophyllum**, is included, are described in the Pen ts'ao under the common name of *"Shui-t'sao"*; all these plants are considered to be edible and are used in medicine.

In South Florida, **Polypodium polypodioides** Hitch., Syn. **Polypodium incanum** Sm., is commonly known as English polypody, Resurrection fern, and Tree polypody and is used by a number of Santeros as *"Helecho del rio,"* or *"Doradilla."* This fern grows on rocks and trunks of trees in the Caribbean Basin. The Plant is reputed to be diuretic, purgative, cholagogue, demulcent and vermifuge.

There are widespread inconsistencies in botanical literatures as to the authenticity of the families **Holoragidaceae** and **Lentiburaceae**. Some taxonomists have chosen to include all plants belonging to the two families, all in either of the two. The problem is further compounded by the misspelling of the family names. W. Keeble Martin (1969) states **Haloragaceae** while Willis (1966 calls it **Haloragidaceae**. I would appreciate receiving feed-back as to the current legitimate name of the family and also, the current status of **Utricaria**. Specifically, I wish to know whether or not **Utricaria** is still retained in the family **Lentibulariaceae**.

OCIMUM BASILICUM L.   Labiatae

Syn. Ocimum americanum L.   **Mint family**

Centers of Diversity: Tropical Asia and Africa, but now a cosmopolite plant. Cultivated in China since 500 A.D., and also now commercially produced in France, Hungary, Morocco, Indonesia and the U.S.A. where California produces a superior quality.

Common/Vernacular Names: *English:* Basil, Sweet basil, Bush basil;*Spanish:* Albaca, Albahaca blanca, Albahacade gallina, Albahaca morada, Albahaca clavo; *Africa:* Rukovi, Manhuwe, Ruridze (Zimbabwe), Efirin wewe (Nigeria), Patmagi (Gambia); *China:* Ai-K'ang, Lo-le, Hsiang-ts'ai

Somatic Chromosome Numbers and Genome Constitution: 2n=48

Description: An annual aromatic herb, 30–90 cm high, commonly cultivated and reproduced from seed. Leaves opposite, petiolate, lanceolate, acute, entire or finely serrate. Stems are squarish, hispid. Flowers small, white, in dense whorls, shortly separated from each other on the terminal branches. Calyx somewhat enlarged in fruit.

Lore, Legend and Romance: This is one of the *"Twenty-one"* plants of the Santeria ceremonial elixer. It is associated with Oggún and Yemayá deities. Oggún corresponds with Geburah of the Qabalistic Tree of Life and is also associated with Ares, the Greek god of war along with the astrological affinity with the planet Mars. Yemayá corresponds with Yesod of the Qabalastic Tree of Life, and is associated with Artemis, the Greek goddess. Astrologically, Yemayá is associated with the Moon.

Sometimes **Ocimum sanctum,** known in Cuba as *"Albahaca cimarrona"* is used as a substitute for **Ocimum basilicum.** Many people mistake the two plants mentioned. This plant is held in high esteem in Cuba and elsewhere in Latin America where it is considered a valued spiritual plant in religious ceremony.

It is revered in ancient tradition. It was sacred to Krishna and Vishnu and it was said to be that every Hindu slept with a basil leaf on his breast. It has the same mildly stimulating properties as its allied species, and has always been used in Indian *"Aruyvedic medicine."*

The basil has a long and varied history and many legends have been told about it. To it have been attributed many potent properties as a talismanic charm. Among the Hindus, basil was one of the most sacred herbs with which they were acquainted. It is usually planted in the garden or courtyard of the Hindu home, where it is worshiped by all members of the family. The pious Hindu invokes the divine herb to bring protection to every part of the body, but above all, to insure children to those who desire them. The plant is considered as every *"good Hindu's"* visa to paradise.

Basil is general regarded as an enchanted flower in Mondavia. It is thought that the flower can cause a spell upon a wayward youth and make him love the maiden from whose hand he grasps a sprig. A similar belief exists among

Italians and Sicilians in our own time. The youths of Sicily wear sprigs of basil behind the ear to denote the fact that they are of marriageable age and romantically inclined. It is given to loved ones as a pledge of fidelity, and in country districts, when a boy wears a sprig behind the ear, a girl may respond by saying, "Baccio carissimo," or "Kiss me, dearest." Baccio is also the common name for basil.

Basil is a crop protector. Some herbs have affinity for specific crops. Basil, for instance, is reported to protect tomatoes, almost as if giving them a wrap-around shield. It generally repels flies and mosquitoes. It keeps pests and disease at bay.

Like the majority of the most fragrant aromatic herbs, basil has been associated with religious or magic rites. In its native country, India, according the Brahmanic religion, it was imbued with the divine essence of the *"Three Brides."* Every family possessed its sacred basil, their protective spirit, to which they made daily offerings of flowers and rice.

From the Renaissance to the French Revolution doctors advocated it for *"cheering the spirit and restoring the humors that compose the blood and for clearing the brain, by causing the watery humors to be discharged through the nose as the qualities of the basil are allies of the body."* In medieval Europe, it was said that if a sprig of basil be left under a stone, it will turn into a scorpion, and if pulled and exposed to the heat of the Sun, it will turn into worms. Pliny recommends it as a cure for epilepsy.

The fact remains that basil has an undeniably sedative and antispasmodic action in addition to its digestive properties. It is therefore, recommended for nervous predisposition, stomach disorders, insomnia of nervous origin, vertigo, migranes, and anger. It is a natural and non-toxic kind of tranquilizer. All the basils are tonic, stimulant, nervine, carminative and disinfectant. They are used by herbalists to improve appetite, allay fatigue and cure arthritis and intestinal catarrh. It is a stimulating and refreshing drink after a hard day's work.

The sap of the fresh leaves acts beneficially on inflammations of the ear (a few drops in the ears); the powdered dried leaves, taken like snuff, is according to Dr. Cazin, *"a pleasant sternutatory."*

In Africa there exists more than 100 varieties of basil and they are used both as a seasoning and as a medicine. It is given to children for worms, to adults for persistent headaches, migranes and for certain rheumatic diseases.

Ocimum basilicum, known as *"Ai-k'ang"* in Peking, is used in the treatment of opacity of the cornea and is commonly called *"I-tzu-ts'ao."* The Pen ts'ao distinguishes three varieties. Peptic and carminative properties are ascribed to it, and the decoction is used to wash ulcers. It is prescribed for vomiting, hiccough and polypus of the nose. The seeds are especially prescribed in diseases of the eyes, and are said to remove films and opacities and to soothe pain and inflammation.

In China, basil is thought of by many authorities to be **Melilotus arvensis,** with the vernacular name of *"Hsun-ts'ao"* or *"Ling-ling-hsiang."* It is quite possible that Chinese botanists often confused the two because of its fragrance and of several resemblances.

Ocimum viride Willd., the species of West Africa, is often called the fever plant of Sierra Leone and is known in Ghana as *"Nonoom."* It is much used

Ocimum basilicum

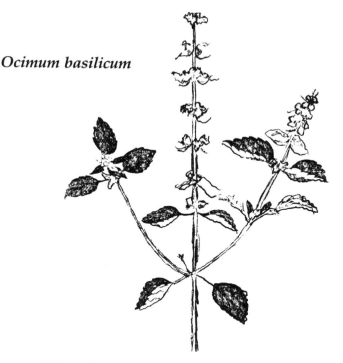

in West African medicine and is often especially grown in villages and sold in markets and is well known as a febrifuge. In many parts of West Africa it is reputed to drive out evil spirits and demons. It is used in Ashanti for fumigation at birth and to drive away spirits. The whole plant may be used as a poultice for rheumatism and lumbago.

In India basil is also used to increase sexual appetite (aphrodisiac). Pasted root is taken in cases of impotence and loss of manhood. It is also used in India in the treatment of gonorrhea. The seed is shaken in water and the slippery beverage is used; the same concoction is used for chronic dysentary, diarrhea and post delivery ailments.

The most common folk remedy used in Cuba is to steep the plant in alcohol, which is then employed as a rub. In El Salvador, the fresh leaves are stuffed into the ears as a remedy for deafness. A decoction of the blooming plant is used in baths to relieve rheumatism and to deodorize the feet. It is drunk as a tonic and aphrodisiac.

The plant varies in chemistry according to the variety and habitat. A Mediterranean type contains mainly cineol, linalol, and methychavicol; the Reunion type contains mainly d-l-pinene, cineole, d-camphor and methychavicol; a Bulgarian type is characterized by methycinna-mate, and a Java type by eugenol. The seed mucilage contains d-glucose, d-galactose, d-mannose, l-arabinose, d-xylose, d-rhamnose, d-galacturonic acid and d-mannuronic acid.

Basil, this strong aromatic herb, is quite appropriately under the influence of Mars, the first planet outside of Earth's orbit, which is associated with high energy and sexuality. A truly royal herb, its name derived from the Greek word for king, *"basileus."*

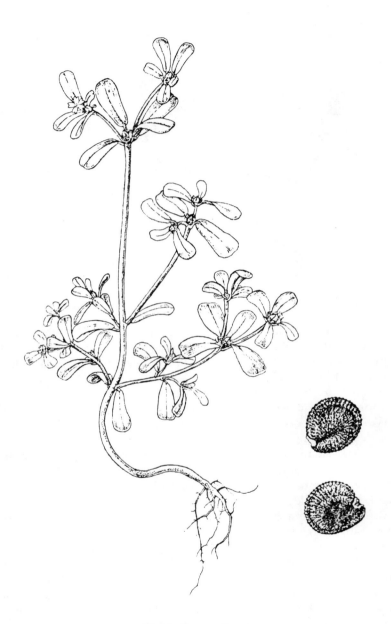

Portulaca oleracea

showing kidney-shaped seeds

PORTULACA OLERACEA L.   Portulacaceae

Purselane family

Centers of Diversity: Africa and Asia; but has now naturalized and become a noxious weed in warmer parts of the globe.

Common/Vernacular Names: *English:* Purslane, Pursley, Pussley, Common purslance, Pigweed; *Spanish:* Verdolago, Porcelana, Verdolaga amarilla, Xucul, Amor crescido; *Africa:* Gbure, Papkuse (Nigeria); *China:* Hsein, Ma-ch'i Hsien

Somatic Chromosome Numbers and Genome Constitution: 2n=(45), 54

Description: An edible, prostrating annual herb with fleshy stems and tiny succulent wedge-shaped green and reddish leaves, rounded at the tip, alternate or nearly opposite. Flowers yellow in terminal involucrate heads, variable in size up to 14 mm across when opening; it stays open in light. Seeds flattish, kidney-shaped and black. Though it is an annual and depends on seeds for reproduction, broken-off bits of stems take root readily and start new plants. Even when hoed, the succulent stems remain alive for a long time. The species is gregarious in disused areas throughout the United States particularly in Southern Florida.

Lore, Legend and Romance: The species is one of the *"Twenty-one"* plants used in the preparation of *"Omiero,"* the sacred elixer of the Santeria religion. The plant is claimed by Yemayá, the Yoruba deity, and is associated with good luck. Yemayá corresponds with Yesod of the Qabalistic Tree of Life and she governs the instincts and the source of vital energy. She is further associated with Our Lady of Regla of the Catholic faith, while Artemis, the Greek goddess is her counterpart. Astrologically she corresponds with the Moon.

In ancient times purslane was considered a protection against evil spirits. Sprigs were strewn about the house to ensure happiness in the home. The bruised leaves placed on the forehead will relieve headache, particularly if caused by heat or lack of sleep.

Purslane, a herb under the rulership of the moon, is an excellent food used in many parts of Africa as both a pot herb (like spinach) and salad herb. It was introduced into Europe as a salad herb. It is sold in markets of Mexico for the same purpose while in Southern Spain it is used as salad and in soups. By and large, the most common use of the succulent herb has been in salads, in which it is particulary nutritious. It was widely cultivated in Europe, and travelers to the New World took specimens with them. Early Americans were surprised to discover that the Indians had no use for it, rooting it out of their corn patches as much as Americans still do.

The plant has been used widely in medicine as a diuretic, antispasmodic, esculent, vermifuge, refrigerant, antiseptic and aperient. The plant and seed are reputed to be vulnerary and antiscorbutic and have been used for sore lips and nipples, and ulcers of the mouth. The decoction of the leafy stems is regarded as laxative, diuretic and vermifugal and that of the raw plant as antiscorbutic in Brazil, Venezuela and on the Yucatan peninsula.

In West Africa, the plant is regarded as good vegetable, with antiscorbutic properties. In Zaire, the plant is used as fodder for cattle and other livestock. The seeds are largely used by the Australian Aboriginal as food. The seeds are said to be vermifugal; the leaves and twigs along with fresh paw paw root (*"Carica papaya"*) are mixed with four pints of water and boiled down to three pints.

In China, no distinction is made between purslanes and amaranths and very naturally so, since the two plants resemble each other in general appearance and habit. Both plants are frequently referred to as *"Hsien."* There is a fairly good description of **Portulaca oleracea** L. in the Pen t'sao, and the plant is said to contain mercury. It is eaten as a cheap, cooling sprig vegetable by the Chinese of all classes. They consider the seeds to be tonic and constructive, and are prescribed in opacities of the cornea and to benefit the intestines.

The entire plant contains the alkaloid norepinephrine, also urea and considerable potassium. It is used as a lotion for inflamed eyes. In Jamaica, the plant decoction is regard as a heart tonic (potassium is a heart regulator). In Trinidad, the herb is taken to relieve palpitations.

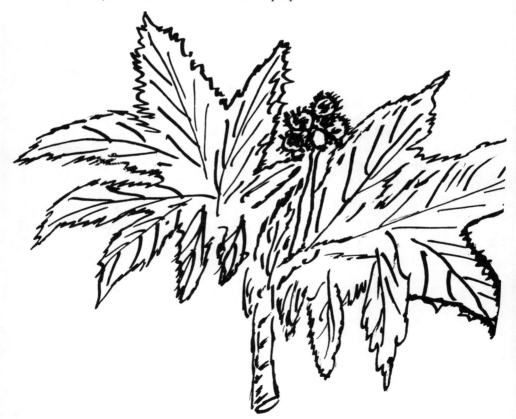

Ricinus communis

RICINUS COMMUNIS L.   Euphorbiaceae

Spurge family

Centers of Diversity: Native to tropical East Africa and India; now a world wide pantropical species; its power as a ruderal plant has been suggested. Cultivated and naturalized in most tropical and sub-tropical areas of the world. In the United States, the plant is common from California to Florida where it forms extensive solid stands. Also from Caribbean countries, Mexico to Peru and Argentina.

Common/Vernacular Names: *English:* Castor bean, Castor oil, Palma Christi, Steadfast, Common ricinus; *Spanish:* Higuereta, Huile mascristi, Higuera del diablo, Cuile ricin, Mascarite, Mamona, Ricino; *Africa:* Adade nkuruma (Ghana), Fude, Hlafuto (Zimbabwe), Zurma (Nigeria), Bafureira (Angola), Ambona (Mozambique); *China:* Pei-ma, P'i-ma

Somatic Chromosome Numbers and Genome Constitution: 2n=20

Description: A tall, quick growing perennial woody shrub or small tree attaining 9–10 m in height with large handsome palmate peltate leaves, divided into 7 or more serrate lobes. It should be noted that the plant behaves as an annual in colder climates. Flowers unisexual, clustered in bunches, terminal, yellowish. Fruits prickly, globose capsule, rather marked in 6 paths. The entire plant is poisonous, containing the toxic protein, ricin, which is most concentrated in the seeds, and a potent allergen. The seeds are also rich in purgative oil that owes its action to a triglyceride of ricinoleic acid.

To an appreciable degree, the plant is resistant to salt and drought and has become an obnoxious weed in Southern Florida, where originally, attempts were made to establish a plantation of these as a possible source of lubricating oil during World War II.

Lore, Legend and Romance: This plant, being one of the ingredients of the *"Omiero,"* the sacred elixer of the Santeria religious ceremony, is claimed by Obatalá, the father of the gods in the Yoruba pantheon. Obatalá as a deity corresponds with the Catholic saint, Our Lady of Mercy. Obatalá who has dominion over diphtheria and headaches, is equated with the Chesed, the plane of love and mercy of the Qabalistic Tree of Life. Obatalá further corresponds with the Greek god, Zeus, and is ruled by the planet Jupiter.

The well known oil produced by **Ricinus communis** L. has been used from time immemorial as a purgative, being known to the ancient Egyptians thousands of years before the Greeks and Romans knew of its virtues. Oil is obtained from the seed by pressure. The seed as well as the poonac contain an alkaloid poison called ricin which, however, does not pass into the oil.

The only species of the genus **Ricinus,** there are, however, numerous varieties of the species, differing in stature, color of foliage, size and shape of fruit and size and color of seeds. As a companion plant, **Rincinus communis** L. is known to protect vine crops from pests. It has a reputation as a fly and mosquito repelling plant and will also rid gardens of moles and gophers.

Its medicinal values are well established; it has been used as a cathartic, galactogogue, and for female complaints. The leaves are galactogogue. The plant contains ricinollein, palnitin, stearin, and myristin. It is poisonous due to the ricin and may even result in death. All parts of the plant can evoke allergic response.

The Chinese value castor oil as a laxative but also use it in cases of difficult childbirth, facial deformities and stomach cancer. The leaves are applied in swellings as a discutient remedy and are given internally as a tussic and expectorant.

In Mexico, the scaled leaves, placed on the breasts of nursing mothers, are claimed to increase milk flow. They are also employed on rheumatic pains and chronic tumors. In Brazil, the leaf decoction is employed in baths to shrink hemorrhoids. The root is taken as a remedy for colic, and in Cuba, is recommended as a diuretic in cases of prostate enlargement. Throughout the world, including parts of Africa, this is known as a powerful galactogogue. In Nigeria the seed is used as a purgative and rubefacient.

Castor oil has a variety of industrial uses, including the manufacture of soap, furniture polish, flypaper, artificial leather and artificial rubber, hair products, some types of cellulose and candles.

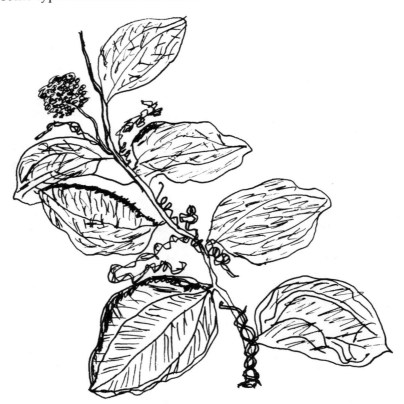

Smilax Kraussiana

SMILAX ORNATA Lem.   Smilacaceae

Lily vine family

Centers of Diversity: Four genera with about 300 species mostly Smilax, widely distributed in tropical and temperate regions. All of these in some way or other have some medicinal properties similar but not identical with the true sarsparilla.

Common/Vernacular Names: *English:* Sarsparilla; *Spanish:* Zarzaparilla; *Africa:* Mandrale (Ghana), Garangurwe (Zimbabwe)

Somatic Chromosome Numbers and Genome Constitution: $2n = 30,32$

Description: A climbing plant characterized by more or less prickly stems and large, ovate, three-nerved leaves found in wild state in the Caribbean Basin and Central America. Some botanists do not separate **Smilacaceae** from **Liliaceae**, from which they differ mainly in habit, mostly diocious flowers and by the confluent anther-loculi. In any case, the group is considerably advance from general stock of the Liliaceae.

Lore, Legend and Romance: Smilax ornata Lem. is claimed by Changó, the powerful god of lightning and thunder. Changó's counterpart is the mystical Saint Barbara of the Catholic faith. Changó corresponds with Tiphareth of the Qabalistic Tree of Life. He also has affininty with the Greek god Helios and comes under the astrological rulership of the Sun. Medicinal properties of sarsparilla are: alternative, diuretic, demulcent, antipsyphilitic, stimulant and anti-scorbutic. It is very useful in rheumatism, gout and skin eruption. An excellent antidote after taking a deadly poison. It increases the flow of urine. It is one of the best herbs to use for infants infected with venereal disease. Before the advent of antibiotics it was felt that children could be cured of venereal diseases with this herb and without the use of mercurials.

All the species of sarsparilla were once used extensively in the treament of syphilis and some skin diseases. It was used, too, in the cure of rheumatism. Nowadays, its chief use is in the making of soft drinks or "minerals." This is because of the somewhat sweetish flavor it imparts to the liquid. The root contains saponins which cause a watery solution to froth when shaken. The drug is often the dried rhizomes of **Smilax ornata** Lem., but rhizomes of other species of Smilax may be used the same way. The dried root of **Hemidesmus indicus** R. Br., belonging to the family **Asclepiadaceae** is used in India for the same purposes and is called Indian Sarsparilla or *"Nagajihva"* in Sanskrit and *"Salso"* or *"Anantnulin"* in Hindi.

Wild sarsparilla, which is **Aralia nudicaulis** is also known as small spikenard, and is used for coughs. The root of wild sarsparilla can make a stimulating *"tea."* A century ago, infertile women would try the old folklore drink made from the bark of common pine, **Physocarpus opulifolius,** Maxim., once believed to encourage fertility. After pregnancy was achieved the root of the wild sarsparilla is collected and used as a stimulant. The plant is believed to be a native American plant as it is not mentioned in either European or Oriental herbals. It is considered a good tonic.

Smilax ornata Lem. was substituted for the true plant which was used in West Africa. **Smilax kraussiana** Meissn. was not available in the New World. The plant is used in similar ways in West Africa as in the Americas. It is reported to be good for venereal diseases. The tuberous roots are boiled and the body exposed under clothing to the vapor for ordering fevers and the acute stages of syphilis and gonorrhea. In South Africa, the eyes are steamed over a root decoction for opthalmia. The young shoots cooked with seeds of cucumber (**Cucumis edulis**) are eaten by pregnant women in Tropical Africa to hasten delivery.

Smilax havanensis Jacq. which occurs in Cuba and other Central American countries is also called *"zarzaparilla."*

SOLANUM NIGRUM L.   Solanaceae

Nightshade family

Centers of Diversity: The plant enjoys worldwide distribution; native region is unknown; at present a cosmopolite, non-tuberous weed which is cultivated. It is sometimes described as a ruderal plant.

Common/Vernacular Names: *English:* Nightshade, Black nightshade, Garden nightshade, Stubby-berry, Hound's berry, Deadly nightshade; *Spanish:* Mora, Yerba mora, Meta gallina, Veneno decuervo; *Africa:* Ikan-yanrin (Nigeria), Saka (Zimbabwe), Mnavu (Swahili); *Asia:* Lung-k'uei, T'ien-p'ao-tsao (China); Ghamai (Hindi), Gurkamai (Bengali)

Somatic Chromosome Numbers and Genome Constitution: 2n=24

Description: A gregarious annual erect herb up to 1 m in height with smooth stems, held in high esteem in Cuba for its medicinal properties. Leaves: smooth, egg-shaped with slightly toothed edges, alternate. Flowers, small, white, clustered on long stalks, axillary, June–Sept. Fruit, small black, globose berry the size of a pea. The plant is found on rich soils in old fields and waste places near settlements throughout the world. The flowers are diaphoretic, narcotic, poisonous and in oil, they are anodyne and discutient. They are bisexual, actinomorphic or slightly zygomorphic, solitary or in unusually cymose inflorescences. The family **Solanaceae** consists of evergreen and deciduous shrubs and vines. They include many economic plants such as potato and eggplant, together with a number of ornamental plants. There are 85 genera with about 2300 species. In the U.S.S.R., steroids (cortisone) are derived from a number of these **Solanaceous** species.

The drug is part of two natural families—**Ranunculaceae** and **Solanaceae.** These two families exemplify relationships which may exist between plants grouped according to natural affinity and their use in medicine. The group may be regarded simply as composed of hyoscymine, atropine and hyoscine. Atropine rarely occurs in the plant as such and when it does, then only in small amounts.

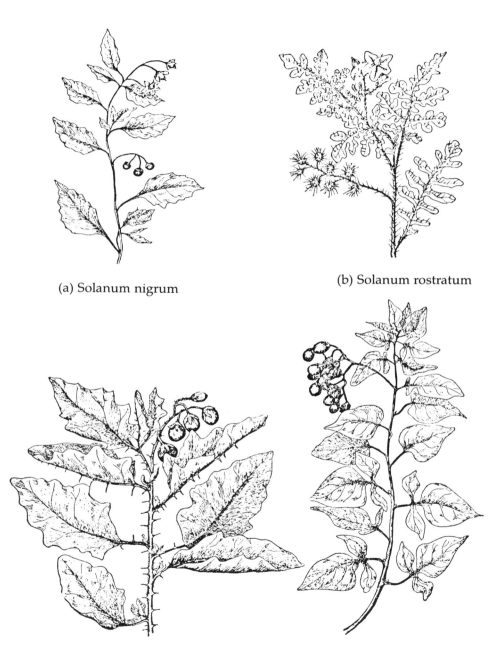

(a) Solanum nigrum

(b) Solanum rostratum

(c) Solanum carolinense

(d) Solanum dulcamara

Other alkaloids occur in plants belonging to the family **Solanaceae** but they do not enter into the group defined above. Thus, the term solanaceous alkaloids, as it is usually used, is rather narrow and excludes substances which would be included if it were of general context. It may be noted that alkaloids closely related chemically to the solanacous ones have been obtained from plants of a quite unrelated family **Convulvulaceae.**

Lore, Legend and Romance: Oggún and Yemayá claim **Solanum nigrum.** It should be noted that the deity Oggún corresponds with the Geburah of the Qabalistic Tree of Life. Ares, the Greek god of war is associated with this deity and it falls under the rulership of Mars. Yemayá, on the other hand, corresponds with the Yesod of the Tree of Life. She is assoicated with the Greek goddess Artemis and is under the influence of the Moon.

In Cuba, the leaves and fruits mixed with almond oil are applied to skin for leprosy, and also for rheumatism. In Mexico and other Central American nations, the leaves are cooked and used as a vegetable where it is claimed that it is effective against bubonic plague. One thing is certain, the Central American countries continue to use the plant as a cure for skin disorders.

In India, the fruits are considered a stimulant, diuretic and febrifuge. It is used for diarrhea, dropsy, hydrophobia and heart disease. Leaf brew is astringent. This is an important ingredient in several Indian medicines. Infusion of the plant is useful in dysentery and other stomach complaints. It promotes urination, the juice of the plant is useful in ulcers and other skin diseases. Hot compresses of leaf are applied on painful, inflamed limbs, and on the scrotum for orchitis and inflammation of the testicles.

In the case of poisoning, it acts as an irritant to the brain and spinal cord, and secondary, upon the circulatory system through the vasomotor system. The irritation seems to be greatest upon the sensory nerves and less upon the motor nerves.

All parts of the plant except the berries contain solanine, solansonine, solanidine, solasodine, solamargine and related glycoalkaloides and alkamines. The fully ripe berries are said to be edible and are made into jam. These should be avoided since the unripe berries are highly toxic.

The plant is reported to have caused death in humans and livestock, but interestingly the leaves are used as "greens" in the West Indies. In parts of the U.S.A. the fruits are used to make pies and jams.

In China, the young shoots are eaten, after boiling and it is considered to be corrective, cooling and tonic to men (virility) and women's menstrual disorders. The stalks, leaves and roots are used in decoctions in wounds, cancerous sores, and as an astringent. The seeds have the same properties and uses as the young shoots.

In Southern Florida and the Caribbean Basin countries a variety of **S. nigrum** is to be encountered. There is **Solanum americanum var. nodiflorum** (Jacq.) Edmonds. It has been suggested that the climatic conditions, including other edaphic factors, affect the concentration of the alkaloids built up by the plants. Also, some human subjects are more sensitive than others to its effect.

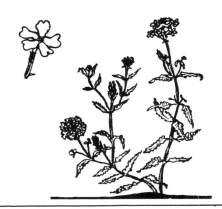

Verbena

VERBENA OFFICINALIS L.   Verbenaceae

Vervain family

Centers of Diversity: Locally found in England and Wales, with a variety native to Chile, Peru and most of the South American countries.

Common/Vernacular Names: *English:* European vervain, Verbain, Holy herb, White vervain, Juno's tears; *Spanish:* Verbena; *China:* Ma-pein-ts'ao, Lung-ya-ts'ao

Somatic Chromosome Numbers and Genome Constitution: $2n = 14$

Description: A herbaceous plant 45-60 cm high with square, tough, hispid stems; leaves opposite; flowers, pale lilac, July–Sept.

Lore, Legend and Romance: This plant is claimed by Yemayá and Oshún. These two deities are given the responsiblity of the care of the hair and liver. Yemayá corresponds with the Yesod of the Qabalistic Tree of Life, which governs the instincts and source of vital energy. She is equated with the Greek goddess Artemis and is astrologically under the rulership of the Moon. Oshún corresponds with Netzach of the Tree of Life. Netzach demands emotional sensitivity in relationships. She further corresponds with Aphrodite, the Greek goddess of love. Astrologically she is under the rulership of Venus.

Whatever certain writers may say, it is the wild vervain offered freely in Nature which possesses the most pronounced virtues. It is, in fact, the wild variety which is *"officinal"* while its sister from the New World is known by botanists as **Lippia citriodora** Kunth., lemon verbena because its leaves are grouped in threes on the stem and because of its delightful lemon aroma. This plant is often confused under the scientific names of **Aloysia citridora, Verbena triphylla, Lippia citriodora** and a common title, *"Yerba Louisa"* of Mexican tradition.

The Santeros and the inhabitants of the Caribbean Basin have been using **Stachytarpheta mutabilis** (Jacq.) Vahl. as their vervain. This plant used to be called **Verbena mutabalis** Jacq. in 1789, but was changed in 1804. This is a small shrub with green ascending leafy branches, up to 2.5 m high; leaves ovate-elliptical. It is generally dispersed on banks, path sides and in open areas in hilly districts. It flowers and fruits most of the year. It is native to Central and northern South America, including Dominican Republic, Trinidad and Tobago and reported from Cuba. Introduced in the Old World tropics, it is interchangeably used with **Stachytarpheta jamaicensis** (L.) Vahl. 1804, Syn. *Verbena jamaicensis* L., 1753.

The local name, porter weed, vervain, is a common weed in disused places, especially in pastures and sandy thickets near the sea. Flower and fruit all year. It occurs in Florida, Bahamas, Mexico to the West Indies, and introduced into the Pacific Islands.

In China, the stalk and leaves are thought to act on blood, relieving congestion, obstruction, dropsical effusions, and hematoceles, and is also accredited with being emmenagogue, anthelmintic with antiscorbutic properties. It is administered in malarial difficulties. The root is considered astringent and is employed in dysentery. The plant is gregarious on the Eastern Seaboard of the United States and is said to be febrifuge, emetic, vulnerary and rubefacient.

Just as **Verbena** spp. differ in outward appearance, so too do they differ in their chemical composition. Analysis has shown that the wild **Vervain officinalis** is by far the richer and more potent. It contains in particular a bitter glucoside, verbanaline, which acts on the liver and is considered tonic, digestive, antineuralgic and febrifuge. It is prescribed for disorders of the liver, particularly jaundice, congestion of the spleen and kidneys. It is an excellent diuretic, and is good for poor digestion, diahhrea, flatulence, gravel, general debility, feverish complaints, painful and irregular menstruation, especially when accompanied by migraine. The plant is used in nervous disorders, epilepsy and asthma; it relieves mental strain and helps cure infectious diseases. It is an efficient vermifuge.

This is one of the important plants of the "Omiero," the sacred elixer of the Santeria ceremony. The plant is used in combination with other plants in spiritual bath for purification of the spirit. It is customary for a sprig to be hung behind the doors to protect the house against evil and negative spirits. Vervain was for a long time the foremost magic herb, so much so that at the end of the 16th century, Mathioli wrote *"...sorcerers lose their senses at the mention of this herb."* The Romans dedicated it to Venus and called it **Verneris herba.** The Druids washed their alters with an infusion of vervain flowers. The plants were sprinkled on the altars of Jupiter in ceremonial rites of love. A crown of verbain was worn as a protection during evocation of demons. The Druids considered this a sacred plant. The leaves were worn on the person for the protection from harm. The plant was venerated in Iran, while in the East it was used as a symbol of enchantment. The Iranians were responsible for the belief that if one smeared the body all over with the juice of the herb, he would obtain anything he might desire, and also be able to reconcile those who were at enmity.

Just as certain herbs are delegated to specific planets, so do astrologers claim that certain plants are in harmony with individual zodiacal signs. Herbs which belong to a particular sign are said to be especially favorable when used by persons born under that sign. Vervain, therefore, is beneficial to persons born under the sign of Cancer.

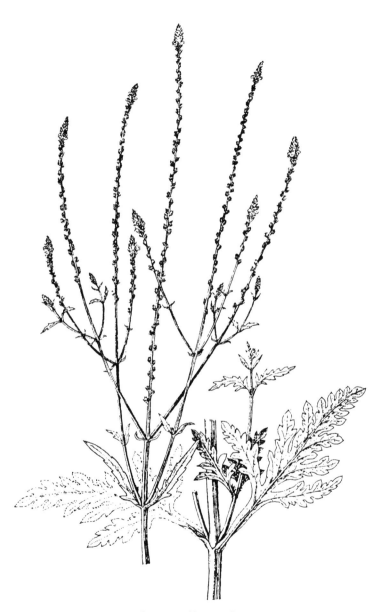

Verbena officinalis

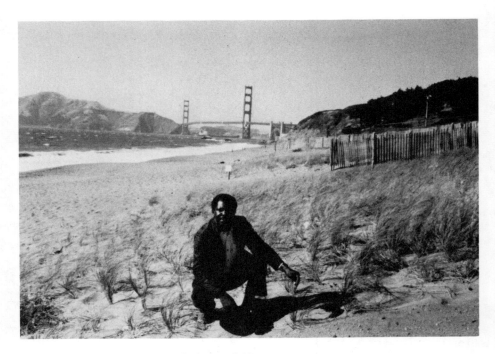

Ammophila arenaria
Grass planting on Baker Beach for erosion control, San Francisco, 1985.

Grass is the forgiveness of Nature—her constant benediction. Fields trampled with battle, saturated with blood, torn with the ruts of cannon, grow green again with grass, and carnage is forgotten. Streets abandoned by traffic become grass-grown like rural lanes, and are obliterated. Forests decay, harvests perish, flowers vanish, but grass is immortal. Sown by the winds, propagated by the subtle horticulture of the elements, which are its ministers and servants, it softens the rude outline of the world. Its tenacious fibers hold the earth in its place, and prevent its soluble components from washing into the wasting sea. It invades the solitudes of deserts, climbs the inaccessible slopes and forbidding pinacles of mountains, modifies climates, and determines the history, character, and destiny of nations. Unobtrusive and patient, it has immortal vigor and aggression. Banished from the thoroughfare and the field, it abides its time to return, and when vigilance is relaxed, or the dynasty has perished, it silently resumes the throne from which is has been expelled, but which it never abdicates. It yields no fruit in earth or air, and yet should its harvest fail for a single year, famine would depopulate the world.

John James Ingalls (Blue Grass)

MONOCOTYLEDONS

ARECA CATECHU L.   **Palmae**

Palm family

Centers of Diversity: Malaya and Sri Lanka and throughout tropical Asia.

Common/Vernacular Names: *English:* Betal nut palm, Areca nut; *Africa:* Mpopo (Swahili); *China:* Ping Lang

Somatic Chromosome Numbers and Genome Constitution: 2n=32

Description: A tall, slender, erect feathery palm attaining 15 m in height. Leaves pinnate; the inflorescence is below the oldest living leaves, monoecious, with the female flowers at the bases of the twigs, the male above. Fruit about the size of a hen's egg, yellow or orange-yellow when ripe. The brown conical seed (nut) is in the shape of acorn, and as hard as date kernels when mature. The plant takes about 6-8 years to come into bearing and continues bearing for at least 25 years or longer.

Lore, Legend and Romance: Among edible palm seeds, the betel nut plays a special role, for it is used in betel chewing, a habit that is adhered to by no less than 200 million people in the world. This habit of chewing **Areca** nut is of great antiquity and is mentioned by Herodotus in 340 B.C.

    The leaf of betel pepper vine, **Piper betel** L., also with the somatic chromosome number of 2n = 32, is wrapped round a slice of roasted betel seed, which contains the stimulating alkaloids and colors the saliva red. Because of the presence of the volatile oil, arecoline (a stimulant) present in **Areca catechu** L., it acts on the central nervous system and induces a state of sexual excitement. Conseqeuently, the betel nut has been employed as an aphrodisiac.

    Sometimes cloves, **Eugenia caryophyllus** (Sprengel) Bullock & Harrison, are used to flavor the betel quid (pan pati), in which chopped Areca nut mixed with lime, folded in a leaf of betel pepper (**Piper betel** L.) is chewed as a masticatory. In this connection, a substitute for **Piper betel** L. in the form of **Piper guineense**, the Ashanti or West African pepper, is sometimes used and the preparation is said to serve as a good substitute for tobacco or alcohol.

    In Sri Lanka, where the tree thrives in the moist low country, up to about 915 m in moist valleys, **Areca catechu** L. trees may also be seen in almost every Sri Lankan's garden. The nut is scraped and applied to ulcers; it also strengthens the gums. It acts as a stimulus on the digestive organs, and is supposed by the inhabitants (who use it habitually) to be preventive of dysentary. The nuts are also used in veterinary medicine, given for worms in animals. The plants are prohibited by the United States Government Agriculture Department.

COCOS NUCIFERA L.   Palmae

Palm family

Centers of Diversity: South East Asia, Indonesia and West Pacific Islands. It is not known whether it comes from South America or Southeast Asia, Indonesia or the West Pacific islands. From its native area it spread to all tropical countries. It has been suggested that sea currents may have helped in the dispersal over small distances (from island groups to island groups), but that man distributed the coconut over the world. It is possible that a secondary center arose in India.

Common/Vernacular Names: *English:* Coconut; *Spanish:* Coco lait, Obi, Cocotero, Coqueiro de Bahia (Brazil); *Africa:* Kokosi, Kube (Ghana), Attagara, Agbon (Nigeria), Mnazi (Swahili)

Somatic Chromosome Numbers and Genome Constitution: 2n=32

Description: A tall, stately tree attaining 30 m in height and up to 60 cm in girth, growing especially well near the seashores. Bole unusually slender, bulbous at the base, often leaning or bowed and giving a picturesque windswept landscape. It has been suggested that the gradually-curved stem appear to be due to heliotropism. Leaves large, composed of a rosette of feather-shaped fronds; pinnate, 5.4 m long and 2 m wide. Flowers small, light yellow in dense clusters, monoecious—both sexes on the same tree. Fruit, a drupe, one-sided, 37 mm long and 30 mm wide, formed from either one carpel or from three joined carpels. The outer layer of the pericarp is fibrous, the inner very hard, the shell of the coconut being sold in the market for various utility purposes. At the base are 3 marks, corresponding to the 3 loculi of the ovary, two of which have become obliterated. Under one of these is the embryo. The thin testa is lined with white endosperm, enclosing a large cavity partly filled with a milk fluid. Although the fruit is called a nut, it is botanically not a nut at all, but rather, a drupe.

Lore, Legend and Romance: Coconut is venerated in parts of the Pacific Islands as an emblem of fertility, while in West Africa it is regarded as a sacred tree and yields a *"holy oil"* much used in religious ceremony. It is the most important of all palms, furnishing the inhabitants of the tropics with practically every requisite, including food, sugar, drink, medicine, palm wine or toddy and alcoholic spirit, fiber, timber, thatch and domestic utensils, in fact as many uses as there are days in the year. Though cultivated in most tropical countries, it is nowhere found in the wild state.

    The coconut shell is used in divination in both West Africa and the Americas. Eight pieces of coconut shell are attached to a chain which has been decorated with beads and *"blessed"* by soaking in a sacred elixer which in the Santeria religion is called *"Omeiro."* These shells are cast by the priest or priestess and the *"prediction"* read according to which side of the coconut shell is faced-up. These coconut shells are often used by the *"Babalawo"* of the Yoruba religion in the divination which is known as *"Ifa."* Sometimes the coconut is replaced by *"cowry"* shells or kola nuts in these divination practices.

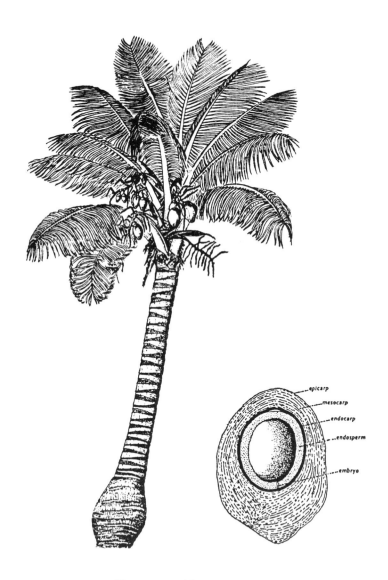

Cocos nucifera

Showing: longitudinal section through a fruit

In Balance with Nature

In the beginning—there was Earth; Beautiful and wild,
And then man came to dwell.
At first, he lived like other animals,
Feeding himself on creatures and plants around him.
And this was called IN BALANCE WITH NATURE
Soon Man multiplied.
He grew tired of ceaseless hunting for food;
He built homes and villages.
Wild plants and animals were domesticated.
Some men became Farmers so that others might become
Industrialists, Artists and Doctors.
And this was called Society.
Man and Society progressed.
With his God-given ingenuity, man learned to feed, clothe,
And protect himself more efficiently
So he might enjoy Life.
He built cars, houses on top of each other, nylon.
And Life was more enjoyable.
The men called Farmers became efficient.
A single farmer grew food for twenty-eight
Industrialists, Artists and Doctors
And Writers, Engineers, and Teachers as well.
To protect his crops and animals, the Farmer produced
Substances to repel or destroy insects, diseases and weeds;
These were called Pesticides.
Similar substances were made by Doctors to protect Humans
These were called Medicine.
The age of Science had arrived and with it came better diet
And longer happier lives for more members of Society.
Soon it came to pass
That certain well-fed members of Society
Disapproved of the Farmer using Science
They spoke harshly of his techniques for feeding,
Protecting and preserving plants and animals.
They deplored his upsetting the BALANCE OF NATURE:
They longed for the GOOD OLD DAYS.
And this had emotional appeal to the rest of Society.
By this time Farmers had become so efficient
Society gave them a new title: Unimportant Minority.
Because Society could not ever imagine a shortage of food
Laws were passed abolishing Pesticides, Fertilizers, and Food Preservatives.
Insects, diseases and weeds flourished.
Crops and animals died. Food became scarce.
To survive, Industrialists, Artists and Doctors
Were forced to grow their own food;
They were not very efficient.
People and Governments fought wars to gain more Agricultural Land
Millions of people were exterminated.
The remaining few lived like animals
Feeding themselves on creatures and plants around them
This was called IN BALANCE WITH NATURE...

John Carew.

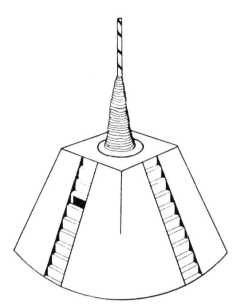

The Dogan people of Mali, West Africa, have understood concepts in astronomy which would have been too advanced for modern astronomers even fifty years ago. Above is the Dogan model of the universe showing the stairs used by the first people and the "gods" to descend to the earth. From: Griaule: **"Conversations with Ogotemmli." (See page 20)**

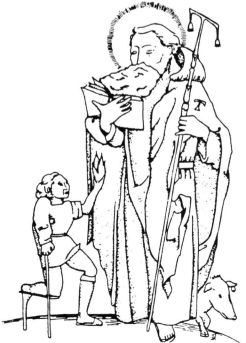

St. Anthony praying for a victim of the gangrenous type disease of ergotism. From a wood cut, 1517

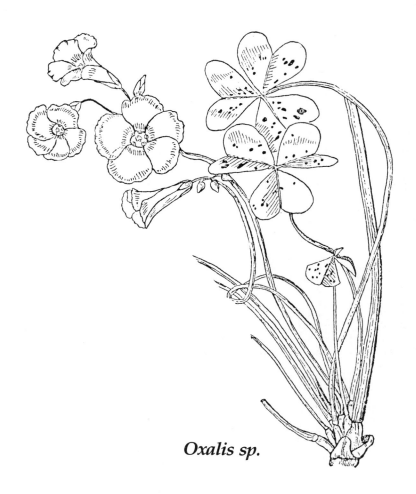

Oxalis sp.

Association of Plants with Deities

The association of a plant with a saint has been recognized since at least the sixth century. Its roots are, of course, in the pre-Christian attributions of plants to members of the pantheons of deities in all cultures. Many plants of economic importance to man were said to have been visible symbols of a deity who, in kindness, sympathy, or generosity, presented the plant to man. Athena became the patroness of Athens for giving the olive to the citizens. Honoring Christian saints with special flowers on their days served to reinforce the flow of religious faith throughout the year. St. Patrick's shamrock (actually an Oxalis) was a Druidic mystic symbol associated with the Celtic sun wheel. The Celtic name *"seanrog"* (little clover) became shamrog and finally shamrock. St. Patrick (390-464 A.D.) took this pagan symbol, pointed out that it really represented Trinity, and subverted its symbolism to the new religion.

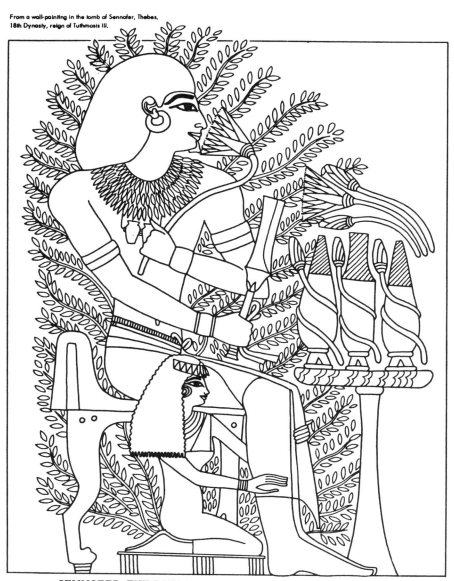

From a wall-painting in the tomb of Sennofer, Thebes,
18th Dynasty, reign of Tuthmosis III.

SENNOFER, THE ROYAL GARDENER, AND HIS SISTER MERIT

The bud or *"cabbage"* at the apex of the stem makes an excellent vegetable and is made into pickles and preserves. The fruit while young contain a pint or more of sweetish watery fluid, a refreshing drink; it decreases as the nut ripens. The kernels are eaten raw, or in curries, milk is expressed from them for flavoring, and oil is extracted by boiling or by pressure. The wealth of many tropical islands is derived from the oil which is expressed from the *"copra,"* the kernels of the palm being first dried before the oil is extracted.

The oil of this palm is applied to the head for cooling. The pulp of young fruits are given in sun-stroke; the root of the palm is said to strengthen the gums. The roots are astringent, though large doses are considered poisonous. The flowers are also considered medicinal. The outer part of the stem is used for toothache and earache.

The more appropriate name for the oil is a *"fat,"* for it is a soft solid at room temperature and in temperate climates, the melting point is about 23.4 degrees C (74 degrees F). The purified extract is variously known as *"coconut butter," "nut butter," "vegetaline"* and *"palmine."* The oil which should be used in pharmaceutical preparations is the product of the first pressing which can be purchased under the name of *"cold pressed"* coconut oil. The *"hot pressed"* oil is used for making candles, soaps and for other industrial purposes. The *"poonac,"* which is the waste product of the expression of the oil, is very valuable in fattening cattle. The outer wood of the stem is called porcupine wood and is used for ornamental articles.*

It is interesting to note that these *"nuts"* can withstand long periods of immersion in the sea. This does not, however, interfere with their ability to germinate later when reaching fertile soil thereafter. By this means, Nature has assured the distribution of the coconut around the world.

In my travels throughout the Caribbean Basin and South Florida, I noted extensive stands of coconut trees stretching for miles which showed signs of complete defoliation. This defoliation and near death is due to the disease known as *"lethal yellowing,"* which is caused by a mycoplasma-like organism which lives within the food-conducting veins of the coconut palm. A mycoplasma is an extremely small cellular microorganism requiring an electron microscope to visualize. Mycoplasmas generally are smaller than bacteria and are sensitive to certain types of antibiotics such as oxytetracycline. I had the pleasure of meeting Mr. Jim Dunaway, a botanist in South Florida who, in cooperation with the University of Florida, has developed an antibiotic substance which is capable of effective control of the disease. The disease has reached epidemic proportions in South Florida. The control of this *"lethal yellowing"* is undertaken in a series of measures: first, by cutting trees in advanced stanges of disease so that they cannot spread the causal agent to nearby healthy trees; secondly, by quarantine of affected areas so that diseased palms are not moved out to areas free of disease; thirdly, by replanting or underplanting with the Malayan Dwarf variety of coconut palm which is known to be resistant to *"lethal yellowing,"* and fourthly, by antibiotic treatment either as a preventative or a curative measure. *"Lethal yellowing"* is an always fatal, highly epidemic disease of coconut palm. This disease seems to be limited to land areas in the Caribbean Basin and South Florida. When

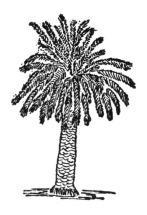

Phoenix canariensis

Pritchardia pacifica

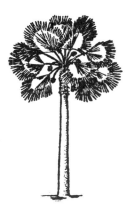

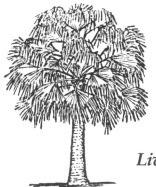

Livistonia chinensis

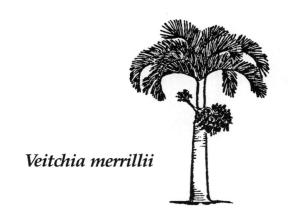

Veitchia merrillii

Howeia spp.

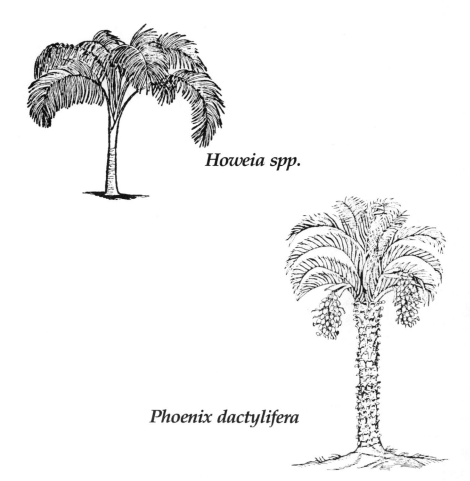

Phoenix dactylifera

the disease was reported in Florida in 1971, it was said to have killed 2,000 coconut trees in the first year and more than 20,000 trees in the first two year span.

The Golden and other Malayan varieties of coconut are known to be disease-resistant strains and as noted above they are being planted in Florida and the Keys in the hope of replacing those disease-riddled stands.

The dwarf coconut palms are a product of mutation, probably originating in Java or Sumatra, from there spreading throughout the world. This variety was imported to Brazil by the Brazilian Minister of Agriculture Miguel Calmon in the 1920's. These few plants formed the basis of the extensive plantations of coconut which form a vital part of the Brazilian economy.

The following list of palms are also susceptible to *"lethal yellowing:"*

PALM	COMMON NAME	PALM GROUP	ORIGIN
Allagoptera arenaria		Cocosoid	Brazil
Arenga engleri	Sugar palm	Caryotoid	Formosa
Arikuryoba schizophylla	Arikury palm	Cocosoid	Brazil
Borassus flabellifer	Palmyra palm	Borassoid	India, Malaya
Caryota mitis	Cluster fishtail palm	Caryotoid	India, Malaya
Chrysalidocarpus cabadae	Cabada palm	ʼArecoid	Madagascar
Corypha elata	Buri palm	Coryphoid	Bengal, Burma
Dictyosperma album	Hurricane or Princess palm	Arecoid	Mascarene Is., Maur
Gaussia attenuata	Puerto Rican Gaussia palm	Chamaedoreoid	Mascarene Is.
Howeia belmoreana	Belmore Sentry palm	Arecoid	Lord Howe Is.
Latania sp.	Latan palm	Borassoid	Mascarene Is.
Livistona chinensis	Chinese Fan palm	Coryphoid	Central China
Mascarena verschaffeltii	Spindle palm	Chamaedoreoid	Mascarene Is.
Nannorrhops ritchiana	Mazari palm	Coryphoid	Afghanistan
Phoenix canariensis	Canary Island Date palm	Phoenicoid	Canary Is.
Phoenix dactylifera	Date palm	Phoenicoid	W. Asia, N. Africa
Phoenix reclinata	Senegal Date palm	Phoenicoid	Tropical Africa
Phoenix sylvestris	Wild Date palm	Phoenicoid	India
Pritchardia affinis	Kona palm	Coryphoid	Fiji Is., Pacific
Pritchardia pacifica	Fiji Island Fan palm	Coryphoid	Fiji Is., Pacific
Pritchardia.thurstonii	Thurston Fan palm	Coryphoid	Fiji Is., Pacific
Trachycarpus fortunei	Chinese Windmill palm	Coryphoid	Cent. E. China
Veitchia merrillii	Adonidia or Christmas palm	Arecoid	Philippine Is.

ELAEIS GUINEENSIS Var. **IDOLATRICA** Chev.   **Palmae**

Syn. Elaeis dybowski Hua   **Palm family**
Syn. Elaeis thompsonii Chev.

Centers of Diversity: West tropical Africa; also a number of semi-wild palms occur in large areas of Africa.

Common/Vernacular Names: *English:* The King palm, Sacred palm, Palmier fetiche; *Africa:* Mchikichi, Miwese (Swahili), Ope Ife, Ogiedi, Ogedudin (Nigeria), Abe ohene (Ghana), Fade, Agoude (Dahomey)

Somatic Chromosome Numbers and Genome Constitution: 2n=32, (37)

Description: A tree which appears everywhere in West Africa and is regarded as a sacred plant. Leaflets joined at the base; fruits large, pericap birch red; nut hard with four or more cores in the endocarp.

Lore, Legend and Romance: The oil of the palm is now used as a medicine, and as a *"holy oil"* in Dahomey.

LODOICEA SEYCHELLARUM Comm. ex J. St. Hill.   **Palmae**

Syn. Lodoicea maldivica (Gmel.) Pers.   **Palm family**

Centers of Diversity: Native to the Island of Seychelles.

Common/Vernacular Names: *English:* Double coconut, Coco-de-mer, Sea coconut

Somatic Chromosome Numbers and Genome Constitution: 2n=

Description: A remarkable dioecious palm attaining 24 m or more in height; its growth rate being 30 cm per annum. Under normal circumstances, the tree does not flower until it is past 30 years of age. When it does, it bears clusters of enormous nuts—the fruits being one of the largest known to botanical science and weighing up to 20–22 kg each; it takes about 10 years to ripen. The nut is two-lobed, rarely three-lobed, and on being sown, takes about two years to germinate.

Lore, Legend and Romance: The seed is undoubtedly the largest known. The fruit, which holds many legends and superstitions is considered a product of the sea, was found floating in the Indian Ocean long before the tree was discovered; hence its French name of coco-de-mer.

   A root decoction or pulverized roots are used by the indigenous people of the islands of Seychelles as an aphrodisiac. The young delicate leaves (decoction) are used for gohorrhea. A fruit kept in a house is supposed to keep evil spirits away from the habitat. The fruits are also employed in religious ceremonies.

   The fruit commands a high price in certain religious and spiritual specialty shops. In San Francisco, I found such a shop which had the fruit available for $1,000.00 each.

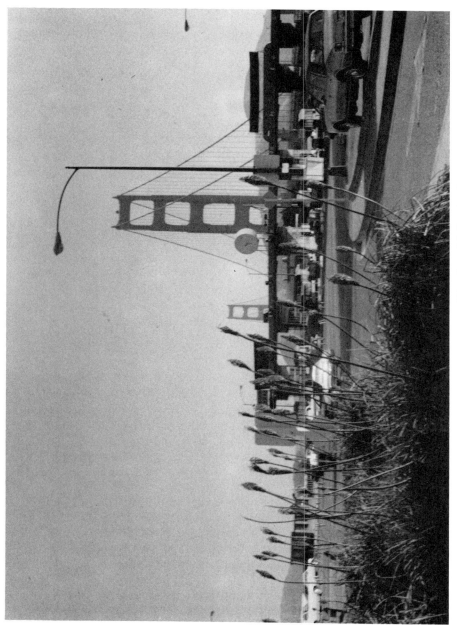

Kniphofia uvaria

Planting at toll gate plaza
Golden Gate Bridge, San Francisco, 1986.

KNIPHOFIA UVARIA(L) Oken   **Liliaceae**

Syn. Kniphofia aloides Moench.   **Lily family**
Syn. Kniphofia alooides
Syn. Tritoma uvaria

Centers of Diversity: South Africa.

Common/Vernacular Names: *English:* Red-hot poker, Touch-lily, Club-lily; *Africa:* Mhandwe (Zimbabwe)

Somatic Chromosome Numbers and Genome Constitution: $2n = 12$

Description: A rhizomatous, hardy, herbaceous perennial 1 m–1.5 m in height. Leaves linear-ensiform, to 1 m long and 2.5 cm wide, gray-green, strongly keeled, margins often rough. Flowers in long, scarlet flame-like spikes, showy in gardens and becoming yellow with age. They begin blooming in Autumn in the United States.

Lore, Legend and Romance: Kniphofia (ni-fóh-fi-a) was formerly known under the generic name of **Tritoma**. It was named in honor of the German professor of medicine, Johann Hieronymus Kniphof. The flowers, which are strikingly beautiful, attract hummingbirds. These flowers are also employed in floristry arrangements.

　　Kniphofia uvaria is considered as a sacred plant by the inhabitants of those areas of the world where the plant is native. Its attractive flowers are offered to the gods.

　　The plant is heat and drought resistant, and does best in climates that are somewhat Mediterranean, with mild winters, such as California. They have been cultivated long enough to give rise to garden varieties with different ranges of sizes and color of flowers. One particular variety worth mentioning is **Kniphofia uvaria var. erecta.** It exhibits a coral scarlet flower with stalks pointing upwards. Another species, though not a variety, that is most appealing from an aesthetic standpoint is the dwarf species **Kniphofia rufa,** a lower gray and with striking yellow flowers with serve as an excellent rock garden material.

　　There are about 70 species of **Kniphofias** in the world and equally twice the number of hybrids. **Kniphofias** are appropriate for planting around pools or ponds or in wild places, as well as for accents in borders or as clumps for striking effects.

THALIA GENICULATA L. Marantaceae

Arrowroot family

Centers of Diversity: Senegal to Nigeria, Sudan, Zaire, and Southwestern Africa. Also in the Americas, Florida to Brazil.

Common/Vernacular Names: *Spanish:* Platinillo, Zolupa; *Africa:* Babadua, Babaoo (Ghana)

Somatic Chromosome Numbers and Genome Constitution: $2n = 12$

Description: A tall, straggling shrub up to 2.4 m high; leaves 40x20 cm, smooth, shining, sometimes unequal-sized at base, lower part of petiole sheating stem, lateral nerves numerous, closely parallel, margin cartilaginous. Flowers white or pinkish-purple, opening only in early morning, often infested with black ants; rhachis articulate, bracts nearly 2.2 cm long, boat-shaped, 2-flowered; fruit 3-sided, yellow-black when ripe, covered with excrescences; aril basal, whitish; seeds mealy.

Lore, Legend and Romance: Parts of this plant are used in the ornamental top of a state umbrella. In olden times, the stems were used as divining-rods in detecting murderers. Leaves are sometimes used for wrapping food. The leaves are used medicinally in Sierra Leone.

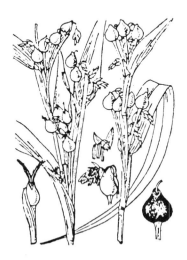

Coix lachryma-jobi

COIX LACHRYMA - JOBI L.

Gramineae (Poaceae)

Grass family

Centers of Diversity: Tropical Asia. Probably first domesticated as a cereal in Indo-China. Cultivated in the tropics but now naturalized and widespread in Africa where it occurs as a weed along streams and ditches, in wet waste places and cultivated fields.

Common/Vernacular Names: *English:* Job's tears, Pearl barley, Adlay;*Spanish:* Santa Maria, Santa Juana, Capin Rosario, Lagrimas de Job, Lagrimas de Cristo, Lagrimas de San Pedro, Capin de Nossa, Cuenta de la Virgen; *Africa:* Boukon, Bonkori, Ewuruwura (Nigeria), Kali bugi (Sierra Leone), Mtasubihi, Mtasbihi (Swahili); *China:* Niao-tuan-tzu

Somatic Chromosome Numbers and Genome Constitution: 2n=20

Description: An annual grass with tough fibrous roots, erect, grooved, leafy stems growing in dense clumps 25–200 cm high. Leaves alternate, linear, lanceolate 10–40 cm long, 2–4 cm wide, pointed at apex, the base more or less indented and clasping the stem, margins rough, flowers are minute.

Lore, Legend and Romance: In the Caribbean Basin, the seed decoction is taken as a diuretic in edema, ascites and pleurisy. In Brazil, the decoction of leaves and stems is taken as a potent diuretic in kidney and bladder troubles, and it is employed as a bath to relieve rheumatism and edema. Colombians take the root decoction to relieve chronic headache. In Cuba and Northern Colombia, it is traditionally believed that wearing the fruits around the neck prevents rheumatism and dental caries and promotes tooth development in infants. Fruits are edible and are used for food.

ERAGROSTIS TEF (Zuccagni) Trotter

Gramineae (Poaceae)

Syn. Eragrostis abessinica Link
Syn. Poa abyssinica Jacq.

Grass family

Centers of Diversity: Native to Ethiopia; introduced through Kew to various British colonies in 1806 from seeds obtained from Ethiopia. Areas of current occurrence include the West Indies, India, Australia, Nepal, Guyana, South Africa, Kenya and later to California.

Common/Vernacular Names: *English:* Teff; *Africa:* Teff (Ethiopia)

Somatic Chromosome Numbers and Genome Constitution: 2n=40

Description: An annual grass 60–120 cm high while under favorable conditions, coming to maturity in 2–3 months. The *"Thaf Tseddia"* is the quick growing variety, while *"Thaf Hagaiz"* the slow growing variety may mature anywhere up to 5 months. Both are distinguished chiefly as white and red in Ethiopia and Erithrea where it is cultivated as an important cereal and elsewhere for forage crop.

Lore, Legend and Romance: The seed, in its country of origin and in Erithrea, is used for making a delicious bread. Injera, an unleavened bread, is usually prepared from Teff, wheat, barley, corn or millet. It is valued because of its high protein content and amino acid balance. A valuable hay and pasture grass, suitable for all kinds of stock. The hay is also used for thatching the roofs of native huts.

An analysis of the grain (red teff) shows: water, 15.2%, albuminoids, 8.2%, starch, 68.1%, oil, 2.8%, cellulose, 2.8% and ash 2.9%.

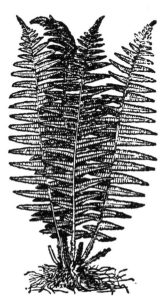

Aspidium filix-mas

ASPIDIUM FILIX-MAS(L.) Schott.   **Polypodiaceae**

Syn. Dryopteris marginalis (L.) Gray   **Common fern family**

Centers of Diversity: From Canada to Alabama and Arkansas and in central and western Carolinas.

Common/Vernacular Names: *English:* Male fern, Basket fern, Knotty brake, Female fern, Bear's paw fern, Male shield fern, Sweet brake, Shield root, Common spleenwort

Somatic Chromosome Numbers and Genome Constitution: 2n=

Description: A perennial, terrestrial fern, cultivated and found in rocky and dense woods throughout North America.

Lore, Legend and Romance: Rhizomes and stipes are used as an anthelmintic, taenicide, vermifuge, astringent for soreness and bruises. It contains an oleoresin and is poisonous due to the oils.

OSMUNDA REGALIS L.

Syn. Osmunda spectabilis Willd.

Royal flowering fern family

Centers of Diversity: This species occurs in swamps and wet places, in the northern and western states of the United States, in the mountains of Southern U.S. and in Caribbean Basin, Mexico to Paraguay, Europe and Western Asia to India and Korea.

Common/Vernacular Names: *English:* Male fern, King's fern, Royal fern, Flowering fern, Fern brake, Flowering brake, Hartshorne bush, Herb Christopher, Saint Christopher herb, Royal Osmund, Buckthorn brake; *Spanish:* Helecho de espigas, Helecho real; *China:* Wei

Somatic Chromosome Numbers and Genome Constitution: 2n = 44

Description: A fern 50 cm to 1.8 m high with hard, scaly, tuberous rhizomes coated with fibers and having a white, mucilaginous core, encountered on acid soils in coastal swamps from New Foundland to Saskatchewan, south to Florida and Texas.

Lore, Legend and Romance: The roots are stimulant, tonic, styptic and mucilaginous. The plant is said to be valuable in female sickness, cough, dysentery, rickets, muscular debility, rheumatism, swelling and indolent tumors. In Cuba, an infusion of crushed rhizome in water is taken as a remedy for liver complaints. Dried rhizome, steeped in hot water is a treatment for leucorrhea and other female troubles.

DICOTYLEDONS

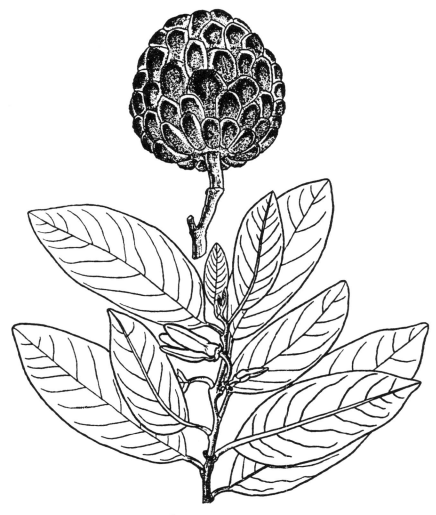

Annona squamosa

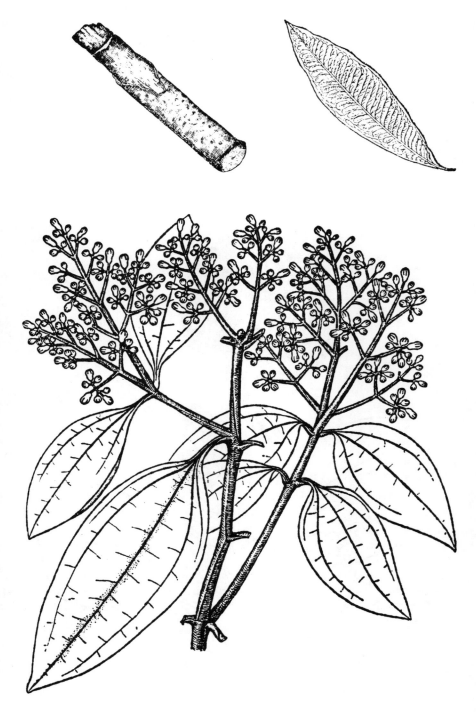

Cinnamomum zeylanicum
Showing stick and leaf

CINNAMOMUM ZEYLANICUM Breyn.	Lauraceae

Laurel family

Centers of Diversity: Native of the moist lowlands of Sri-Lanka and South India. Cultivation started in Sri-Lanka in 1770 and now cultivated in several countries including Burma and India and to a lesser extent in South America and the West Indies.

Common/Vernacular Names: *English:* Cinnamon; *Spanish:* Canela; *Africa:* Mdalasini (Swahili); *Asia:* Dalchini (Hindi), Dalchirii (Gujarati), Darushila (Sanskrit)

Somatic Chromosome Numbers and Genome Constitution: $2n=24$

Description: A small to medium-sized evergreen tree up to 15–18 m in height. Leaves opposite and sub-opposite, strongly 3-nerved from base to near apex, shiny adaxially, somewhat glaucous abaxially, drying yellowish-brown, glabrous, ovate to elliptic-lanceolate, rounded at the base and up to 15 cm long. Flowers in lax axillary inconspicuous terminal panicles, yellowish. Fruits very nearly black, fleshy berry, 1-seeded, ovoid.

Lore, Legend and Romance: This plant is also called Canela in Spanish and is sometimes used instead of Canela winterana in the preparation of *"Omiero."* The characteristic aroma and taste of this plant is due to the presence of a volatile oil consisting of cinnamic aldehyde mixed with resins. This oil can now be produced synthetically and like the natural substances, it is used by the food industry for sweets , liqueur, drugs and perfume industries. The branches of 3–5 years' growth are cut down at the end of the rainy season, and the bark ripped up longitudinally with a knife and gradually loosened until it can be taken off. The slices are then exposed to the sun and as they dry, they curl up into quills, in which they form cinnamon for export.

Due to this volatile oil, cinnamon behaves as a carminative and antiseptic and by virtue of the tannins present, it acts as a mild astringent. In India and Sri-Lanka, the dried inner bark which constitutes the drug is used in diarrhea, nausea and vomiting. It is also commonly used as a condiment. The scientific name **Zeylanicum** refers to Ceylon, the old name of Sri-Lanka, where the true indigenous species occurs.

In Brazil the Canela as a vernacular name is used for a number of species of the **Lauraceous** genera, namely: **Ocotea, Nectandra** and **Cryptocarya.**

According to Purseglove (1968), it is doubtful whether cinnamon bark was used by ancient Egyptians in embalming, as is stated in some works. The plant is generally believed to have reached Egypt and Europe by 5th century B.C. and was known to Herodotus, being brought by Sabaens from India or Sri-Lanka to Southern Arabia, which became the center of the spice trade; the traders concealed the true source of these spices.

DISTEMONANTHUS BENTHAMIANUS Baill.　　Caesalpiniaceae (Fabaceae)

Pea family

Centers of Diversity: West Africa; Sierra Leone to Gabon.

Common/Vernacular Names: *English:* African Satinwood, Yellow Satinwood; *Africa:* Bonsamdua, Anyen-dua (Ghana), Ayan, Amurinkogun (Nigeria);

Somatic Chromosome Numbers and Genome Constitution: 2n=

Description: A slender tree up to 37 m high and 3 m girth; bole slightly bent, cylindrical, butressed. Leaves pinnate, leaflet 20-28, 10x4 cm, ovate-lanceolate, alternate, acuminate, with numerous conspicuous lateral nerves; flowers in loose panicles, creamy-white and red or pinkish; sepals 5, pinkish brown and unequal, Feb.–July.

Lore, Legend and Romance: This tree has various superstitious uses in West Africa, in addition to being a useful timber. The leaves, bark, and roots are ingredients in the brasspan ceremony of making a new shrine in Ashanti; it is a much venerated magic tree in Sierra Leone.

The sapwood is narrow, white and the heartwood dull yellow or light brown when dry. The powdered bark, mixed with redwood powder (padouk) in water, is used in Tropical Africa for skin diseases. It is given in enemas.

PROSOPIS SPICIGERA L.　　Mimosaceae (Fabaceae)

Pea family

Centers of Diversity: Northern India.

Common/Vernacular Names: *English:* Sami tree

Somatic Chromosome Numbers and Genome Constitution: 2n=28, 52, 56

Description: A medium-sized thorny tree of the arid regions of Northern India. It is a close ally of the American mesquite, **Prosopis juliflora** (Sw.) D.C., known in the Caribbean Basin as *"Cashaw."* The plant grows gregariously.

Lore, Legend and Romance: This is the main fuel of the Punjab. Because of its enormously long tap root, which has been measured and found to be as much as 25 m long and penetrating vertically up to 19.5 m, it is able to exist under conditions of extreme aridity. Gum exudes from the stumps of cut stems and branches and from other wounds. The gum is very brittle and occurs in small angular fragments of yellowish color, sometimes in ovoid tears about 5 cm long. Internally an amber color, but taking on a frosted appearance on the outside. With water it forms a tasteless mucilage.

The bark and seed are astringent. Bark brew is taken for colds, catarrh, cough, asthma, gout, piles and worms. This is a highly regarded and sacred tree of the Hindus, those of Northern India in particular.

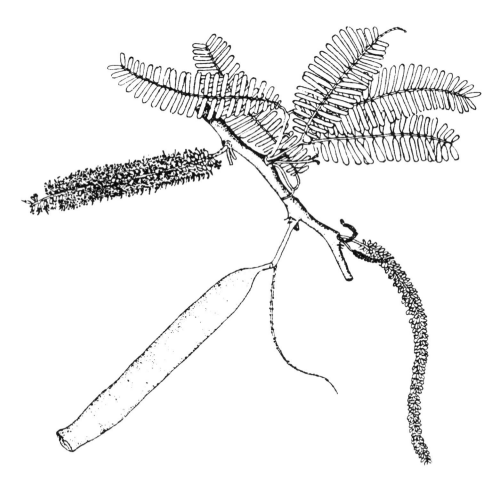

Prosopis juliflora

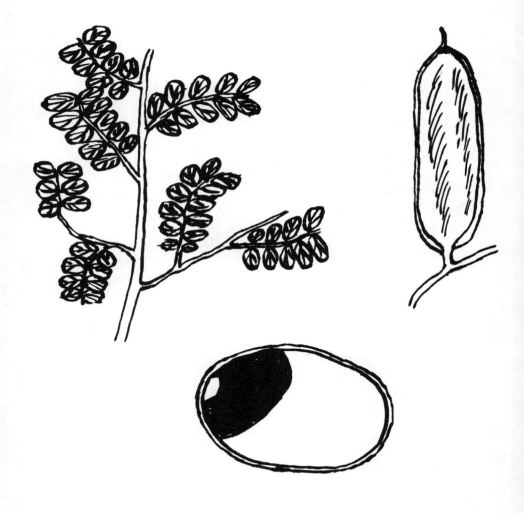

Abrus precatorius
showing fruit pod and seed

The Sami tree's close relative in Africa is **Prosopis africana** Taub., with a synonym of **Prosopis oblonga** Benth. The species occurs from Senegambia to Zaire and then to Sudan and Uganda. **Prosopis africana** Taub. is known in Ghana as *"Prekese"* and *"Lungbung"* while in Nigeria it is called *"Ayan"* and *"Kiriya."* This spreading tree is about 18 m high with slightly buttressed lower bole and open crown with drooping foliage resembling **Tamarindus** spp. Flowers yellowish, fragrant, in dense axillary racemes 5–10 cm long, Mar.–May. Fruit up to 50 x 35 mm, black or brown-purple, shining, stout, roughly cylindrical, pericarp thick, brown, powdery; seed loose and rattling, up to 10, nearly 18 mm long, shining with a thin line around margin. The seeds are used for food in Nigeria in much the same way as those of **Parkia** spp. (*"Igba"*).

The bark of the roots contains tannin while that of the stem contains up to 16% tannin and is used in tanning. The root decoction is used for toothache while the bark has been used as a dressing or in making a lotion for wounds.

ABRUS PRECATORIUS L.   Papilionaceae (Fabaceae)

Pea family

Centers of Diversity: Native of India, the plant has now been introduced and naturalized practically throughout the tropics and sub-tropical regions of the world, including Southern Florida where it behaves as though it is a native on the oolitic soils.

Common/Vernacular Names: *English:* Indian licorice, Love bean, Lucky bean, Weather vine, Prayer bean, Seminole bead; *Spanish:* Peonia de St. Thomas, Cain ghe, Jequerit, Liane reglisse, Graines reglisse rouges et noires; *Africa:* Bope (Zimbabwe), Titi (Zambia), Damma-bo, Anyen-enyiwa (Ghana), Mkamdumwe (Swahili); *China:* Hsiang-su-tzu, Hung-tou

Somatic Chromosome Numbers and Genome Constitution: $2n = 22$

Description: A salt tolerant climbing shrub with string-like greenish stems curling counter-clockwise around objects and plants, gregarious in thickets and in secondary regenerations in rather dry areas. Leaves alternate, pinnate 5–13 cm long; leaflets 15–20 pairs. Flowers pale pink in dense, axillary racemes. Fruit a dehiscent pod, pubescent, ripening brown and exposing up to 8 seeds per fruit. Seeds decoratively scarlet and tipped with a black spot at the hilum.

Lore, Legend and Romance: This plant is known as Indian licorice, in India its scarlet and black seeds are made into prayer beads or rosaries. They are also used as weight measures. Another interesting bit of romance is added to this remarkable plant becuase the famous Kohinoor diamond was weighed by means of these pretty seeds.

According to A. Hyatt Verrill in his *"Wonder Plants and Plant Wonders,"* (1939), some plants are regarded as weather *"prophets"* because they can accurately predict or give an indication of the weather. One such plant, and the most important of them all is **Abrus precatorius** L. The plant was actually grown at the author's alma mater near London at the Royal Botanic Gardens, Kew, England. Its weather forecasting abilities were noted.

This plant is in harmony with the astrological sign of Virgo and comes under the rulership of Mercury, Wednesday being the day for using it. All parts of the plant, especially the seeds, are poisonous. The seeds contain two poisonous principles which when extracted and mixed are known as abrin (a toxalbumin) and abric acid, a glycoside. Chemically, abrin is related to ricin (of **Ricinus communis** L.) and in action behaves like snake venom. Like snake venom, it is ineffective on the blood if taken internally. As boiling destroys the poison, the seeds have been eaten as food occasionally, e.g., in Egypt. The leaves and roots contain glycyrrhizine, hence its name *"liquorice plant."* It should be pointed out here that the root of the plant has been used as a pleasant demulcent as well as an excellent cough remedy.

In India, the seeds are used as an abortifacient and in cases of nervous debility; pasted seed is used as an aphrodisiac and is applied on skin diseases, leprosy, and paralytic limbs. Seed oil rubbed on the scalp promotes hair growth. The root is emetic, leaf juice is taken in cases of gout, choked throat and hoarseness. Seed and root are toxic in heavy doses.

In the Caribbean and tropical South America, an infusion of the leaves, flowers, stems or roots is taken for sore throat or cough remedy. The Bahamians use the leaf decoction as a febrifuge. In Trinidad the leaf or vine decoction is taken as a remedy for influenza, tuberculosis and fever. Cubans consider the root decoction beneficial for heart problems, flatulence, hernias and burns. A seed infusion has been employed in Brazil to treat trachoma, however, the practice was abandoned as too dangerous.

The seeds are much used by the Santeros in their religious works. There is widespread belief in the Caribbean Basin and South America that chains of this seed worn around the neck of an infant assures good luck protecting the child from illness.

In West Africa, seeds are often used as necklaces and rosaries, and had at one time been used as a gold weight by the Ashantis. The Arabs use the plant for malaria and considered it to be conducive to sleep; it is effective in kidney and bladder troubles though dangerous when used in excesses. On the Ivory Coast the pulp of leavy stems is applied to wounds and cuts as a styptic. When eaten, it allays gastro-intestinal pains, acts as an aphrodisiac, and is said to help in confinements. Root preparations are considered strongly diuretic and are prescribed for gonorrhea. Abrin acts strongly on the conjunctiva, hence oculists use it for trachoma. A paste prepared from the seeds, with salt, is applied to boils by the Yorubas. The seeds are used in East Africa for venereal diseases and urinary troubles.

In China, where the plant occurs in South China, the seeds are taken as medicine and are said to *"permeate the nine cavities of the body and expel every sort of evil effluvia from heart and abdomen."* It is diaphoretic, expectorant, antiperiodic, and destroys every sort of visceral or cuticular worm.

As attested to by A. Hyatt Verrill (1939) this plant is unquestionably an accurate weather predictor. I should, however, point out that a number of plants indigenous to diverse areas around the world have been known to serve as weather *"prophets."* **Abrus precatorius** is among the most important of those known to date. The efficacy of this phenomenon has been well documented from the field trials at the Royal Botanic Gardens, Kew, England.

An established plant *"told"* ot the impending weather variations in advance on several occasions, prior to the scientists in the Government Weather Bureau.

Although the East Indians have long known of the seemingly mystic powers of the plant, and its amazing ability to foretell weather, electrical disturbances, and even catastrophies, yet it was not known to the outside world until about 50 years ago, when Professor Nowack, the Australian scientists, astonished his fellow scientists by proving that the magic plant could predict weather two days in advance. His demonstration was so convincing and was considered of so much importance that the Prince of Wales (later King Edward VII of England) arranged for Baron Nowack to go to England and establish the strange plant weather bureau at Kew.

The plant is known to be extremely sensitive to magnetic and electrical conditions, even when at a great distance, and any approach of atmospheric or other disturbances is indicated by the movement of the leaves of the plant. Again and again, Professor Nowack *"beat"* the trained meteorological experts by means of weather-plants, even predicting cyclonic disturbances and earthquakes. But the greatest feat of the astounding plant was its forecast of a catastrophe which no human weather *"prophet"* could have foretold, for the plants at Kew actually predicted a fire-damp explosion in British mines which caused the loss of many lives.

BAPHIA NITIDA Lodd.   **Papilionaceae**

Pea family

Centers of Diversity: West Africa; Sierra Leone to Cameroons. Cultivated formerly as a source of red dye. Now it is only cultivated as an ornamental.

Common/Vernacular Names: *English:* Camwood, Bread leaf tree; *Africa:* Dwene, Aboloobaatso (Ghana), Igi-osun, Ufiye (Nigeria)

Somatic Chromosome Numbers and Genome Constitution: 2n=44

Description: A shrub or small tree up to 9 m high and 45 cm in diameter; branchlets usually glabrous; leaves 13–20 cm x 5–8 cm, oblong, elliptic or ovate, acuminate, base rounded, petiole over 2.5 cm long; flowers white with yellow spots, sweet scented, usually 1–4 together, Jan.–July, Sept.; fruits glabrous, 50 x 15 mm, pointed at ends, seeds 1–2.

Lore, Legend and Romance: This is the earliest of the West African dye woods and was exported mainly from Sierra Leone, but later the West Indian logwood, **Haematoxylon campechianum** L. largely replaced it, and now it is obtainable in quantity from African Padauk (**Pterocarpus soyauxii** Taub.). **Baphia nitida** Lodd. has certain sacred and superstitious uses, including that of the dying of sacred objects. It has been said that the red dye, placed on the forehead of a man during a particular ceremonial dance, indicates that he has killed a man or a leopard.

A paste prepared from this tree is rubbed on the body by Yoruba honey-hunters to prevent bee-stings. On the Ivory Coast, the powdered leaves are much used for venereal diseases, either in palm-wine, or as a dietary supplement. The leaves or sap obtained by heating them is applied to parasitic skin diseases.

Haematoxylon campechianum L., a native of Central America, belongs to **Leguminosae** and is commonly called *"Campeche wood"* or the West Indian *"logwood."* The tree has a thorn-covered trunk. The plant has been introduced into Brazil very successfully.

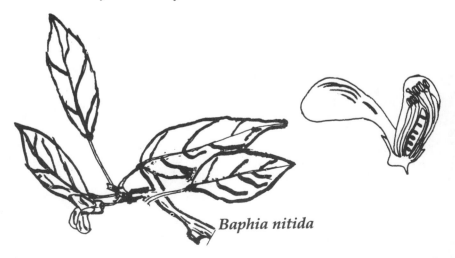

Baphia nitida

BUTEA FRONDOSA Koen ex Roxb.   Papilionaceae (Fabaceae)

Syn. Butea monosperma Kuntze.   **Pea family**

Centers of Diversity: Native of India and Pakistan.

Common/Vernacular Names: *English:* Flame of the Forest, Parrot tree; *Asia:* Palas, Tesu, Dhak (Hindi), Khakro (Gujarati), Palasha (Sanskrit)

Somatic Chromosome Numbers and Genome Constitution: 2n = 18

Description: A salt tolerant small to medium-sized tree to 15 m high, especially sacred to the Brahmins in India. This deciduous tree, found chiefly in the mixed or dry deciduous forests of Central and Western India, is most common in the plains or lower regions of hilly environs. The bark is grey, rough and the trunk is crooked with upright branches. Leaves compounded with 3 broad-oval, leathery leaflets to 2.4 m long, downy and bronze when young, dull and ugly when old. Flowers, scarlet and orange, exceedingly beautiful, massed along the ends of the branches from late Jan. to Mar. Seed pods flat, 10–20 cm long, containing 1 flat brown seed 3.2 cm long. The name monosperma refers to the single seed.

Lore, Legend and Romance: The tree is considered purgative, anthelmintic, vermifuge and rubefacient; it is taken for destroying all sorts of intestinal worms, piles, haematemesis, hemorrhage, and for increasing micturition (diuretic) and menstrual flux (emmenagogue). The leaf is febrifugal and promotes sexual excitement (aphrodisiac). The gum is taken orally in diarrhea and rubbed on sprained and inflamed limbs. Bark is antidote to snake poisoning. Flowers and buds are astringent and diuretic. When incisions are made in the bark, a juice exudes and dries to form a gum. The red colored gum, called *"Bengal Kino,"* or *"Butea gum,"* contains tannins, is a best treatment for roundworms. The tree is highly valued as a host tree for the lac insect, Tachardia lacca Kerr.

CAJANUS CAJAN (L.) Millsp.   Papilionaceae (Fabaceae)

Syn. Cajanus indicus Spreng.   **Pea family**

Centers of Diversity: Native to Africa. Wild and naturalized plants have been found there. Spread to India where a secondary center arose; now a pan-tropical plant where it has naturalized itself and spread to the sub-tropics as well. Seeds have been found in Egyptian tombs of the XIIth Dynasty and it was cultivated there before 2000 B.C., by which time Egypt had established trade relations with tropical Africa to the south and Syria to the east.

Common/Vernacular Names: *English:* Pigeon pea, Gungo pea, Congo pea, Cajan pea, Red gram, Yellow dahl, Angola pea, Christmas pea, Arhar of India, Tur of India; *Spanish:* Abavante, Cachito, Frijol chino, Garbanzo folso, Pois Congo, Chicharo de Paloma, Cajun, Gandul; *Africa:* Atii, Atiyi (Ghana), Waken turawa (Nigeria), Mbaazi (Swahili); *China:* Shan-Tou-ken

Somatic Chromosome Numbers and Genome Constitution: 2n=22, 44, 66

Description: A drought resistant bushy shrub to small tree up to 3.5 m in height behaving more like a straggler, with a deep root system which permits good growth under semi-arid conditions with under 75 cm of rain per year. Leaves compounded; leaflets bifoliate, elliptical and pubescent. Undersurface of leaves strikingly silvery-tomentellous. Ribbed twigs and branchlets also armed with grey velvety hairs. Flowers yellow to orange-yellow, borne in short axillary and terminal clusters. Fruits in a capsulate seed pod, ripening brown, containing almost spherical smooth seeds. Seed is green when immature but on maturity may assume any combination of colors from white, yellow to red or black.

Lore, Legend and Romance: The seeds are a source of nutritious food in West Africa, and are used in soups in Ghana. The flowers are reputedly beneficial in bronchitis, coughs and other respiratory troubles. A decoction of 20–40 grams of leaves boiled in one liter of water is used to bathe swellings, wounds, sores and skin diseases and is also used as a vaginal douche. Boiled leaves as a *"tea"* may be taken every morning by women who haven't had babies and want to become pregnant. It is also drunk by pregnant women for 7 to 8 months to promote an easy delivery. It is also a remedy for menstrual cramps and leucorrhea and may be employed as an eye lotion to dispel inflammation. In Jamaica, the leaves are boiled with ashes, salt, root of Coconut (**Cocos nucifera**) and bark of the **Zanthoxylum mortinicense**, and the decoction is held in the mouth to relieve toothache. In some countries in the Caribbean Basin, a leaf decoction is an antidote for fish poisoning. The leaves are sometimes boiled with leaves of mango (**Mangifera indica** L.), and the *"tea"* taken to overcome dizziness.

In China, the woody root varying from the size of the little fingers, to mere rootlets is the part used in medicine; it is said to be anthelmintic, sedative, expectorant and vulnerary.

Both mature and immature seeds are staple food in the Bahamas, Puerto Rico, Trinidad, Panama and India. They are a good source of protein and are considered an excellent food when eaten with rice as is customary in those tropical countries.

The plant serves as a host to Liriomyza sativa, the vegetable leaf miner, a pest that ravages most economic crops in South Florida. In Africa, too, the plant is a host to silkworms (Dalziel). This is the plant bearing the seeds that furnish the **pulse** so well known in India as dahl. The young leaves are eaten in Indonesia, either raw or cooked in food. The raw unripe seeds contain about: water 67.4 per cent; protein 7.0 per cent; fat 0.6 per cent; carbohydrate 20.2 per cent; fiber 3.5 per cent; ash 1.3 per cent.

ERYTHRINA CORALLODENDRON L.   Papilionaceae (Fabaceae)

Pea family

Centers of Diversity: Indigenous to Jamaica, Haiti and Puerto Rico. Cultivated in Bermuda, the Bahamas, Cuba, Southern Mexico and Brazil.

Common/Vernacular Names: *English:* Baumortel, Bean tree, Immortel, Judas tree, Jumbie bead, Devil's tree, Lent tree; *Spanish:* Abre a corail, Bico de papagaio, Bucare espinoso

Somatic Chromosome Numbers and Genome Constitution: 2n = 42

Description: A deciduous shrub to small tree up to 15 m in height. Leaves trifoliolate. Flowers attractive, coral-red or blood-red, in clusters measuring 30 cm long. Fruit a typical legume up to 25 cm long and 1.5 cm wide; constricted between the seeds, which are entirely scarlet or sometimes with a black area covering about 1/3 of the seed.

Lore, Legend and Romance: This plant is venerated by Santería adherents who believe that benevolent spirits dwell in the plant, especially during the flowering period when the plant is completely leafless.

It is a substitution for the African species **Erythina senegalensis** DC., the coral flower of tropical rain forests of West Africa, where in Ghana it is known as *"Osurokasoro"* meaning "heaven remains up." This decorative West African plant is sometimes grown for sacred purposes.

A decoction of roots and bark is generally used for baths, often with lemon juice, spices and Guinea grains for bronchial troubles, coughs, pneumonia, jaundice and gonorrhea, in much the same manner as **Erythrina corallodendron** is employed in the Caribbean basin.

ERYTHRINA SENEGALENSIS D.C.   Papilionaceae (Fabaceae)

"Sacred Plant"   **Pea family**

Centers of Diversity: West Africa; Senagambia to Cameroons.

Common/Vernacular Names: *English:* Coral Flowers; *Africa:* Osurokasoro, Akoble, Zanzambuli (Ghana)

Somatic Chromosome Numbers and Genome Constitution: 2n=42

Description: A medium-sized, soft-wooded tree up to 15 m (usually much smaller) with rough, spiny bark; branches brittle, slash yellow; leaves with 3 leaflets 15 x 13 cm (central leaflet largest), lanceolate to broadly ovate, glabrous or nearly so, sometimes with prickles on midribs. Flowers in lax racemes, large and scarlet, when leafless, standard, petal folded flat (Dec–Mar); pods nearly 13 cm long, constricted between seeds, becoming twisted; seeds red, smooth, shining.

Lore, Legend and Romance: The plant is grown for sacred purposes and is a well-known medicinal plant among Africans inhabiting the savannah regions. The roots are used for venereal diseases. A decoction of the powdered bark is given to women after childbirth in Guinea. The pounded bark and leaves in soup, are used in Ghana for sterility in women. The wood is chewed as an aphrodisiac.

LONCHOCARPUS CYANESCENS (Schum. & Thonn.) Benth   Papilionaceae (Fabaceae)

Pea family

Centers of Diversity: West Tropical Africa

Common/Vernacular Names: *English:* West African indigo, Yoruba indigo; *Africa:* Njassi, Elu (Nigeria); Akase, Amati (Ghana) Msumari-mwitu (Swahili).

Somatic Chromosome Numbers and Genome Constitution: 2n=44

Description: A shrub or woody climber over 6 m in height; branchlets silky when young; leaves pinnate, 4-5 pairs, ovate or elliptic, 50 x 25 mm, lateral nerves about 5 pairs, leaves turning blue-green on drying. Flowers in panicles, 30 cm long, reddish or bluish-white, sweet-scented, May–June; much frequented by insects. Pods flat, indehiscent, 100 mm x 10 mm, turning bluish-black on drying; seeds 1-5, standing out prominently.

Lore, Legend and Romance: Crushed leaves are made into balls, then fermented and dried. To obtain the actual indigo, the yellow liquor in the fermenting pot is strained and aerated, the process changing it first to green and finally to blue. The blue coloring extracts, chiefly from young leaves are used in Nigeria for dying traditional clothes.

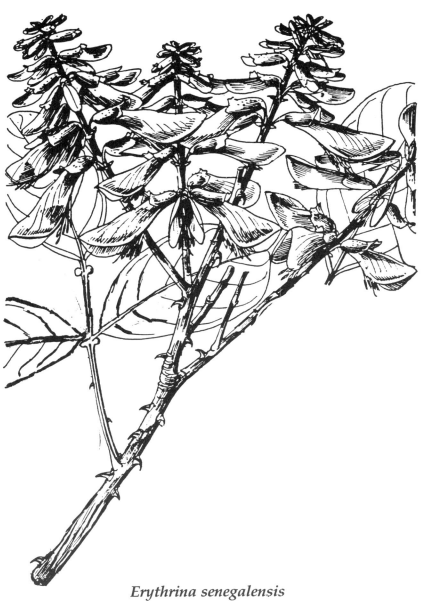

Erythrina senegalensis
[After Irvine]

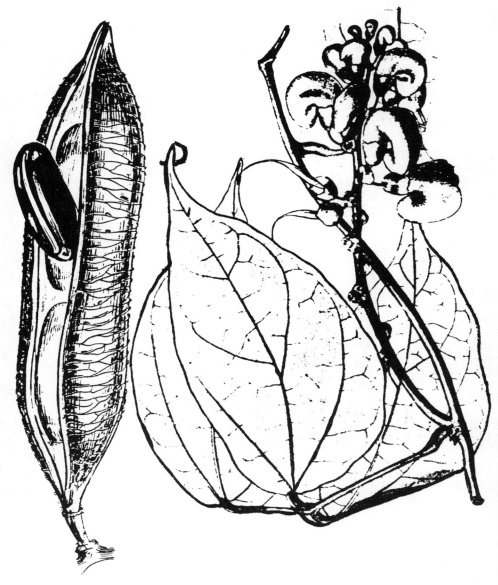

Physostigma venenosum
(showing fruit pod & seed)

A decoction of root and leafy stems are drunk by women after childbirth in Ivory Coast. The washed roots, boiled with other herbs, are a cooling stomachic in Ghana.

The plant's closest relative, **Lonchocarpus utilis** Smith, a native of Peru, is used in the same manner as in West Africa by the Peru Indians. It, too, has a chromosome number of 2n = 44. It is cultivated as a source of rotenone.

PHYSOSTIGMA VENENOSUM Balf.   Papilionaceae (Fabaceae)

Pea family

Centers of Diversity: West Africa; Sierra Leone to Cameroon and then to Zaire

Common/Vernacular Names: *English:* Ordeal bean, Calabar bean; *Africa:* Osamanntew *("spirits marbles")* (Ghana); Esere (Nigeria)

Somatic Chromosome Numbers and Genome Constitution: 2n=

Description: A twining woody climber up to 6 m or more in height. Leaves trifoliolate, 15 x 10 cm, 3-nerved at base, central leaflet broadly ovate, laterals obliquely ovate and unequal-sided, base rounded, acuminate. Flowers zygomorphic, purple, in axillary drooping racemes, Aug. Fruit, dehiscent pod, narrowed at ends, 15 x 5 cm, yellowish-brown, glabrous, seeds few, ellipsoid, over 2.5 cm long, one sided nearly straight, the other grooved by depressed hilum.

Lore, Legend and Romance:

There are many plants which have traditionally been shrouded by a cloak of mystery and superstition and conveying a lore and legend which boggle the imagination and arouse skepticism about the efficacies of these plants. One of the most fascinating plants in this category is **Physostigma venenosum,** known as the *ordeal bean* or the *Calabar bean* because of the availability of the fruits of the plant in the Calabar Province of Nigeria as well as the prolific use of the plant by the indigenous people in the area.

These powerful people, the Efiks, a nation of Ibibio speaking people, inhabit the coastal area of Nigeria around the Niger Delta at the estuary of the Cross River and the Calabar River, these waterways also known as the *Oil Rivers.*

The Efiks were a clever, domineering group of merchants who established themselves in the slave trade with the Europeans early on at the beginning of building of trading posts along the coast of Africa in the late 15th century. One of the first European settlements was around Sao Tome and Fernando Po, islands just off the coast and away from the swamp lands.

The Efiks became very rich and influential due to their trade in human beings for the American colonies and palm oil for Europe. Along with their wealth came political power which they used to terrorize the inhabitants and subdue any dissent. The authoritarian kings of the Efiks, known as the *Obong*, established secret societies called *Egbo* or Leopard societies. This society was responsible for enforcing laws, settling disputes, declaring wars and arranging peace pacts with neighbors. There were many levels of this society, each of which had a very distinctive costume and social responsibility.

The religious and recreational functions of the Leopard society pervaded the entire society. In their fervor to enforce the law, these *Egbo* administered a potion made with this Calabar bean to people who were suspected of wrong- doing or *witchcraft* and thereby subjecting these persons to the *poison ordeal*.

The beans of the leguminous plant would be crushed and mixed with water. The suspect would then be forced to drink this mixture and according to legend, the guilty would die of poison while the innocent would regurgitate the mixture, hence, proving his innocence.

The *Egbo* exploited their position in society with the threat of this *poison ordeal*; The *Egbo* almost always were senior members of the councils of government and religious organizations. They used their positions to insure dominance over the populace. They would administer heavy fines and punishments to individuals who caused Society members any personal inconvenience or distress.

One account of such a *poison ordeal* appeared in the American Association for African Research, publication no.2, 1958, based on the early writings by a British medical officer, William Daniell. In this account, a Calabar man sneaked aboard a moored ship belonging to Dr. Daniell. He asked for asylum and protection from his master, an *Egbo* merchant. The man wished to escape captivity as he was accused of being a *free mason* (which meant witchcraft at the time). The *Egbo* merchant had asked the servant to *chop nut* which meant that he should eat the Calabar beans to prove his innocence. The servant was afraid to *chop nut* because of the effects he had seen on others who had ingested the *ordeal bean*. The servant described the victim of the *poison ordeal* as *foaming at the mouth* with spasmodic body convulsion like movements.

Diviner's Chain

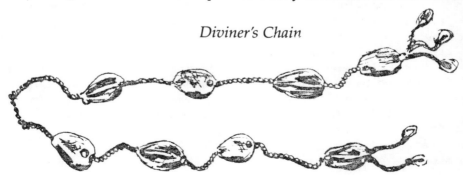

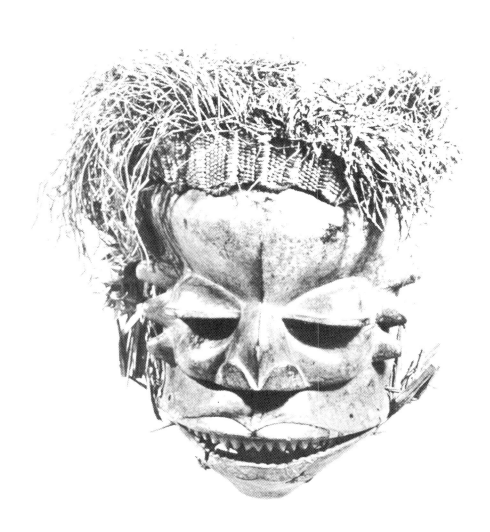

IBO SPIRIT MASK

This *Egbo* merchant took ill shortly after he had last punished the servant by severe beating; this made the merchant suspicious of the servant's use of witchcraft as reprisal for the severe punishment which he had endured; the servant therefore feared for his life.

The alkaloid component of the Calabar bean, **physostigmine** or **eserine**, has a profound effect on the spinal cord, causing paralysis of the legs and asphyxia, and in large doses, paralysis of the heart, leading to the death of the victim. This alkaloid is used extensively in ophthalmic medicine.

In the old traditional cultures, religion and authority went together;hence, the king was expected to set the religious example. Because such power and authority was vested in the kings, their autocracy inevitably led to abuses. The widespread belief in supernatural forces led the king toward seeking answers through any available method such as oracle divination. As a result of this practice, the kings and priests developed very sophisticated methods for discerning the truth.

The Efiks used several forms of divination. They believed that the Calabar bean, or *esere*, possessed the power to reveal truth and destroy witches. There were distinctions between divination, oracle and ordeal. Divination was used to discover/uncover information through the use of metaphysical, intuitive, and psychic medium. In Yorubaland, the kola nuts and cowrie shells were used as an oracle and in divining or uncovering hidden information. But the Efiks believed that the *esere* could be used to discover hidden truth in the *ordeal*, to obtain information about the accused, that person had to subject himself to dangerous bodily injury or even death to prove his innocence or guilt.

The seeds contain about 48% starch and 23% albuminoides, and an alkaloid—physostigmine or eserine—employed in opthalmic medicine. Other alkaloids present are eseranine, eseridine, calabarine, and physocenine, the latter having a strong mytotic action (Kerharo and Bouquet). As a poison it is a powerful sedative on the spinal cord, causing paralysis of the legs, and death by asphyxia, and in large doses, paralysis of the heart. Doses of small pieces of crushed bean, in a little water, is used on the Ivory Coast for edemas.

In recent psycho-physical studies it has been established that certain emotions bring about definite chemical changes in the body. One hypothesis to explain the phenomenon of the Calabar bean is that of the emotion of *"fear"* manifested in the guilty party. The body chemicals produced in the high emotional state of *"fear"* probably, in combination with the alkaloid of the Calabar bean, brings about the spinal or heart paralysis which culminates in death.

There is a whole new field of modern medicine known as *"Psychoneuroimmunology"* which relates emotional states of mind with physiological functions and attempts to explain how these emotional changes bring about physical dysfunctions. Although this is a *"new"* concept in Western medicine, ancient medicine men have long known that the first *"cure"* in any disease is the healing of the emotions or the *"spirit"* of an individual. In *"Ifa Therapeutics,"* which is native also to Nigeria, the remedies are both physical and metaphysical, or relating to the cure of the mind or *"spirit"* which is called the

"Odu" or *"head"* in Yorubaland. Ifa prescriptions are based on the attributes inherent in herbs, roots, animals, birds and minerals associated with the different *"Odus"* or *"heads."* The *"Ifa Priests,"* who are also the doctors, must not only know the many recitals (chapters) of the Holy Book of *"Ifa,"* in bringing about the cures for his patients, he must also be an Anatomist, a Naturalist, a Botanist, a Psychologist, a Chemist and a Diviner before he can claim to be fully qualified *"Ifa Priest."* (*'Ifa,"* Akin Fagbenro Beyiodu, 1940.)

In the traditional medicine of China, the basis of the entire medical paradigm is the theory of *"Emotions and Disease."* This medical model relates the emotions of joy, worry, grief, anger and hate to the functioning or dysfunction of certain internal organs. The author has observed that these relationships to Chinese Medicine correspond closely with *"Odus"* of Ifa Therapeutics. Hence, once again we see that the ancient medical practitioners were far advanced in medical knowledge; it behooves all serious medical practicioners of the West to take a somber look at these traditions.

Another leguminous plant, though belonging to the subtribe **Caesalpini-aceae,** is known and widely used as an ordeal treatment by the inhabitants of Tropical Africa. The scientific name of this plant is **Erythrophleum guineense** G. Don, with the common English names of Ordeal tree, Red water tree, Sasswood, Sassy bark. It is known in Ghana as *"Apotrodum"* (meaning poison tree) and in Nigeria as *"Erun-obo,"* while in Swahili it is called *"Mbaraka."* This tree is known in Zimbabwe as *"MuSande,"* where it is gregarious in the Eastern District Kloofs and forests.

This is a tree attaining 30 m in height and 3 m in girth. Its centers of diversity range from Senegal to Cameroons and then south to South Central Africa. Crown spreading and dense, buttresses slight and blunt, bole usually slightly bent. Leaves alternate, about 10 per pinnule, 5 cm long and 3 cm wide, ovate-elliptical with blunt apex, glabrous. Inflorescens a panicle of spike-like racemes. Flowers small, cream, scented, Jan.-Feb., July. Pod broad, flat, woody, about 12.5 cm long and 5 cm wide, slightly curved, opening without scattering seeds, June. Seeds 5-10, hard, with twisted funicle.

The bark contains gum-resin and a certain amount of tanning and has been used for tannin or as a red dye. It has been reported that it contains a yellow or red resin containing a red coloring matter which is the decomposition product of an alkaloid. It dyes leather brown or violet red, turning dark purple later. The whole tree, especially that of bark and root, is extremely poisonous and has been described as one of the virulent poisonous plants of Tropical Africa. It forms the basic ingredient in the *"sassy bark ordeal"* used by the Krus of Liberia and other coastal tribes stretching to Malawi in Southern Africa. As the poison was highly soluble, the bark was boiled and the resulting *"red water"* was drunk. Innocent persons vomited the poison but the guilty failed to do so and usually died!

The poison is due to an alkaloid erythrophleine (traces 6–7%), the physiological effect is said to resemble that of digitalis and has been adopted in medicine for the treatment of heart disease and spasmodic asthma. It can be used as a local anesthetic, like cocaine.

In Sierra Leone, the charred bark is used, mixed with clay, in the treatment of rheumatism. In Cameroons, the crushed bark is applied to the fugitive swellings of Filaria, a nematode worm. It is applied to the swellings after being painted with the latex of **Alstonia congensis.** The Krobos of Ghana grind the dried bark and sniff the powder for faintness and headaches. The bark has been used with other substances, as an ordinary poison, and is probably never used alone. It is used as an arrow poison by the Tiv of Nigeria, and has been identified with **Strychnos** as an ingredient in arrow poisons among the Central African Pygmies.

CHLOROPHORA EXCELSA (Welw.) Benth.   Moraceae

"Sacred Tree"   **Fig or Mulberry family**

Centers of Diversity: Ivory Coast to Angola, Congo, Central and East Africa including Mozambique.

Common/Vernacular Names: *English:* Iroko wood of commerce, African oak; *Africa:* Odum (Ghana); Iroko, Loko (Nigeria)

Somatic Chromosome Numbers and Genome Constitution: 2n=

Description: A large tree up to 50 m high and 10 m in girth, exuding dirty white latex, almost unbuttressed and unbranched up to 21 m. Crown, dense and dark; crown of female tree more spreading, with bole thick and unbranched up to 24 m or more; roots a characteristic bright red with yellow lenticels; flowers, male and female on separate trees, dioecious; male Jan.–Feb.; female Mar.–April.

Lore, Legend and Romance: Barter at the Herbarium, Kew, states that trees were kept in the male pantheon of the Yorubas. In Ghana and Nigeria, the tree is regarded as sacred and as one of the plants credited with furnishing souls of the newborn. The household god of the Ibo of Nigeria is always carved from a solid block of Iroko. The bark is an ingredient in the brass bowl used by the Ibo in the ceremony of making a new shrine.

The tree yields a valuable timber of strong, moderately hard, very durable and of fairly open grain. This wood is sometimes erroneously described as African teak. The bark is sometimes considered an expectorant. It is an ingredient in mixtures used in a hip-bath for venereal sores and as a wash for chancre. The bark infusion is used in Zaire as a purgative; in Ghana it is used for coughs. The crushed bark, in water or palm wine, is drunk for heart troubles, lumbago and general fatigue. A leaf decoction is used in Sierra Leone as a wash for fevers.

A phenolic substance, a derivative of resorcinal, with fungicidal properties known as Chloropherin is isolated from the wood.

In Cuba and elsewhere in the Caribbean basin, where the use of Iroko is necessary in Santería works, a substitute has been found in an indigenous plant of the region which belongs to the same family—**Moraceae.** The scientific name of this plant is **Chlorophora tinctoria** (L.) Gaudich. ex Benth., Syn. **Morus tinctoria** L. The common name of this plant in English is Faustic tree, while the plant is known in Cuba and other Spanish-speaking countries as *"Fustete."* This is a tree, often with spreading and drooping branches, up to 20 m high.

FICUS CAPENSIS Thunb.   **Moraceae**

"Sacred Tree"   **Fig or Mulberry family**

Centers of Diversity: Senegal to Cameroons and throughout Tropical Africa. Also in South Africa and Cape Verde Islands.

Common/Vernacular Names: *English:* Fig, Cape Fig; *Africa:* Doma, Koomli-agbomitso (Ghana), Kuyu, Kuya-pasi (Zimbabwe), Mkuyu (Swahili)

Somatic Chromosome Numbers and Genome Constitution: $2n = 26$

Description: A common shrub or tree up to 18.2 m high, with milky white latex turning darker. Crown cylindrical, extending almost to the ground. Leaves alternate, petiolate, ovate or ovate-elliptic, slightly cordate or shortly cuneate at the base, apex obtuse or shortly acuminate, margin coarsely repand and obtuse dentate, smooth, glabrous or somewhat hairy below, especially on the nerves; texture fairly thin. Figs borne on woody, panicled, leafless branches on the main stem, obovoid or obovoid-globose, glabrous, with a prominent ostiole at the apex, pinkish green and fleshy when ripe, sometimes with darker blotches. Edible when not ant-ridden.

Lore, Legend and Romance: In Sierra Leone, the bark is eaten with cola nut and the inner bark is sometimes chewed with cola nuts to quench thirst. This tree is much used on the Ivory Coast and is considered diuretic and aphrodisiac, and is often used for sterility, probably because of its numerous fruits. The root decoction is used as an enema, and the latex of young shoots is drunk as a cure for gonorrhea. The tree has various sacred uses on the Ivory Coast. The young leaves in palm soup are used by nursing mothers in Ghana to promote a copious flow of milk.

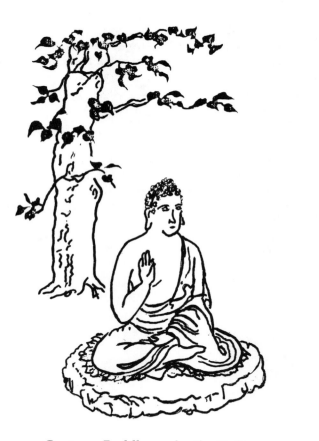

Gautuma Buddha under the Bo Tree—

Ficus religiosa, the Buddha *"Tree of Life"*

FICUS RELIGIOSA L.   Moraceae

"Sacred Tree"   **Fig and Mulberry family**

Centers of Diversity: Sri-Lanka and India

Common/Vernacular Names: *English:* Peepul Tree of India, Bo Tree of Ceylon, Pipal Tree of India, Sacred Fig; *Spanish:* Alamo; *Asia:* Aswatha, Aracha (Sri Lanka)

Somatic Chromosome Numbers and Genome Constitution: $2n=26$

Description: A tree up to 30 m high, erect with smooth, light grayish-brown bark and compact head; leaves deciduous, up to 15 cm long, somewhat heart-shaped with prolonged, very slender "drip-tip;" Flowers purple, 12 mm across, borne in pairs. Fruits and leaf buds edible.

Lore, Legend and Romance: The most sacred tree of India and Sri Lanka, being venerated by the Buddhists as well as Hindus. Devout worshippers will not act or injure the smallest seedling or branch of this tree.

    The specimen at Anuradhapura, Sri Lanka, is probably one of the oldest historical trees in the world, having been brought from India as a young plant in 288 BC. When a Bo tree is in a dangerous position, or seedlings grow spontaneously, as they frequently do, in the crevices of buildings, bridges, etc., a non-Buddhist person must be found to deal with the offending tree or plant. This scion which was planted in 288 B.C. died in 1971.

    The leaves and twigs are laxative. The fruit is digestive and is taken in asthma and for sterility. A brew prepared from bud, fruit and roots excites sexual function according to Indian tradition.

    The use of **Ficus religiosa** goes back to the Spartan times when species of fig was known to form part of the daily menu, and both Greeks and Romans thought that it conferred bodily strength upon the consumers. **Ficus religiosa** has been found depicted on a seal—probably of the first millenium, with animal heads issuing from the stem.

    The fig of the Bible, **Ficus carica**, was also a sexual and fertility symbol because of its large number of seeds, but because this fruit could be dried for storage, its role as a food staple was well established (Numbers 13:23). Rabinical scholastics suggest that the fig was the *"Tree of Knowledge;"* this suggestion has much merit as any of the other plants suggested for their role. As a plant used in allegory and parable, figs appear many times as a symbol of peace (I Kings 4:25), good vs. evil (Jer. 24:1-8), literally analogy wherein *"All thy strongholds shall be like fig trees"* (Nar. 3:12) and parable (Luke 13:6-9; Matt. 21:18-19; Rev. 6:13).

    Ficus carica ($2n = 26$) was cultivated for thousands of years. Its principal gene center is Southeast Asia, and has spread to Asia Minor, Mediterranean countries and Western Europe. In Egypt figs were already cultivated in 4000 B.C.

    Ficus religiosa has the reputation of being the tree under which the Gautuma Buddha sat in meditation for forty days until he received enlightenment. He thus attained *"Nirvana"* in the shade of this tree at Magadha in India.

FICUS THONNINGII Blume — Moraceae

"Sacred Tree" — **Fig or Mulberry family**

Centers of Diversity: Senegal to Cameroons, and widespread in Tropical Africa.

Common/Vernacular Names: *English:* Fig; *Africa:* Gamperoga (Ghana);

Somatic Chromosome Numbers and Genome Constitution: 2n = 26

Description: A medium-sized, low branching tree up to 12 m high or more, beginning life as an epiphyte; aerial roots in dense masses. Trunk fluted with combination of former adventitious roots; bark grey, smooth, latex white, some branches erect, crown spherical. Produces abundant resinous latex. The fig "fruits" are not edible.

Lore, Legend and Romance: This is a sacred tree in parts of Nigeria. An infusion of decoction of the bark is used in Ghana for sore throats and colds. On the Ivory Coast, the bark of the tree is used as an ingredient in the cure for poison. In Northern Ghana, **Ficus thonningii** Blume is generally considered to be a male by the inhabitants while **Ficus polita** Vahl. is regarded as female.

MIRABILIS JALAPA L. — Nyctaginaceae

Four O'clock family

Centers of Diversity: Widely distributed in the warmer parts of the world and occurring in West Africa.

Common/Vernacular Names: *English:* Four o'clock plant, Marvel of Peru, False jalap; *Spanish:* Buenas tardes,Belle de Nuit *Africa:* Kinuka-jio (Swahili); *China:* Tzu-mo-li, Yen-chih

Somatic Chromosome Numbers and Genome Constitution: 2n=(54), 58

Description: An ornamental plant 61 x 122 cm high, perennial; may be propagated by seed or division of tuberous roots. Flowers, white, or yellow variegated, last only for a night, opening in the evening (hence the name, four o'clock plant) and withering the next morning.

Lore, Legend and Romance: The roots, leaves and sometimes the whole plant is used for various medicinal purposes in India, for colds and fever and as a laxative. The leaves are also used as a vegetable; the powdered seeds are used as cosmetic in Japan and also in Cuba.

In West Africa the plant is highly venerated as a fetish plant and is believed to possess magical powers. This is one of the first plants my father pointed out to me when I was at the age of 7 years; he insisted that I know how to recognize it by its flowers which almost always open fully at 4:00 pm Greenwich Mean Time.

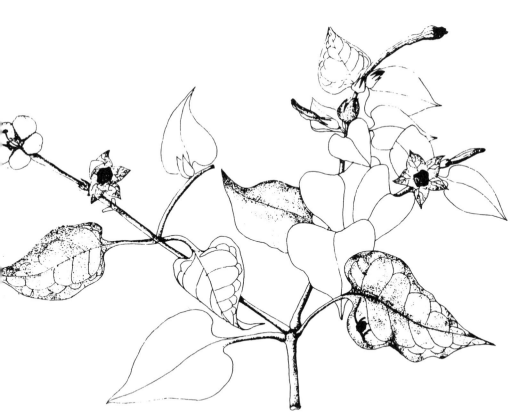

Mirabilis jalapa

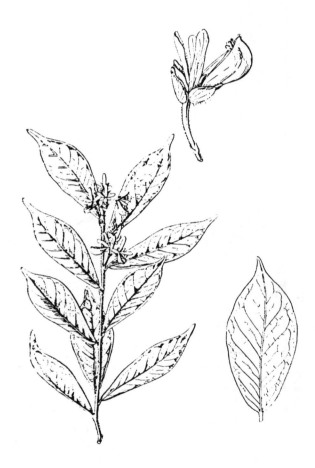

Carpolobia lutea

CARPOLOBIA LUTEA G. Don   Polygalaceae

Polygala or Milkwort family

Centers of Diversity: Indigenous to West Tropical Africa; gregarious around Lagos and Abeokuta environs.

Common/Vernacular Names: *Africa:* Oshun-shun (Nigeria); Otwewa (Ghana)

Somatic Chromosome Numbers and Genome Constitution: 2n=

Description: An evergreen shrub to small tree growing up to 6 m high. Leaves alternate, deep green, variable in shape, ovate, oblong-elliptic, obovate, up to 20 x 10 mm; flowers, whitish-green, July–Aug. Fruits pendent in axillary clusters of 2–3, bluntly angled, orange, glossy. Seeds, generally one, sometimes 2–3, surrounded by juicy pulp.

Lore, Legend and Romance: The wood is very hard, resists the white ant, and is used for house posts and walking sticks. The Yorubas prepare a decoction of the bark, and apply externally and internally as a cure for rheumatism. The fruits are sweet and edible.

STERCULIA COLORATA   Sterculiaceae

Chocolate or Cola nut family

Centers of Diversity: Indigenous to the dry region of the eastern province of Sri Lanka.

Common/Vernacular Names:

Somatic Chromosome Numbers and Genome Constitution: 2n = 40

Description: A moderate-sized tree, to 15 m high, in dry arid regions of Sri Lanka. The plant, however, is able to thrive in moist habitats. The species is very conspicuous in the landscape during February and March when its orange-scarlet flowers appear in profusion. This almost always coincides with the dry season.

Lore, Legend and Romance: This is one of the sacred plants of the Veddahs, an aboriginals of Sri Lanka, who sing odes to it!

STERCULIA SETIGERA Del.   Sterculiaceae

Syn. Sterculia tomentosa Guill. & Perr.   **Chocolate or Cola nut family**
"Ritual Costume"

Centers of Diversity: Senegal to Nigeria and widespread in Tropical Africa.

Common/Vernacular Names: *Africa:* Adodowa, Pullipunga (Ghana); Da, Kandi gum (Sudan)

Somatic Chromosome Numbers and Genome Constitution: $2n = 40$

Description: A small tree to 15 m high and 30 cm girth or more, with a small and fairly sharp buttress, sap watery, yielding a white gum; branchlets velvety; leaves up to 20 x 20 cm, roughly 3–5 lobed, lobes acutely long-acuminate, base almost overlapping, cordate, light green, and soft, downy on both surfaces; flowers when leafless, pale green with reddish lines within, on short stalks along stems, style curved and conspicuous, Dec.–Mar. Fruits are in follicles up to 12.5 cm long, boat-shaped, pointed, greenish velvety, usually produced in clusters of 4–5; seeds about 10, purplish, with yellow aril, seated on bosses with brown irritating hairs.

Lore, Legend and Romance: Fiber from the bark is used in ritual costumes among other uses. The gum is an occasional ingredient in prescriptions for venereal discharges, and the macerated gummy bark is used for catarrh.

    The seeds are chewed or ground for use in soup in times of famine. The tree yields an edible tragacanth-like gum which is used especially in Sudan. It is partly soluble in water and is used in Europe for dying silk fabrics.

    The bark owes its properties mainly to a gum composed of lacturonic acid, rhamnosis, and lactose, and it includes 16% acetic and 3% catechic tanin. The seeds with dates are supposed to help fecundity in cattle.

    The watery sap is very refreshing to thirsty travelers. In the eastern Sudan, this gum is called "da" or "kandi gum," and is similar to that of **Sterculia cinerea.** In Western Sudan, the people use it in food in place of Baobab leaf when the latter is unobtainable.

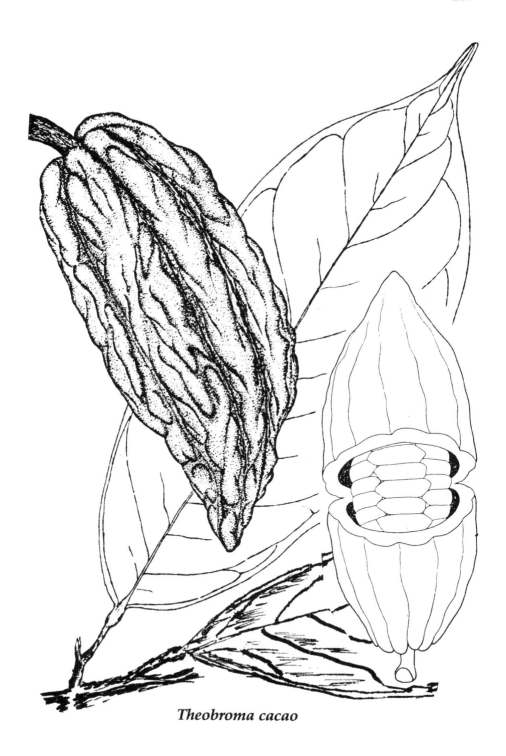

Theobroma cacao

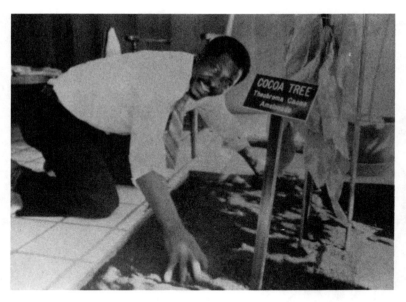

The author planting **"Theobroma cacao"** in the atrium of the Guittard Chocolate Company, Burlingame, CA. (below) Terrill Timberlake, Vice President with Anthony Andoh, planting **"Amelonado"** variety of **"Theobrama cacao."** April, 1984.

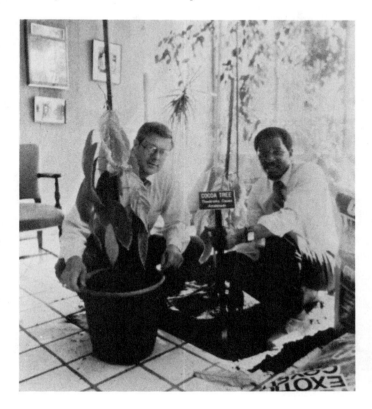

THEOBROMA CACAO L.   Sterculiaceae

Chocolate or Cola nut family

Centers of Diversity: Primary gene center is in the vicinity of the *"upper waters of the Amazon,"* where the greatest range of variation in natural population exists. Cocoa has been cultivated since ancient times in Central America, from Mexico to the southern Costa Rican border, possibly for over 2,000 years. It has been introduced into some warmer parts of the world, such as Bahia, West Indies and West Africa. Only in Mexico was domestication of the cacao completed by the Maya; the theory of divine origin and its use as currency would appear to support this view, as it is unlikely that a wild tree would be held in such high esteem. Elsewhere cacao was wild or semi-domesticated.

Cuatrecasas (1964) described 22 **Theobroma** species, all of which are found in the tropical South and Central America. Relative isolation of cacao populations and their original parentage resulted in the development of two more or less uniform groups distinguished as Criollo (**Theobroma cacao** L. **subsp. cacao**) = **Theobroma sativa** (Aubl.) Ling. & LeBey, and Forastero (**Theobroma cacao** L. subsp. **sphaerocarpum** (Chev.) Cuatr.) = **Theobroma sphaerocarpum** Chev. The Criollo is located in Central America (Central American Criollo) and North Colombia (South American Criollo). The Forastero can be divided into Upper Amazonian Forastero, indigenous to the Upper Amazon basin and the Lower Amazonian Forastero also named and found in Guyana. The Trinitario is a recently originated hybrid swarm of Criollo from Central America and Amelonado.

The word "cacao" is often used for the tree and its parts and the word "cocoa" for the products of manufacture. In this account the word "Cocoa" is used throughout, both for the tree and its products.

Common/Vernacular Names: *English:* Cocoa, Cacao; *Spanish:* Cacao, Cacao amarillo, Cacao morado, Cacoyer; *Africa:* Mpow-dua (Ghana)

Somatic Chromosome Numbers and Genome Constitution: 2n=16, 20, 26

Description: A small to medium-sized tree attaining 6–8m in height, and forming the lowest story of the evergreen tropical rain-forest. It usually grows in groups along river banks, where it may often stand for 6 months in water, but the water must be running to supply the necessary oxygen. Its status as an under-story tree led to the belief that cocoa must be grown under shade, but, as with many other economic crops, the natural environment where it grows in competition with many other species does not necessarily give the best conditions for growth and high yield when cultivated; heavily shaded wild cocoa often carries little fruits.

Leaves large and simple, oblong shaped; red when young. Flowers actinomorphic, hermaphrodite, small and yellowish, produced on the trunk and branches. Fruits indehiscent, bright yellow or red, containing a number of reddish seeds embedded in a whitish pulp. Pods 15–22.5 cm long by 7.5–10 cm across and containing seeds usually called beans, from 25–60 in number. The fruit is usually considered a drupe, but is commonly called a pod.

The tree thrives at elevations between 304.8 and 609 m, with an evenly distributed rainfall of 187–200 cm. It has a long tap-root, and requires deep and well-drained soil, light shade and shelter from strong winds.

Lore, Legend and Romance: Southern Bahia is the center of Brazil's cocoa production, and a very considerable part of its economy depends on the cultivation of cocoa. A recent introduction to Ghana, it has been a great source of income for the country. The variety almost exclusively grown there is the Amelonado which has yellow pods.

The genus **Theobroma** was formerly called **Theobromodes.** The crop is of ancient cultivation in Central America and the Indians believed it to be of divine origin; hence, the generic name **Theobroma** given by Linnaeus, meaning the *"food of the gods."* Well-to-do Indians made a thick beverage by pounding roasted cocoa beans with maize and capsicum. The beans were also used as a currency; 100 beans would buy a slave. Tribute to the Aztec emperor from the lowland people was made in cocoa beans. Large quantities were found in Montezuma's palace when he was defeated by Cortez in 1519.

Propagation is by seeds which are sown fresh. Sometimes propagation is by budding. The limits of cultivation are 20 degrees North and South latitude, but the bulk of the crop is within 10 degrees North and South latitude. It is grown mainly at low elevations, usually below 305 m, but is cultivated up to 1220 m in the Venezuelan Andes and 915 m in Colombia. The optimum temperature range is 35–46 degrees C., with small seasonal and diurnal range. Rainfall in the cocoa belt varies from 1–2.5 m, but most cocoa, without irrigation, is grown with a rainfall above 1.3 m.

The ground should be forked over once a year and light pruning carried out three times per year. Excessive pruning can be injurious and exposes the leaves and fruit to insect attacks, especially the *"mosquito blight,"* Helopeltis.

Harvesting is a long and delicate process; the pods should be cut off, not pulled or torn off and the seeds are placed in a wooden box or cement-lined tank to undergo *"sweating"* or fermentation for three to four days; the beans are turned over and washed daily. Afterwards they are spread out to dry in the sun during the day and covered with sacks at night. The entire process takes approximately one week.

The average tree produces 70–80 pods, but under ideal conditions, some trees have been known to produce 300 or more pods.

In the preparation of cocoa powder, the cured beans are subjected to processes of roasting, nibbing, grinding and heating. The butter-like fat of the beans is extracted and used in medicine and cosmetics; its melting point is a little below body temperature. This oil of **Theobroma** is known as Cocoa butter. To make chocolate, further ingredients, such as sugar, mild and aromatic substances are added and all ingredients are ground into a paste. Inferior chocolates are often made of or adulterated with nuts and various vegetable fats. Shea butter is a greenish-yellow fat, solid or semi-solid at room termperature. It is obtained from an African tree **Butyrospermum parkii** (G. Don) Kotschy, a member of the family **Sapotaceae**. The fat is used commercially as a substitute for cocoa butter in the manufacture of chocolate. It is used locally in place of butter. The cocoa shell (testa) is used in stock feed or as a mulch; it is a source of theobromine, shell fat and vitamin "D."

Several mulches have been used in different parts of the garden in the past few years. Cocoa bean hulls (cocoa shells) have been used extensively since 1952, both alone or mixed with saw-dust. The latter is the preferred way of using them (2/3 cocoa bean hulls, 1/3 saw dust), applying a layer 5–10 cm deep. The hulls help to color the saw-dust and the saw-dust helps to break up the cocoa hulls which when used alone are apt to cake and become moldy. Cocoa hulls supply a small amount of nitrogen. The lilacs and viburnums, when applications have been liberal, have made considerable foliage growth and looked much healthier after use of this mulch. The strong smell of chocolate disappears in a week or so after the cocoa hulls are applied. Care should be exercised when using cocoa shells as mulch. When fully saturated with water, they will heat up on warm days and because of this, precaution is taken to keep them about 30 cm from the trunks or basal branches of the plants. A mold grows through them quickly in warm weather, but as far as can be determined, this is not harmful to the plants.

As the cocoa shells come from the factory, they are extremely light and dry and are very easily applied. In every ton of cocoa shells there are only 11 kg or less of water. Even more important, there are 24.5 kg of nitrogen and 0.85 kg of organic matter. Hence, cocoa shells can be considered not only as mulch but as a fertilizer as well, since some commonly-sold fertilizers have less nitrogren. Cocoa shells have a pH of 5.5; phosphorous content in 1.1% and potash, 3.7%.

Cocoa shells as mulch are being used increasingly in California landscape schemes in recent years. As a mulch it gives a uniformly pleasing brown color immediately after application, though it turns black after several months. In California, the author has grown diverse landscape plants using cocoa shells as mulch and had also employed the shells in the construction of Japanese and Rock Gardens. The following are some of the plants the author grew using cocoa shells with notes on their effects:

Mahonia lomariifolia
Erica melanthera "Pink heather"
Pieris japonica variegata
Crassula argentea
Festuca ovina glauca
Nandina domestica "Wood's Dwarf"
Pinus mugo
Cotoneaster dammeri "Coral Beauty"
Rhododendron "F.D.R."
Phyllostachys aurea
Dianthus spp.
Polygala dalmasiana
Elaeagnus clemsonii aurea variegata
Cedrus deodora pendula glauca

There were at least four species of molds that invaded the planting beds, although they in no way appeared to harm the plantings. One particular planting which did not thrive was Pieris japonica variegata.

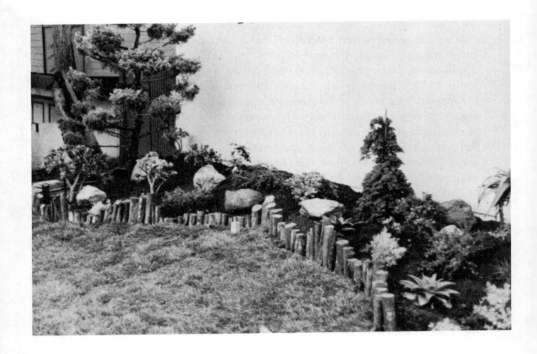

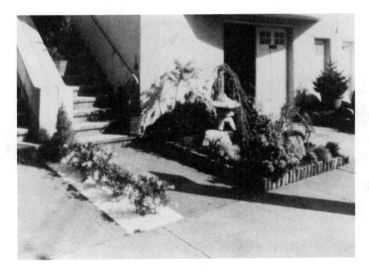

Rock garden with cocoa shell mulch

There are two distinct groups of cocoa, the Forastero (foreign) and the Criollo (native), and Calabacillo (small calabash). The last named, formerly regarded as a form of Forastero, is now considered a distinct type.

The typical Forastero has a thick and deeply furrowed bottle-necked pod, and is red or reddish-yellow. This is usually a prolific tree, bearing numerous large, rounded, purplish seeds. Due to cross-pollination, however, this type has become very variable. Some of the best varieties of Forastero are *"Cundeamar," "Amelonado," "Ocumare," "Verdilico"* and *"Cayenne."* The Criollo type, known in Ceylon as *"Caracas"* or *"Red Ceylon,"* is distinguishable by its smaller, thin-shelled and red pods with rather globular seeds which are usually white in section; these were formerly much valued and commanded a high price. The tree is of a rather delicate nature and though once the principal variety grown in Sri Lanka, it is now almost extinct there. The **"Calabacillo"** has usually a small and roundish pod with smooth skin, the beans being flat and dark purple in section. *"Amelonado"* is the variety chiefly grown in West Africa. This variety gives the best yield under varying conditions. Other species are: **Theobroma pentagona** or *"Alligator cacao"* and **Theobroma angustifolia**, *"Monkey cacao."*

Cocoa is one of the three most important hot beverages, the other two being tea and coffee. Cocoa has a high nutritive value, and is mildly stimulating, since it contains a certain amount of alkaloid caffeine, though considerably less than coffee.

Theobromine is extracted from the cocoa bean husk. It is a lower homologue of caffeine and isomeric with theophylline found in tea. It is thought to be present in the unfermented seeds but which is developed by hydrolysis of glycoside during the fermenting process. In its action, theobromine resembles caffeine but its effect on the central nervous system is much less than caffeine, while its action on muscle and kidney is more pronounced. It is often prescribed along with digitalis. The alkaloid theobromine is a more powerful diuretic than caffeine and there is a derivative, diuretin, which is prescribed to relieve edema in diseases of the kidney and heart. Chemically the seeds contain 40–60% solid fat, 0.9–3% of the alkaloid theobromine, 2.5% of sugar and a small amount of caffeine.

Cocoa beans, obtained from a canoe off Central America, were taken by Columbus to Europe as a curiosity. The Spaniards did not appreciate the Indian method of preparation, but soon learned to make it palatable by mixing the ground roasted beans with sugar and vanilla; exports to Spain in this form soon began, Cortez recognizing its possible commercial value. Later the unprocessed dry beans were exported and the first chocolate factories were opened in Spain. Cocoa beverage became popular in Italy and France early in the 17th century and soon afterwards in Holland, Germany and England. Chocolate houses appeared alongside coffee houses and were used as clubs. At this time cocoa was very expensive, and consumption was limited to the wealthy classes.

In 1828 van Houten, a Dutch manufacturer, invented a method of expressing much of the fat from the bean, thus making it more palatable and digestible. References to defatted cocoa were published in France in 1763 and in Italy in 1769. The fermented beans were roasted, when water and acetic acid were driven off, and the characteristic aroma of chocolate was produced. In the manufacture of milk chocolate, discovered by M.D. Peter in Switzerland in 1876, dried or powdered milk was incorporated.

After the arrival of the Spaniards cocoa spread rapidly in the New World. Criollo cocoa, presumably from Central America, was taken to Venezuela and Trinidad, introduced into the latter in 1525. Jamaica, Haiti, and the Windward Islands became important producers and there were extensive plantations in Jamaica when the island was captured by the British from Spain in 1655.

The variability of **Theobroma cacao** decreases as one goes further down the Amazon from the center of origin on the slopes of the Andes and self-compatible trees are encountered. The *"Amelonado"* forms of Amazonian Forastero with dark purple cotyledons were taken into cultivation in Bahia in Brazil. These were introduced by the Spanish and Portuguese to islands in the Gulf of Guinea in the 17th century. One or a few *"Amelonado"* pods were taken to Ghana in 1879 from Fernando Po and gave rise to the large West African industry. There is evidence that cocoa was grown at mission stations in Ghana before this date.

Cocoa was introduced into Southeast Asia by the Spaniards (Philippines in 1670) and the Dutch in the 17th century. The Germans took it to Samoa and New Guinea in the 18th century. Uganda obtained seedlings from the Royal Botanic Gardens, Kew, in 1901.

The general names used are based on Venezuelan terminology, namely, *"Criollo"* meaning native, and *"Forastero,"* meaning foreign, and *"Trinitario,"* meaning native of Trinidad.

"Gurana" or Brazil cocoa is derived from the seeds of **Paullinia cupana** H.B. & K., and belongs to the family **Sapindaceae**; the seeds contain about 4% caffeine.

Quetzalcoatl, the god of the air of the ancient Mexicans, who presided over commerce and the useful arts, was said by the Toltecs to have predicted the coming of the Spaniards to Mexico. This tradition aided the Spaniards in their invasion. A beneficent deity, Quetzalcoatl was finally superseded by the terrible Aztec god of war. The legend of Quetzalcoatl was magnificently depicted in frescoes at Dartmouth College at Hanover, New Hampshire. These murals were painted from 1932–34 by Jose Clemente Orozco, a Mexican artist, who showed the destruction of the Indian civilization by the Spaniards. These murals are so moving that they can be understood by anyone, whether they are familiar with the legend or not.

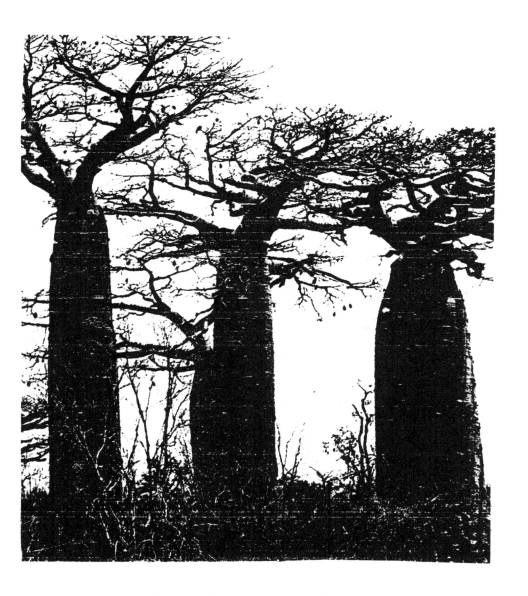

Adansonia madagascariensis

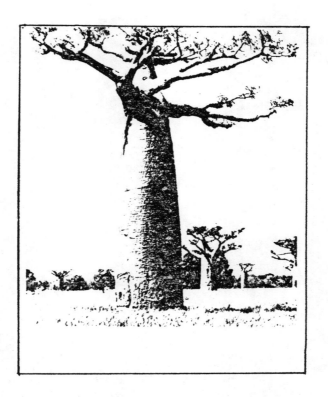

Adansonia digitata

ADANSONIA DIGITATA L.   Bombacaceae

"Burial Place for the Dead"   **Bombax family**

Centers of Diversity: Indigenous to the drier parts of tropical and sub-tropical Africa, Senegambia to Zimbabwe; now introduced into many parts of the tropical and sub-tropical countries around the world with a number of trees growing in Southern Florida.

Common/Vernacular Names: *English:* Baobab tree, Cream of Tartar tree, Monkey Bread tree, Upside-down tree; *Spanish:* Baobab, Mapou africain, Mapou estranger, Mapou zombi; *Africa:* Dade, Adido (Ghana); Komo, Mungu, Vuku (Zimbabwe); Mbuyu, Mkuu-hapingwa (Swahili)

Somatic Chromosome Numbers and Genome Constitution: 2n = C144

Description: A low spreading tree with a grotesquely swollen bole, attaining up to 48.8 m in height and 30 m in girth. It dominates the plains of tropical Africa, from the West Coast along the southern edge of the Sahara to Southern Africa where it is gregarious on the low veldt. Leaves digitately 5–foliolate, leaflets obovate, acuminate, up to 12 x 5 cm,. entire or denticulate nearly glabrous below during the rainy season, otherwise deciduous. Fruit massive, indehiscent, yellowish-brown tomentose, 50 cm long, cucumber-shaped (monkey breads), pendulous on long peduncle. Seed embedded in a dry pith; flowers large and white, May–July, smell of melons and are pollinated by bats.

Lore, Legend and Romance: Such giant trees as the **Adansonia digitata** L. are estimated to have an age of 1000 years. Adanson was probably over-generous when, in 1750, he attributed an age of 5,150 years to a specimen at the mouth of the Senegal River. The plant yields a white, semi-fluid gum from its massive trunk when wounded. This is odorless and tasteless and somewhat resembles gum tragacanth. It is more or less insoluble in water and has an acid reaction. With age it becomes reddish-brown.

    Remarkable for the great age and girth to which it attains, the acid pulp is made into a cooling drink, the leaves are dried and pulverized for soup; in fact, the whole tree and all of its parts fill many needs, especially of the desert people.

    This is an esteemed and sacred tree of many nations of African people, particularly those of the veldts.and savannah regions, where the tree is held to be possessed of a soul or the spirits of the ancestors.

    The trunk with age becomes decayed and hollowed out in the center, forming a storage for water, sometimes holding as much as 938 liters. It is supposed to be one of the longest-lived trees in the world. Wood soft and spongy; inner bark fibrous. The white gourd-like fruits are spongy, farinaceous, acid and edible. In Southern Africa, the bark is used in making mats and rope. Young plants are eaten in Southern Africa as spinach.

    Nearly all of the tree's parts are useful, particularly the fruits, both pulp and seeds being edible, the shell forming fuel whose ash is handy as a potash manure and for making soap. The pulp contains pectin, pectic, malic and free tartaric acids, potassium acid tartrate, glucose and reducing sugars with

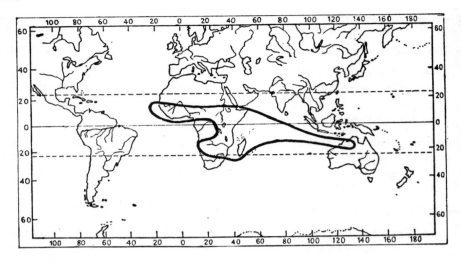

Ecological limits of the genus *Adansonia* seem to indicate that the land masses of Africa, Madagascar, and Australia were at one time joined.

mucilaginous matter. The seeds, widely used as food, are prepared sometimes by roasting, sometimes by soaking and fermenting in much the same way as those of **Parkia**, and taste like almonds.

The bark contains the active principle, adansonin, and is known in French Antilles and in India as a quinine substitute in periodic fever and has been so used in South Africa. Such medicinal uses are dependent on its refrigerent and diaphoretic properties rather than on its astringent effect. Adansonin, which is an alkaloid, is said to be an effective antidote to **Strophanthus** arrow poison. The leaves contain potassium acid tartrate, common salt and tannin, and are therefore astringent. They are used in Sierra Leone as a prophylactic against fever during the rainy season; it is also used to check excessive perspiration. In some parts of West Tropical Africa the tree is associated with the burial place for the dead.

I should point out that there are a number of plants occurring outside of Africa which have close botanical affinity with **Adansonia digitata**. There is the Australian Baobab, botanically known as **Adansonia gregori** and sometimes known in some areas of Australia as *"Gouty-stem tree"*. Its dry acidulous pulp is eaten by the Australian aboriginals.

Stranger looking than even the **Adansonia digitata** are **Adansonia madagascariensis** and other seven species endemic to arid regions of Western Madagascar. Oddly enough, the species occurring in Australia have much affinity with the African Baobab.

BOMBAX BUONOPOZENSE P. Beauv. **Bombacaceae**

Syn. Bombax flammeum Ulbr. **Bombax family**
Syn. Bombax angulicarpa (Ulbr.) Bakh.

Centers of Diversity: Native to Tropical Africa; Sierra Leone to Gabon.

Common/Vernacular Names: *English:* Red-flowered Silk tree; *Africa:* Okuo, Kyankobin, Akron-kron, Agudese, Vaboga, Kuntunkuni (Ghana); Pompola, Kuriya (Nigeria); Nguwe (Sierra Leone)

Somatic Chromosome Numbers and Genome Constitution: $2n = c.72$

Description: A large tree to 36.5 m high and 3 m girth; buttressed with round flanges, bark of young trees especially in savannah, thick and corky, fissured and spiky. Young leaves pubescent, differing from older ones; digitately compound, leaflets 6–7, sessile or subsessile, obovate to oblanceolate, up to 15 x 6.5 cm, lateral nerves prominent, 12 or more pairs, leaves fairly long, acuminate, base cuneate, petiole to 15 cm long; flowers appearing before leaves, opening wide, deep red on young trees, sometimes orange-red on older, borne separately; calyx over 12 mm long, cup-shaped, yellow-green, leathery (Nov.–April). Fruits brownish-black 12.5 cm long, pendulous.

Lore, Legend and Romance: The sapwood is dirty-white. The bark yields a gum resin and a reddish-brown dye used for hunter's clothes. The Ghanaian name for the dye, *"kuntunkuni,"* is applied also to various species of **Bombax, Lannea** and ***Terminalia spp.*** Immature fruits are made into beverage and used in parts of West Africa. The young tender leaves, dried and pulverized makes a good pot herb.

The bark, leaves and flowers are chiefly used as an emollient. A decoction of ground leaves forms a warm bath for fever, especially for children. Women use pounded bark to increase lactation. Yorubas use a bark concoction as an effective emmanagogue.

The Mano of Northern Liberia often make contact with ancestors through Ma, a wooden mask, part fetish and part symbol of Poro, a secret society connected with initiation, or at an annual sacrifice made at the foot of Bombax in sacred groves.

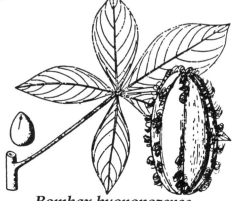

Bombax buonopozense
showing fruit and seed

CEIBA PENTANDRA(L.) Gaertn.   Bombaceae

Syn. Eriodendron anfractuosum DC.   **Bombax family**
Syn. Bombax pentandra L.

Centers of Diversity: Native of Tropical America, now distributed throughout the tropics. Native and cultivated from Cuba to Barbados and from Southern Mexico to Peru and Brazil. Gregarious also in Tropical Africa.

Common/Vernacular Names: *English:* White Silk Cotton-tree, Silk Cotton-tree, Kapok Tree; *Spanish:* Arbol de Algodon, Bois coton, Bonga, Ceiba de Garzon, Cabellos de Angel, Sumauma (Brazil); *Africa:* Onyina, Gongu (Ghana), Akpe-ege, Egungun (Nigeria)

Somatic Chromosome Numbers and Genome Constitution: 2n=72, 80, 88

Description: A deciduous or partly deciduous tree up to 40 m high, with or without prickles on the trunk and branches; trunk buttressed; leaflets 5–8–(15), lanceolate to oblanceolate, acutely acuminate, cuneate and sessile at base, 10–20 cm long, 3–4 cm broad, glabrous; pedicels about 3 cm long; calyx 1–1.5 cm long, glabrous; petals 2–4 cm long, silky-villous outside; capsule 10–30 cm long, flowers Jan.-Feb.; seeds subglobose, 4–6 mm in diameter. Fruits in March.

Lore, Legend and Romance: Toxopeus (1950) believed that the Kapok tree originated in an area which was later divided by the Atlantic Ocean (Atlantis?). Therefore, this species is native to both Tropical America and Africa. He based his conclusion mainly on the great variability of this plant and on the high frequency of dominant inherited characteristics of the species in these two continents. However, Bakhuizen van der Brink (1933) and Chevalier (1949) thought that seeds may have come from America in prehistoric times and that later introduction increased the variability. Its chromosome numbers suggest a polyploid origin and if this supposition is correct the Kapok tree can only have arisen in that area where its parents occur. As all other **Ceiba** species are restricted to America, this could also indicate an American origin.

    In the West Indies, the root decoction is taken as a diuretic. In Cuba, the leaf decoction is taken internally and used for baths. People in Trinidad also use the leaves for bathing and also as poultices on erysipelas and sprained or swollen feet. In Mexico, the bark is applied on wounds and the decoction of the inner bark is emetic, diuretic and antispasmodic.

    In West Africa the tree is highly venerated and esteemed for spiritual purposes. Sacrifices are often placed under this tree as it is believed to house *"spirits."*

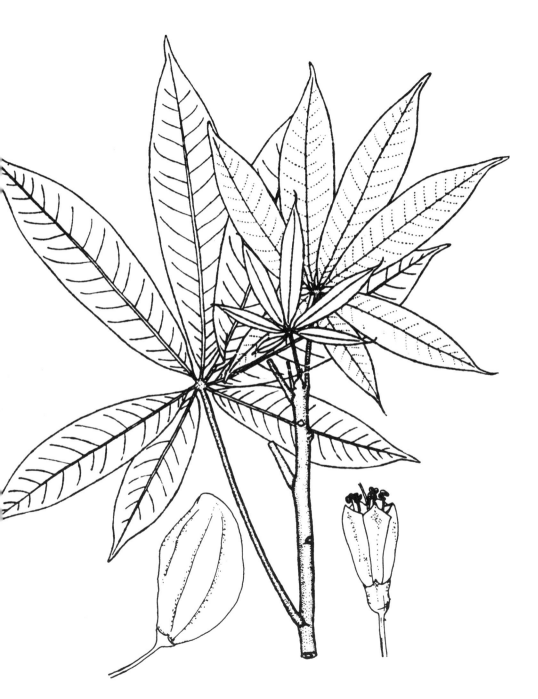

Ceiba pentandra

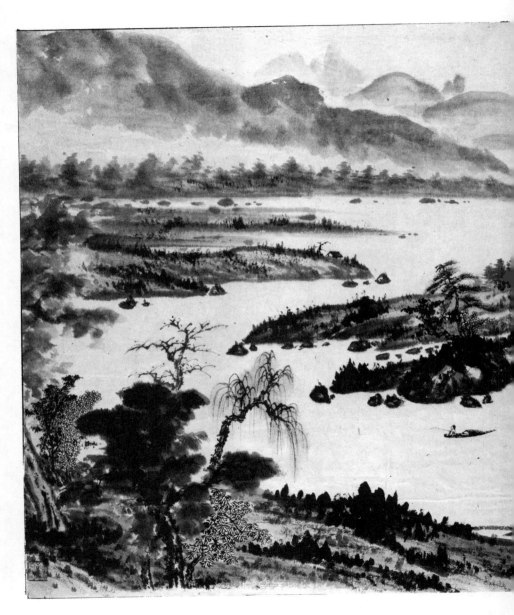

Painting by Dr. Andrew Tseng

MALVA SYLVESTRIS L.   Malvaceae

Mallow family

Centers of Diversity: Native to Europe where it is cultivated as a medicinal crop and also used as an ornamental plant.

Common/Vernacular Names: *English:* High mallow, Country mallow, Cheese flower, Pancake plant, Ground dock; *China:* Chin-k'uei, K'uei

Somatic Chromosome Numbers and Genome Constitution: 2n=42

Description: A biennial plant 60–90 cm high usually grown as an annual. Leaves 5–7.6 cm wide, folded triangular. Flowers purple-rose, summer. Fruit spreading, carpels, reticulate, usually glabrous.

Lore, Legend and Romance: The species has a remarkable adaptation to diverse ecosystems around the world; probably the early vegetable *"k'uei"* mentioned in Chinese literature. At present, it is a weed in China. In the United States, it can be found growing in the Central and Western North Carolina where another variant, **Malva sylvestris var. mauritiana** has arisen. This variety grows to about 1–1.4 m high with purple flowers coming into bloom in summer. In the Carolinas the seeds of **Malva sylvestris** and its variety are treated as pectoral.

    The emollient qualities make them helpful for skin irritations and insect stings. The fresh, young leaves and whole seed pod are edible. The latter is often referred to in country places as *"cheese."* In countries where crop failures often bring famine, the mallows are an important subsistence food. The roots may be boiled, or steamed, then pan fried with butter or oil and onions. Any plant of the family **Malvaceae**, usually the marshmallow or hollyhock, the roots and leaves are boiled and drunk to increase the milk in nursing mothers, speed delivery, ease pain of urination and serve as an antidote to poisons. An infusion of **Malva coccinea** was used by the Arikara Indians of Michigan to control post-partum hemorrhage. In France, the confectioners paste, *"pate de guimauve,"* is made from the roots of marshmallows. But the marshmallows sold in the United States are made from flour, gum, and egg album and contain no mallow.

    Mallows have been used medicinally from the earliest times by the Arabs, the Greeks and the Romans and are used today as food and medicine by herbalists everywhere.

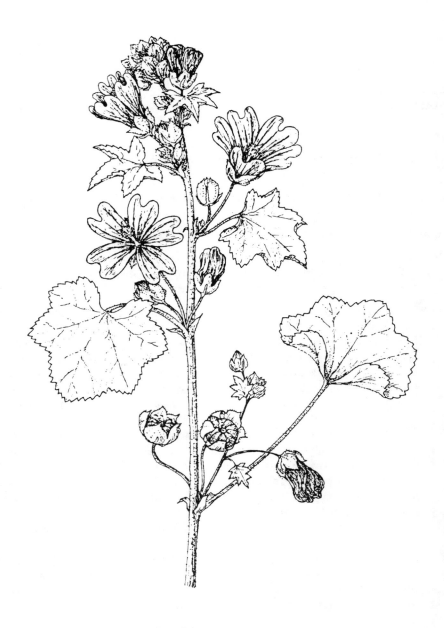

Malva sylvestris

MALVA VERTICILLATA L.

Syn. Malva crispa L.
Syn. Malva mohileviensis Graebn.
Syn. Malva pamiroalaica Ibj.

Mallow family

Centers of Diversity: East Asia. It was an early Chinese domesticate there. About 500 A.D. it was then an important vegetable with several varieties like purple and white stemmed, large and small leaves. During the 7th–10th centuries the cultivation in China declined.

Common/Vernacular Names: *English:* Winter mallow, mallow; *China:* Tung hsien-ts'ai, Tung-kwei-tzu

Somatic Chromosome Numbers and Genome Constitution: 2n=c.84, c.112

Description: A biennial herb up to 60–75 cm in height. Stems erect with bristle hairs. Leaves alternate, with long petioles, pubescent on both sides; leaflets palmate, obtuse-rounded at the apex; margins crenate, with 5–7 main ribs. Flowers 2 cm wide, actinomorphic and hermaphrodite; carpels smooth, angles square, sepals enlarged in fruit. Blooms in late spring through to early fall; small red flowers clustered at the axils. Fruits capsulate.

Lore, Legend and Romance: The cultivation of this plant declined in China and in the late 1800's, it was observed in remote areas. Introduced to Japan where it is now a weed. Cultivated in Europe as a medicinal crop, and almost naturlized in the British Isles. This plant has been described as **Malva crispa** being a cultigen of **Malva verticillata.**

The family **Malvaceae**, the word being derived from the Greek *"malake"* meaning soft, as the plant heals and soothes. As a family it comprises nearly 1000 species of herbs, shrubs or trees with alternate, often palmately lobed stipular leaves and hermaphrodite flowers. The family contains some genera of great economic importance and includes such groups as **Malva, Hibiscus, Urena, Gossypium, Lavatera, Abutilòn, Malope, Kitaibelia, Althaea, Anoda, Goethea** and **Pavonia.**

The members of this family are distributed from the tropics to the Arctic the numbers decreasing as they go north. All species are emollient and demulcent in varying degrees, and some are expectorant and diuretic. They contain starch, mucilage, pectin, oil, sugar, asparagine, phosphate of lime, glutinous matter and cellulose. The mallows, **Malva** spp., the subject of this study and a familiar name in the United States and Western Europe, are useful in treating sore throats and laryngitis, and as a soothing demulcent for the lining of the stomach. However in many developing nations, besides its medical, aesthetic and industrial uses, it forms a basic diet in their food. In South Central Africa, a *"square meal"* is never complete without **Abelmoschus esculenta,** *Syn. Hibiscus esculenta* , the okra, which forms an important relish in Zambian dishes. It is known as *"Delele"*—and it goes very well with their *"Nshima"* and *"Kapenta,"* a maize porridge and dry small fish.

Malva verticillata has recently been promoted as a diet drink which supposedly helps with weight reduction. What can be said is that it encourages increased peristalsis of the large intestine. It is reported to help mobilize excess fat in the large intestine.

ELAEOPHORBIA DRUPIFERA Stapf.   Euphorbiaceae

"Sacred Tree"   **Spurge family**

Centers of Diversity: Guinea to Zaire.

Common/Vernacular Names: *Africa:* Akane, Tredzo (Ghana), Boto (Liberia), Gopo (Ivory Coast)

Somatic Chromosome Numbers and Genome Constitution: 2n=

Description: A tree up to 15 m high with copious white latex. Leaves over 20.5x10 cm, fleshy, oblanceolate to obovate and strap-like, sometimes indented at apex; margins entire. Flowers greenish-white, male flowers numerous, female flowers subsessile, solitary Jan.–May; fruit over 2.5 cm long, a fleshy drupe, yellow when ripe.

Lore, Legend and Romance: In parts of both Ghana and Ivory Coast, this plant is sacred. The latex is poisonous and dangerous to the eyes; may cause incurable blindness. It causes considerable swelling if rubbed on the skin. The latex is taken internally as a purgative, with eggs or cereal pap, or with palm nuts in soup. It is used on the Ivory Coast as a fish poison. It is either applied direct to water or placed in shells or calabashes in the water, where it stupefies fish quite readily.

EUPHORBIA BALSAMIFERA Ait.   Euphorbiaceae

"Superstitious use"   **Spurge family**

Centers of Diversity: Mauritania to Nigeria, also in Canary Islands, probably its original home.

Common/Vernacular Names: *English:* Balsam Spurge; *Africa:* Jiri-yung (Ghana), Aguwa, Kagua (Nigeria), Kweche, Mpangara (Swahili)

Somatic Chromosome Numbers and Genome Constitution: 2n = 42

Description: An erect shrub up to 2.1 m high, with white latex; semi-secculent, forking branches, stems glabrous, thick and fleshy when old; older stems wrinkled; leaves slightly fleshy, crowded near ends of twigs only, linear or linear-lanceolate, up to 10 cm long, shortly pointed, nerves inconspicuous; flowers and fruits small and inconspicuous.

Lore, Legend and Romance: This tree is planted in villages for superstitious reasons and for medicinal purposes. The latex is placed in carious teeth to relieve toothache and to loosen teeth for easier extraction.

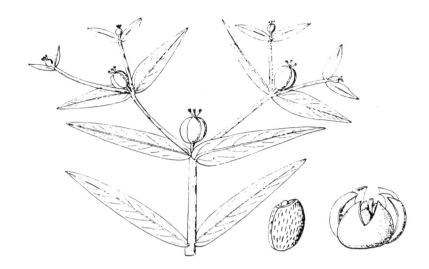

Euphorbia lathyris
showing fruit and seed

EUPHORBIA LATERIFLORA Schum. & Thonn.　　　　　　**Euphorbiaceae**

"Charm"　　　　　　　　　　　　　　　　　　　　**Spurge family**

Centers of Diversity: Sierra Leone to Nigeria.

Common/Vernacular Names: *Africa:* Nkamfo-barima (Ghana), Kweche, Mpangara (Swahili)

Somatic Chromosome Numbers and Genome Constitution: 2n = 20,40

Description: A shrub up to 1.5 m high; latex white; many small, succulent, erect, green, glabrous branches, lax and hanging, leafy when young, up to 4 cm long, linear-lanceolate, 1-nerved; male and female flowers produced separately, each female flower on a long stalk; fruit 3-celled.

Lore, Legend and Romance: A common hedge shrub, it is planted as a *"charm"* by farmers to protect their crops. The plant is thought to be disliked by snakes, hence, its use in hedges. It is sometimes planted for superstitious purposes in Ghana.

It is a drastic purge and is used chiefly for syphilis. A decoction of the plant is taken in Sierra Leone as a blood purifier.

PHYLLANTHUS EMBLICA L.   **Euphorbiaceae**

Syn. Emblica officinalis Gaertn.   **Spurge family**

Centers of Diversity: Tropical Asia. Cultivated both in the Old and New Worlds for its fruits.

Common/Vernacular Names: *English:* Emblic, Myrobolan; *Asia:* Aola (Hindi), Amlake (Bengali), Amran (Gujarati), Amlika (Sanskrit)

Somatic Chromosome Numbers and Genome Constitution: 2n=28, 98

Description: A small to medium-sized deciduous tree up to 7.6 m high with graceful feathery foliage; native to Sri-Lanka, India, Malaysia and China. Commonly found in wild, open patana land of Sri-Lanka at elevations up to 1.2 kilometers. The round, green acid fruits are about the size of marbles, have a comparatively large kernel and are made into a much esteemed preserve. Male and female flowers borne on the same tree, flowers pale green, usually in small dense clusters below the leaves. Fruits, Nov.–Feb.

Lore, Legend and Romance: The fresh fruit juice is highly astringent, diuretic, carminative and a mild laxative. The fresh juice is taken internally in gonorrhea, jaundice, dropsy, anemia, indigestion, dysentery, painful micturition, menorrhagia, uterine hemorrage, vaginitis, cough, hiccough and nausea. Seed with honey is an excellent remedy for leucorrhea. Fruit juice or bark brew taken regularly maintains balanced biliary, phlegmatic and flatulentic order. This plant is highly esteemed in Indian pharmacopoeia.

The fresh or dried fruits constitute the drug. The fruits are one of the three constituents of the well known Indian preparation, *"Tripha"*; the other two ingredients being *"Bahera"* (**Terminalia bellirica**) and *"Harra"* (**Terminalia chebula**). *"Triphala"* is used as a laxative and in the treatment of enlarged liver, piles, stomach complaints and pain in the eyes.

Emblica fruits are a good liver tonic; raw fruits are cooling and a mild laxative. A fermented liquor made from the fruits is considered useful in indigestion, certain heart complaints and colds. It is a very rich source of vitamin C, and is valuable in diseases caused by deficiency of vitamin C, like scurvy.

OCHNA AFZELII R. Br. ex Oliv.   Ochnaceae

"Walking Stick for Priests"   **Ochna family**

Centers of Diversity: Guinea to Cameroons; also in Sudan and Uganda.

Common/Vernacular Names: *Africa:* Okoli Awotso (Ghana), Mchonga-makana (Swahili)

Somatic Chromosome Numbers and Genome Constitution: 2n=

Description: A shrub or small tree, sometimes up to 12 m high; leaves elliptic to lanceolate, acuminate, up to 12.5x4 cm; flowers white with yellow anthers, usually produced before the leaves are fully developed, sepals turning greenish and finally to pink or red; seeds black, on red torus.

Lore, Legend and Romance: The wood is used for walking sticks by priests. The fruits are said to be edible. The seeds are oily.

SHOREA ROBUSTA Roth.   Dipterocarpaceae

Syn. Vatica laccifera W. e A.   **Dipterocarp family**

Centers of Diversity: India and Southeast Asia.

Common/Vernacular Names: *English:* Sal tree, Saul tree, Dammar, Rock tree; *Asia:* So-lo-mu (China), Lal dhuma (Cambodia)

Somatic Chromosome Numbers and Genome Constitution: 2n = 14

Description: The tree is extremely common in many parts of Central and Northern India where it is often the dominating tree in the forests. It is valued for its timber. The resin is aromatic and of pale creamy-yellow color, a bit opaque; it generally occurs in stalactitic form.

Lore, Legend and Romance: The flowers are much sought after for floral offerings at temple shrines. This diptocarp tree of India, described in the *"Kuang-chun-fang-pu,"* grows in Cambodia. The frankinscense-like resin is known as *"Tu-nou-hsiang"* in China. It is a source of resin for making varnishes. Dammar, the resin, is collected from the holes through the bark, 3–6 months after the holes are first made. In India, it is used for caulking boats and for use as incense for burnt offerings.

ARCTOSTAPHYLOS UVA-URSI (L.) K. Spreng   Ericaceae

Heath family

Centers of Diversity: At home in Scotland where the flowers appear as soon as the snow melts. In the United States, however, some botanists believe the plant to have its native habitat from San Mateo County, California, north to Alaska. The author has observed the plant to be gregarious in other northern latitudes.

Common/Vernacular Names: *English:* Bearberry, Kinnikinic, Meal berry, Hog cranberry, Mountain box, Bear's grape, Creashak, Sanberry; *Spanish:* Manzanita

Somatic Chromosome Numbers and Genome Constitution: 2n = 52

Description: An evergreen prostrating plant, attractive and widespread, with thick, shiny leathery leaves reminiscent of its cousins, the **Rhododendrons** and **Azaleas,** they all having a shared common ancestry. Common on stony moors in Scotland, Yorkshire and Western Ireland and elsewhere on the European mainland. Reaches a height of 15 cm; flowers attractive, urn-shaped, pink colored in June, in terminal racemes or panicles, pink to pinkish-white, succeeded by bright red berries. Foliage turns red in winter. The reddish branchlets contrast with small bright green leaves that take on a bronze tone in fall.

Lore, Legend and Romance: The leaves of bearberry known as *"Uvae ursi folia"* contain tannins as well as characteristic glycosides. The drug thus has astringent and diuretic properties. It is administered in the form of an infusion where it is used in the treatment of such diseases as urethritis and cystitis. Dried leaves are made into tea and used as a mild disinfectant in urinary disorders.

Usually found growing in sunny acid soils, the Manzanitas, as they are known in the Americas, will tolerate poor soils which can be gritty, providing there is adequate drainage. They object to lime in the soil and require little attention and scarsely need summer watering once established. Propagation by cutting.

There are approximately 70 species of **Arctostaphylos** occurring throughout the world. All of them are evergreen and either a prostrating shrub or small tree. It has been recorded elsewhere that **Arctostaphylos pungens** Kunth. is the true Manzanita of California.

In the Caribbean basin, Central and South American countries the common/vernacular name *"Manzanita"* is generally ascribed to a number of diverse plants which includes the following:

1. **Crataegus pubescens** Steud., Syn. **Crataegus stipulosa** Steud., family **Rosaceae**
2. **Brysonima crassiflora** HBK, family **Malpighiaceae**
3. **Malpighia glabra** l., family **Malpighiaceae.** This plant is often confused with **Malpighia punicifolia** L., the cultivated Barbados cherry.
4. **Colubrina greggii** S. Watson, family **Rhamnaceae**
5. **Malvaviscus arboreus,** family **Malvaceae**
6. **Syzygium jambos** Alston, Syn. **Eugenia jambos** L., family **Myrtaceae**
7. **Ehretia tinifolia** L., family **Boraginaceae**

VISMIA GUINEENSIS (L.) Choisy   **Guttiferae**

Syn. Vismia leonensis Hook. f. **var. macrophylla** Hutch. & Dalz.   **Garcinia or Mangosteen family**

Centers of Diversity: West Africa; Guinea to Cameroons. Also in the Americas, Southern Mexico to Brazil.

Common/Vernacular Names: *Spanish:* Achiotillo, Palo de Mayo, Palo Vangre, Sangrillo; *Africa:* Okosoa-nimmaa, Bombaga, Agboti (Ghana)

Somatic Chromosome Numbers and Genome Constitution: 2n=

Description: A shrub to small tree up to 15 m high and 1 m girth, exuding a copious resinous, reddish-yellow latex, which turns red on exposure to air. Leaves and inflorescences are covered with very small stellate hairs; leaves 10-12.5x3.75 cm, acuminate, elliptic, to elliptic-lanceolate, opposite, rusty-stellate, hairy beneath, and black-gland-dotted, lateral nerves about 10 pairs; flowers small, feathery, petals greenish-yellow with red stripes, inflorescences shorter than leaves (Mar.–June, Sept.). Fruits are in cymes, small berries with persistent styles (Jan.–Mar., June–Oct.).

Lore, Legend and Romance: The oily resin extracted from the boiled bark mixed with palm kernels makes an ointment which is used in Liberia as a *"superstitious ordeal."* The pounded yellowish-red resin makes an ointment for craw craw. The sap is applied to circumcision wounds in Sierra Leone.

An infusion of young leaves is purgative and used for abdominal complaints in women. The young leaves, with guinea-grains, cure sore throat. In Columbia, the latex is employed as a resolutive and drastic purgative. Brazilians take the latex as a purge, as a remedy for urinary troubles and as a febrifuge; they also apply it in the case of skin affliction. Also in Brazil, the latex (Goma lacre) is used as a food coloring.

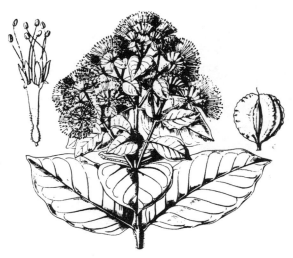

Combretum racemosum
showing flower and fruit

COMBRETUM HYPOPILINUM Diels   Combretaceae

"In Sacred Groves"   **Combretum family**

Centers of Diversity: Native to drier fringes of Tropical Africa; Senegambia to Cameroons, Ubanji-Shari.

Common/Vernacular Names: *Africa:* Urinli (Ghana), Jan-ganye (Nigeria)

Somatic Chromosome Numbers and Genome Constitution: 2n=

Description: A medium-sized tree attaining 9–12 m in height. Leaves elliptic to oblong-elliptic, slightly acuminate, undersurface covered with soft hairs. Flowers, Jan.–Feb., April; stamens creamy white; fruit winged, velvety, purplish-brown.

Lore, Legend and Romance: The tree yields a gum. It is common in Tengani sacred groves. A root decoction is used for stomach ache, the gum for toothache in Gambia, and the leaves are used there as a purge. Also in Nigeria, the gum is used to plug carious teeth.

In south Florida, Caribbean Basin, Cuba and elsewhere in the region, because **Combretum hypopilinum** do not occur there, the people use a substitute, **Combretum laxum** Jacq., commonly called in the Anglophone countries *"Red Withe"* and in the Spanish speaking countries as *"Bejuco de Berraco."* This is a climbing shrub to 15 m or more high, young twigs, petioles and veins of leaf beneath rusty-tomentose; leaf blade oblong-elliptical, acuminate, cuneate to rounded or auriculate at the base, up to 25 cm long and 11 cm broad; racemes dense, up to about 6 cm long in axillary or terminal panicles; fruits 3–4 cm long. Flower and fruit in Jan.

Mention should be made of **Combretum primigenum** Mar. & Engl. There is a *"Herero"* myth which ascribes the origin of man to this plant. The species is regarded with reverence and all Hereros and Ovambos who come in contact with it take a bunch of leaves and rub their forehead with it, saying, *"I greet thee, O my father! Grant me a prosperous journey!"*

OCTOKNEMA BOREALIS Hutch. & Dalz.   Octoknemaceae

"Sacred Tree"

Centers of Diversity: Guinea to Ghana. (Some botanical authorities ascribe Octoknema borealis to the family Olacaceae.)

Common/Vernacular Names: *Africa:* Wisuboni, Abodwe (Ghana)

Somatic Chromosome Numbers and Genome Constitution: 2n=

Description: A large tree of evergreen forests up to 33.5 m high and 2 m girth with straight long bole, buttresses low. Leaves 25x10 cm, lateral nerves 6–9 pairs, petioles about 2.5 cm long. Flowers small, yellowish green, in crowded axillary racemes, over 5 cm long with stellate hairs (Feb.). Fruits are less than 1.5 cm long, subglobose with broad persistent calyx-lobes at tip, in small, almost sessile clusters, with rather hard husks and small seeds.

Lore, Legend and Romance: Bees seem to favor living in this tree, and Liberians watch the tree carefully for honey. The bark is ground and rubbed on the skin as a remedy for fever.

LEEA GUINEENSIS G. Don   Leeaceae

"Sacred Plant"

Centers of Diversity: Throughout Tropical Africa.

Common/Vernacular Names: *Africa:* Okatakyi (Ghana), Koukoissa (Ivory Coast)

Somatic Chromosome Numbers and Genome Constitution: 2n=

Description: An erect or sub-erect shrub up to 2–4 m high, exuding watery sap when broken; leaves bipinnate, petioles swollen, leaflets 18x7.5 cm, opposite, oblong-elliptic, acuminate, base rounded, margins shallowly toothed; flowers small, globular, orange with white centers in glabrous cymes, Feb., July–Aug. Fruits red turning purple-black, depressed globose, 10 mm diameter on red stalks; seeds 6, grooved, 6 mm long.

Lore, Legend and Romance: The foliage, flowers, and fruits are highly ornamental. The fruits are said to be edible. This plant is sacred in Ivory Coast. The roots and seeds are used medicinally in Ghana and make a purgative drink.

    The roots, boiled with red peppers, are used for gonorrhea in Nigeria, where a cooling root decoction is also a sudorific.

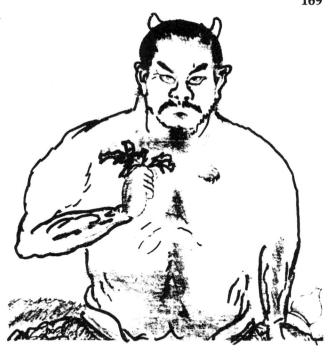

Sheng Nung, The "DIVINE CULTIVATOR"
The legendary founder of Chinese medicine was said to have discovered the curative
properties of herbs (circa 2700 B.C.)

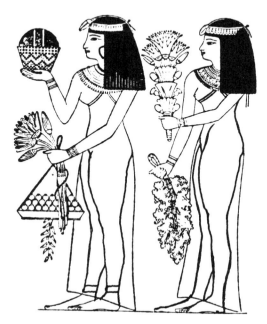

Egyptian Bearers with Fruits, Flowers and Herbs—Great Pyramid of Cheops—circa 2500
B.C.

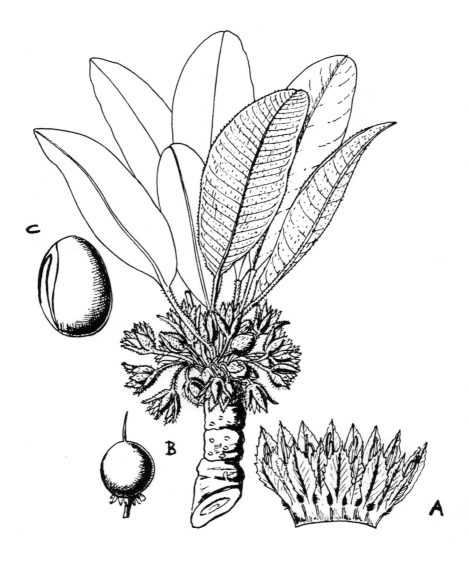

Butyrospermum paradoxum
showing (a) flowers, (b) fruit and (c) seed

BUTYROSPERMUM PARKII (G. Don.) Kotschy   Sapotaceae

Syn. Butyrospermum paradoxum (Gaertn. f.) Hepper spp. Parkii   **Sapodilla family**
Syn. Vitellaria paradoxa (Gaertn. f.) Karite

Centers of Diversity: Semi-wild in the savannahs of West Africa; gregarious from Senegambia to Uganda.

Common/Vernacular Names: *English:* Shea butter tree; *Africa:* Nkudua, Yokuti (Ghana); Emi-emi, Kadanya (Nigeria)

Somatic Chromosome Numbers and Genome Constitution: 2n=24

Description: A small deciduous tree, commonly confused with **Lophira alata** but with a spreading habit; height up to 12 m, bole 1.5–1.8 m in diameter; bark thick, fissured both longitudinally and horizontally, in squares like crocodile skin. Slash, red with milky juice. Leaves clustered at the ends of shoots, 25x7.5 cm, oblong or obovate-oblong, glabrous. Flowers, creamy white, sweet scented, in terminal clusters and attracting bees, Dec.–Feb. when the tree is leafless. Fruits—a shiny brown with a large hilum, ellipsoid in shape, thick rind and large white kernel, 25 cm long, Mar.–April, June.

Lore, Legend and Romance: An African sapotaceous species, the so called Shea tree, produces seed from which a fat, similar to butter, is obtained (*"Shea butter"*). The product prepared by the indigenous people is actually used as butter. In Guinea as well as in the interior of West Africa this tree is a substitute for palm oil of the coastal regions. There it is the most important fat-producing plant for food and illumination; indeed, the only one of real importance. This butter is exported to Europe for industrial uses. This plant is gregarious in the savannah areas of West Africa where it is often protected and inherited.

In Brazil a similar product, derived from the fruits of **Caryocar villosum** (Aubl.) Pers., family **Caryocaraceae**, commonly known in Brazil as pequia, a large tree of the Amazon region. The fruits reach the size of oranges, and contain the hard seeds nested in a fatty mass from which the product may be extracted by means of heated presses. The product closely resembles the *"Shea butter"* and is used locally for the same purposes as well as for preparing soap. The fat is called *"manteiga de pequia"* (*"pequia butter"*). The fat could be exploited industrially in the same way as African *"Shea butter".*

Besides this butter, the seeds of **Caryocar villosum** themselves yield 70% of another, much finer fat which is recommended for the preparation of cosmetics. Yet a serious obstacle stands in the way of recovering this latter fat; the outer shell of the seed is endowed with a great number of sharp thorns which point inward. In the process of cracking the seeds, these thorns splinter and may cause wounds in the human skin.

There is the other **Caryocar nuciferum** L. native to Brazil and Guyana; a tall tree cultivated in the West Indies for its edible *"Suari nuts."*

Butyrospermum parkii was named in honor of Mungo Park, who first showed that the Sudan Toulou (Bambouk), i.e., *"shea butter,"* came from the **Butyrospermum parkii.**

In commerce, *"shea butter"* is used in soap and candle-making, also in the manufacture of butter substitutes. When extracted it is known as *"shea oil"* in Europe. Its main use by the locals is in cooking. If carefully prepared and clarified it is a good substitute for lard. The oil is used as an illuminant, as a pomade for cosmetic application to the hair, though it does have a certain odor. It is also made into soap by using certain plant ashes. The residual meal, after extraction of the butter, is used by the Dagombas of Northern Ghana as a water-proofing material on the walls of their huts.

A reddish, gummy substance *"gutta shea,"* is obtained by tapping the bark. The bark decoction is drunk as a medicine by the Nankanis of Northern Ghana, who also use it in bathing children. A bark decoction is drunk on the Ivory Coast, and also used in baths and sitz-baths to facilitate delivery. The roots, root bark and latex are also used medicinally.

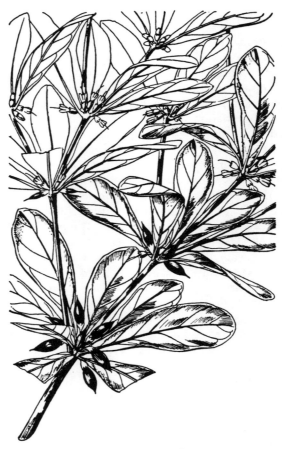

Synsepalum dulcificum
[after Irvine]

| **SYNSEPALUM DULCIFICUM** Daniell. | **Sapotaceae** |

Syn. Sideroxylon dulcificum A. Dc.   **Sapodilla family**

Centers of Diversity: Gregarious in West Africa: Nigeria, Ghana, Sierra Leone and Benin.

Common/Vernacular Names: *English:* Miraculous Berry; *Africa:* Asaa, Abrewe (Ghana); Abayunkun (Nigeria)

Somatic Chromosome Numbers and Genome Constitution: 2n=

Description: A slow growing shrub to small tree up to 2 m high. Leaves glabrous below, obovate to obovate-oblanceolate, in clusters near ends of branchlets; petioles in clusters near ends of branchlets, very short. Flowers brown, in small axillary subsessile clusters, June–Aug. Fruits to 2 cm long, red, 1-seeded, nearly glabrous, Jan. Propagation is from seed.

Lore, Legend and Romance: The fruits when ripe and fresh are singularly sweet and have a peculiar property of imparting a sweet taste to anything bitter, sour or acrid in character—lime juice, vinegar, unripe fruit and quinine. In West Africa, the locals use the ripe fruits to sweeten palm wine.

| **CLAUSENA ANISATA** (Willd.) Hook. f. ex Benth. | **Rutaceae** |

"Sacred Plant"   **Rue Family**

Centers of Diversity: West Africa; Guinea to Angola and widespread throughout Tropical Africa.

Common/Vernacular Names: *Africa:* Sesadua (i.e. *"Spirits Tree"*), Samanyobli, Ayira (Ghana); Ata pari obuko (Nigeria)

Somatic Chromosome Numbers and Genome Constitution: 2n=18, 36

Description: A shrub to small tree up to 6 m high. Leaves pinnate, strongly anis seed scented, leaflets 15 or more, pellucid-dotted, rather pubescent below, especially on nerves. Flowers, white or cream, numerous, small, in inflorescence up to 23 cm long, Jan., Mar., July; fruits small, ellipsoid, 13 mm in diameter, shining blue-black drupes, June (Nov.)

Lore, Legend and Romance: This plant is commonly hung in houses or put on fires to keep away mosquitoes and evil spirits; and in Ashanti it is used for making a new shrine, being itself supposed to possess a spirit. The Peki Ewes of Ghana use the stems as a chewstick, the wood is used for smoking fish. It is reported that the plant is very palatable to elephants. The pounded roots, with lime and Guinea grains, are applied to rheumatic and other pains in Nigeria, where also the leaves are considered anthelmintic. The leaves are burnt in Ghana to drive ghosts from haunted houses, hence, the vernacular name, *"Sesadua."*

FAGARA XANTHOXYLOIDES Lam.   **Rutaceae**

"Magic Uses"   **Rue family**

Centers of Diversity: Cape Verde to Nigeria.

Common/Vernacular Names: *English:* Candelwood. Africa: Okanto, Xetsi (Ghana); Mjafari, Mtata (Swahili)

Somatic Chromosome Numbers and Genome Constitution: 2n=????

Description: A shrub growing to a small tree up to 15 m high and 1.5 m girth; trunk grey with large woody thorns falling later, and then covered with thick corky and woody thorns only on older branches, twigs very thorny; leaves pinnate, with 3–4 pairs of shining, aromatic leaflets, elliptic to oblong, obtuse, entire, 10 x 4 cm; rhachis with recurved thorns, thorns on midribs belows, releasing aroma when crushed. Flowers small, numerous, white in dense terminal panicles Dec.-Mar. Fruits are brown, splitting into two, with one shiny blue-black seed within, having a spicy taste.

Lore, Legend and Romance: In Ghana, post-delivery pains are relieved by an extract of this root in combination with Yam. The pulverized seed, root-bark and bark are made into a poultice and applied to rheumatism and swellings.

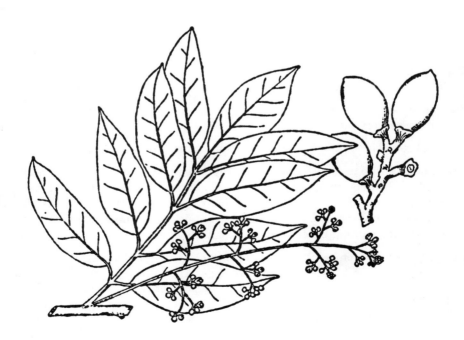

Canarium luzonicum

COMMIPHORA SPP.   Burseraceae

Balsam family

Centers of Diversity: From Northern Ethiopia to Southern Arabia.

Common/Vernacular Names: *English:* Myrrh; *Africa:* Mbambara, Mpambara (Swahili); *China:* Mo-yao

Somatic Chromosome Numbers and Genome Constitution: 2n = 26

Description: A shrub to medium-sized tree attaining 10 m in height.

Lore, Legend and Romance: Burseraceae as a family is distinguished from the closely related **Rutaceae** and **Simaroubaceae** by the presence of special resin ducts in the bark. The balsam family consists of tropical trees and shrubs in both hemispheres, quite a number of which are of some economic importance. Frankincense comes from **Boswellia carteri** Birdw., which is indigenous to Northern Somalia and Southern Arabia. In classical times frankinscense was known from Mesopotamia to Egypt, and was carried over to Greece and Rome.

    The Bible generally associates frankinscense with myrrh, a rubber-like resin of the genus **Commiphora**, which grows in the same ecosystem as **Boswellia** and comprises some 160 species. The chief sources of myrrh are: **Commiphora abyssinica, Commiphora molmol** and **Commiphora schimperi**; all ranging from 3 m to 10 m high and distributed in the region from Ethiopia to Arabia. Myrrh is a medicine as well as an incense. A tincture of myrrh is used as a local application in various forms of stomatitis and also in tooth-paste. In antiquity, myrrh was used for embalming corpses. Nowadays, the largest part of the harvest goes to India where it is turned into incense.

    Mecca balsalm, another medicament, which is often added as ritual unguent and oils, comes from **Commiphora opobalsamum**, Engl., a small shrub from Somalia and Arabia. Unlike frankinscense and myrrh, it does not coagulate freely, but begins to flow when the tips of the branches are broken off.

    Elemi resins are obtained from several members of the balsam family. Manila elemi is obtained from **Canarium luzonicum**, Pili tree, Philippines. African elemi from **Canarium schweinfurthii** of tropical and West and Central Africa; American elemi is from **Protium icicariba**, Brazil, with more than 80 spp. and is the largest genera in this family, comprising altogether 600 spp. in 20 genera.

    Commiphora opobalsamum Engl. is said to yield the balm of Gilead, but according to MacMillan, **C. opobalsamum**, Mecca balsam, the Balm of Gilead and myrrh are all common names for the same plant, **Commiphora myrrha**, though I have not come across this name anywhere except in MacMillan (p. 364).

    Cleopatra, we have been informed through history, was able to seduce even the most unlikely male of her day. She is credited with having used a *"fatal fragrance"* which made men succumb to her wishes. This fatal fragrance has been found to contain nothing more than a fragrant incense, which when

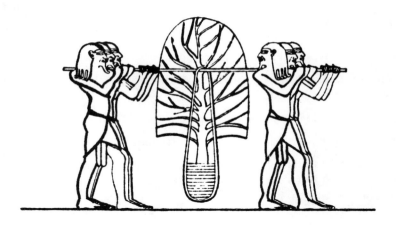

Queen Hatshepsut's Punt Expedition: Transporting a Myrrh Tree

burned in the right setting, was conducive to peace and quiet and promoted amorous behavior leading to romance.

It is a recorded knowledge that her chambers were filled with beautiful odors, where rare incense was burned all the time. Furthermore, it was her custom to anoint her body with fragrant oils so that those who might enter her chambers would believe that they were near a beautiful flower. It is no wonder that Mark Antony was drawn to her exotic chambers to become enslaved by her physical charms.

Some authorities of ancient antiquities give the mixture of incense which Cleopatra used in her day as follows: myrrh, sandalwood, orris root, winter's bark, olibanum tears and wood base. Of course we are all aware nowadays that incense is soothing and quieting to some individual's nerves and can be used to achieve extraordinary feats in the areas of psycho-sensory perceptions; an example being alluring, seductive, sensuous, carefree and meditative. It is generally agreed that incense can cast a spell or set a mood for a variety of activities.

Some botanical authorities of the Bible are of the opinion that the Balm of Gilead mentioned in the Holy Book may have been mastic, the resinous exudation from **Pistacia lentiscus** belonging to the family **Anacardiaceae**. Myrrh, as we know it, is an oleo-gum-resin, a substance between a resin, which is soluble in alcohol but not water and a gum which is soluble in water but not alcohol. It can be used as a mild disinfectant and as a stimulant to mucous membranes. It is a mild carminative and acts as a mild stimulant. In China, **Commiphora myrrha** is used medicinally, in reducing swelling and localized pain. Conditions most generally used for are: traumatic injuries and pain, carbuncles, abscesses and sores, pains in the chest and abdomen region, rheumatism, amenorrhea and dysmenorrhea.

COMMIPHORA AFRICANA (A. Rich) Engl. Burseraceae

Syn. Balsamodendron africanum Arn. **Balsam family**

Centers of Diversity: East Africa

Common/Vernacular Names: *English:* African Bdellium, African Myrrh, LeBaumier Bdellium; *Africa:* Oanka (Somali); Narge (Ghana); Bazana (Nigeria); Mbambara (Swahili)

Somatic Chromosome Numbers and Genome Constitution: 2n = 26

Description: A small tree up to 6 m high with fragrant bark and leaves; branchlets reddish-purple; leaflets trifoliolate, obovate, 5 x 2.5 cm, margins toothed. Flowers red, Feb.

Lore, Legend and Romance: One of the sources of African myrhh or *"bdellium,"* a drug resembling the true myrrh, **Commiphora myrrha** and other **Burseraceous** species. It is the gum-resin which is obtained largely in Senegal and Ethiopia.

 The wood is burned and used for fumigating the clothes of women suffering from the beri-beri disease.

COMMIPHORA MYRRHA Engl. Burseraceae

Syn. Balsamodendron myrrha Nees. **Balsam family**

Centers of Diversity: Northern Ethiopia to Southern Arabia, tropical Africa and Asia.

Common/Vernacular Names: *English:* Myrrh; *Africa:* Mpambara (Swahili); *China:* Mo-yao

Somatic Chromosome Numbers and Genome Constitution: 2n = 26

Description: A small tree resembling a low-spreading cedar.

Lore, Legend and Romance: This plant is mentioned in Egyptian papyrus as far back as 2000 B.C. Myrrh has a spiritually distinct aromatic substance. It is still used today, as in ancient times, as a basic ingredient of incense in Catholic churches. An oleo-resin from the stems and shoots are used for medicine and embalming. It is antiseptic and acts as an astringent, and for this reason, has been used for thousands of years as a mouthwash and tooth powder. It helps to strengthen the gums and harden loose teeth. It increases blood circulation and is good for all mucous membranes. Taken internally, it acts as a blood purifier and is reputed to increase the number of white blood cells. It is said to neutralize the uro-genital tract, and for this reason is often used as a douche.

 The Bible generally associates frankinscence with myrrh; both species were highly valued spiritually as it was one of the gifts from the Wise Men to the Baby Jesus at the celebration of his birth. It is associated with the highest spiritual attainment of man, that of the Sage, or Wise Man; it is also associated with the number 9 and the sign Aquarius.

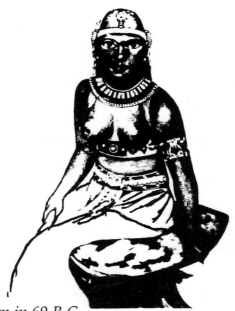

Cleopatra—Born in 69 B.C.
This black queen of Egypt was beloved by Julius Caesar then later, Mark Antony.
Cleopatra used her romances to protect Egypt from the brutality of the Roman Empire

AZADIRACHTA INDICA A. Juss.   **Meliaceae**

Mahogany family

Centers of Diversity: A native of the dry region of Irrawadi valley in India. Introduced into the tropics of Africa and Asia.

Common/Vernacular Names: *English:* Nim tree, Neem; *Spanish:* Margosa (Portuguese); *Asia:* Nim, Nimba, Limbro (India), K'u Lien (China)

Somatic Chromosome Numbers and Genome Constitution: 2n=28

Description: An evergreen, drought-resistant, tall, erect tree up to 24.4 m in height. Flowers creamy white, scented. Fruit a drupe, pale yellow, seed surrounded by fleshy pulp; leaves pinnate.

Lore, Legend and Romance: This plant is much used medicinally. The seeds contain a deep yellow, acrid oil of repugnant taste and garlic-like smell used in India as an anthelmintic and for wounds and skin diseases. The oil is also used for rheumatism. Dried root, leaves and stem bark constitute an important drug in India, Sri Lanka and neighboring countries. The bark is a bitter tonic, astringent and antiperiodic. In West Africa, the root and leaf decoction is used for fever. Seeds are ground and applied to snake bites in Ghana. The fruit is a purgative.

This is yet another plant where much confusion has arisen over the correct ascribed name. Different botanists call it by different names. Synonyms have always been given as **Melia indica** Brand., **Melia japonica** Hassk., and **Melia parviflora** Moon.

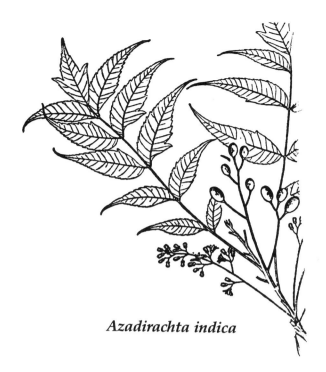

Azadirachta indica

MELIA TOOSENDAN Seib. et Zucc.   **Meliaceae**

Mahogany family

Centers of Diversity: Endemic to woody areas of Szechuan, mainland China, and no attempt having been made to introduce it to cultivation outside its native habitat. This species is relatively unknown in those areas where the following species occur: **M. azaderach, M. azaderach var. umbraculiformis, M. dubia, Azadirachta indica.**

Common/Vernacular Names: *China:* Chuan-lien-tze, K'u Lien.

Somatic Chromosome Numbers and Genome Constitution: $2n = 28$

Description: A tree attaining 10 m or more in height.

Lore, Legend and Romance: The stem and root bark are used as medicine (Cortex meliae or Radix meliae). It has no odor but tastes very bitter. The bitter taste component is the crystalline alkaloid, margosine. In addition, there are neutral resins and tannins present. The latter is the main component which is effective in treating parasites. There is about 0.02–0.43% of toosendanin. It is used as an ingredient in insecticides manufactured for agricultural purposes.

In China, **Melia toosendan** is an ingredient of a herbal mixture known as *"Lan-wei-ching-chieh-tang"* where it is known to possess the ability to inhibit the growth of organisms often seen in the intestinal tract and to detoxify their endotoxins. The plant in combination with other herbs has been used successfully in gallstone cases where no surgery was necessitated. The principle was to induce peristalsis of the gall bladder so as to expel the stone.

BLIGHIA SAPIDA Konig   **Sapindaceae**

Soapberry family

Centers of Diversity: Indigenous to West Africa, Senegambia to Gabon, introduced and cultivated in Jamaica for its edible fruits, but rare or absent in many of the West Indian islands. The plant is also grown in South Florida.

Common/Vernacular Names: *English:* Ackee, Vegetable brain, Akee; *Spanish:* Seso vegetal, Akee, Aki, Abre á Fricasse; *Africa:* Ankye-fufuo, Adza (Ghana); Bwinga, Ishin (Nigeria)

Somatic Chromosome Numbers and Genome Constitution: 2n=32

Description: A medium-sized evergreen, polygamous tree attaining over 20 m in height. An attractive shade tree, especially when in fruits. Leaves pinnately compound, light green, semi-deciduous; leaflets opposite or subopposite, elliptical to oblong-ovate, shortly acuminate, 6–18 cm long, up to 7 cm broad. Flowers whitish and fragrant about 4.5 mm long. Fruit campanulate, 3-lobed pod up to 10 cm long, yellowish to bright red; poisonous until fully ripe when pod naturally splits open in three parts exposing three oblong black seeds with soft yellow arils.

Lore, Legend and Romance: The seeds are always poisonous. Akee poisoning, which causes vomiting, has resulted in casualties in Jamaica and southern Florida. When fresh and firm, the arils may be eaten raw but are commonly cooked and are exceedingly popular in Jamaica. Fried, it is a great delicacy in the West Indies. The fruits give a good lather when rubbed in water and are used by the Krobos of Ghana in washing clothes to fix colors. The dried husks and also the seeds are burned and the ashes used in making soap, as they are rich in potash of good quality.

The tree has certain uses in magic, and is considered sacred in parts of the Ivory Coast; the bark-pulp is used as a linament for edema and intercoastal pains, and seasoned with Guinea grains and ginger, is eaten to allay orchitis. The bark, ground with **Capsicum** peppers, is used in Ghana as an overall body stimulant.

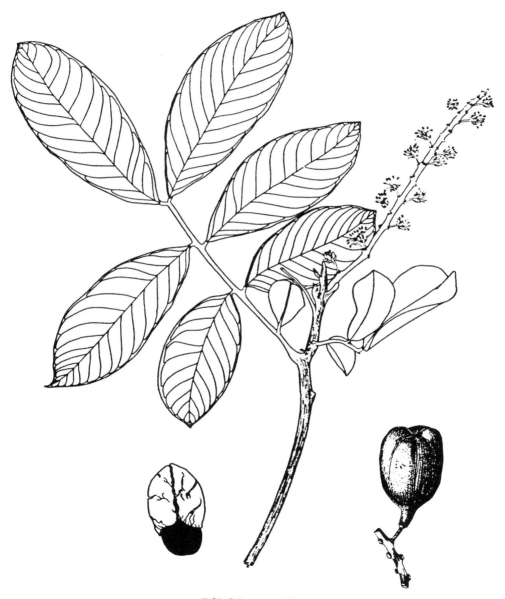

Blighia sapida
showing flowers, a fruit and seed with aril

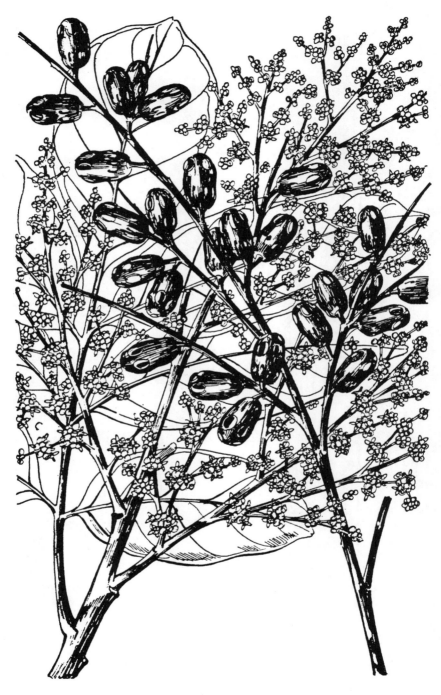

Pseudospondias microcarpa
[after Irvine]

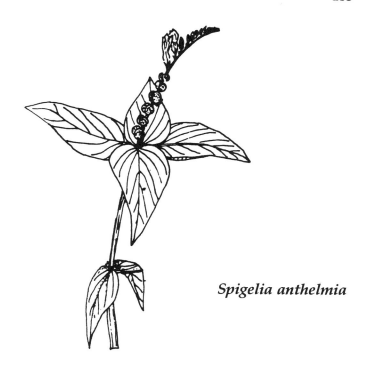

Spigelia anthelmia

PSEUDOSPONDIAS MICROCARPA A. Rich) Engl. **var micricarpa**

Anacardiaceae

Sumac or Cashew family

Centers of Diversity: Senegambia to Zaire; Angola, Sudan, Uganda and Tanzania

Common/Vernacular Names: *Africa:* Akatani, Mamia (Ghana)

Somatic Chromosome Numbers and Genome Constitution: 2n = 32

Description: A tree up to 30 m high; buttressed at base, crown spreading, sometimes with a crooked, irregular, even fluted bole. Leaves pinnate, up to 45 mm long, 6 pairs of alternate to sub-opposite leaflets, with terminal leaflet 20 x 10 cm slightly cuneate. Flowers numerous and small, white and sweet-scented, in lax terminal panicles (Jan.–Feb., June–July). Fruits 4-celled, nearly 2–5 cm long, in clusters on hanging stalks, red or bluish black when ripe, resinous, particularly when unripe; seed large, embedded in pulp, often disseminated by birds. Fruits are edible.

Lore, Legend and Romance: This tree is supposed to be narcotic to those who sit or sleep under it, hence its Ghanain name, *"Kataw'ani"* i.e., close your eyes, and is therefore regarded with awe and suspicion.

The pulp bark with water in palm-wine is drunk on the Ivory Coast as a purgative or diuretic, the resin from the trunk being used the same way. The resinous bark is used in Liberia for jaundice and eye disease.

DESFONTAINEA SPINOSA Ruiz & Pav.   Loganiaceae

Logania family

Centers of Diversity: In the mountains of the Andes; Peru and Southern Chile, where it is commonly referred to as the Lake Country.

Common/Vernacular Names: *English:* False Holly

Somatic Chromosome Numbers and Genome Constitution: 2n = 14

Description: An evergreen shrub up to 1 m in height, native to the Andes of Peru and Chile. Leaves opposite; leaflets elliptic-oblong, to 9 cm long, spiny-toothed resembling the leaves of holly. Flowers in axils, 5-merous, corolla tubular, scarlet and yellow, 4 cm long. Fruit, a berry.

Lore, Legend and Romance: The only species in the genus, this rather attractive plant lends itself as a potential aesthetic and landscape material. Its holly-like leaves and the red flowers it produces makes it an attractive container grown small shrub that could grace partially-shady patios. The plant is a recent introduction to Horticultural Science and it is cultivated on the Pacific Coast.
  Predictions have been made that this plant of the future could potentially displace **Rhododendron** spp. or at best, steal some of the romantic attention which is bestowed on certain members of these **Ericaceous** plant group.

SPIGELIA ANTHELMIA L.   . Loganiaceae

Logania family

Centers of Diversity: Native to tropical America, now generally distributed in the tropics of both hemisphere.

Common/Vernacular Names: *English:* Pink weed, Worm grass; *Spanish:* Yerba de Lombrices

Somatic Chromosome Numbers and Genome Constitution: 2n = 48

Description: An erect annual herb 5–40 cm high; stems glabrous, leaves broadly lanceolate, long, acute. tapered to base, scarbidulous above, puberulous-setulose on veins beneath; flowers white with magenta stripes on either side of the midline of lobes; fruits 2-lobed, scalywarted.

Lore, Legend and Romance: This esteemed plant is utilized in the Santería religion during initiations. It is also used medicinally as an anthelmintic.

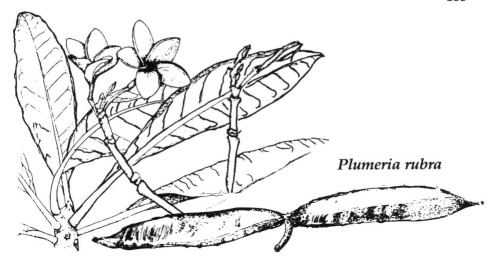

Plumeria rubra

ALSTONIA BOONEI DeWild. **Apocynaceae**

Syn. Alstonia congensis Engl. **Dogbane family**

Centers of Diversity: Senegambia to Zaire, Sudan and Uganda.

Common/Vernacular Names: *Africa:* Osen-nuru, Onyame-dua; (*"sky god's tree"* *Ghana); Ahun, Akpe (Nigeria)*

Somatic Chromosome Numbers and Genome Constitution: 2n=

Description: A large, fast-growing tree attaining 40 m in height and 3.5 m girth at breast height and having high, narrow buttresses. It exudes a characteristic white, milky latex. Leaves in whorls of 4–7 at each node, 25 x 7.5 cm, elongate-oblanceolate, rounded to acuminate, with prominent parallel lateral nerves almost at right angles to midrib. Flowers small and white, in lax grey-puberulous terminal cymes, Nov.–Feb. Fruits paired, long, thin follicles up to 45 cm long; seeds 0.5 cm long with brown floss.

Lore, Legend and Romance: This is an esteemed and venerated plant of West Africa where, in Ghana, it is to be encountered in every compound in Ashanti. An altar is erected to the Sky God in the shape of a forked branch cut from the tree. The Ashanti name for the tree Nyame dua meaning God's tree. The tree is considered to be a slow, sure poison, which shows itself in a progressive loss of strength, followed by languor and emaciation shortly before death (Kerharo and Bouquet).

   The wood is used in Ghana for wooden shoes, carving toys, images, *"devil masks,"* and general household utensils. A bark decoction is used after childbirth to assist the delivery of the placenta. The latex is used by Bakwiri women of Cameroon Mountains to encourage lactation (Dalziel), and it is also a well known antidote to **Strophanthus** poisoning. The plant is used on the Ivory Coast for gonorrhea where also, the bark, macerated in water with spices, is widely used for fevers. The leaves are used externally for rheumatism. An infusion of the bark is drunk for snake-bite and arrow poison.

PLUMERIA RUBRA var. ACUTIFOLIA Bailey

Apocynaceae

Syn. Plumeria acutifolia Poir
Syn. Plumeria acuminata Ait.
Syn. Plumeria obtusa Lour.

Dogbane family

Centers of Diversity: Native of Mexico and South America. Cultivated in the tropics as a medicinal tree. Commonly planted near Buddhist temples in Sri Lanka.

Common/Vernacular Names: *English:* Temple tree, Mexican Frangipani, Graveyard flower, Pagoda tree, Spanish Jasmine; *Spanish:* Atabaiba rosada, Atabaiba, Flore de Cuervo; *Africa:* Mbono wa kizungu, Mjinga (Swahili)

Somatic Chromosome Numbers and Genome Constitution: 2n=36

Description: A low, spreading, semi-succulent, milky tree or large shrub, introduced into Sri Lanka. The highly scented flowers are greatly esteemed as a temple offering. The tree is almost or quite bare of leaves in the dry season, when it bears large heads of white yellow-centered and highly fragrant flowers, followed occasionally by a few bifurcated pods. Leaves are deciduous, lance-shaped 5 cm wide and up to 35 cm long in clusters at the ends of branches. Grown from seed or large cuttings, dried before planting and inserted in wholly sandy medium to assure good drainage.

Lore, Legend and Romance: This is considered one of the better perfume yielding flowers of the world. The root-skin and plant latex are strongly laxative. The latex is applied to obstinate ulcers, scabies and skin diseases. A thin and blunt branch-end kept in the uterine passage causes abortion.

This plant has been reflected in many photographs and paintings of early English colonial homes in the tropics. The wives of the colonial governers and officials were often depicted having *"tea"* under these fragrant-flowered trees.

TABERNANTHE IBOGA Baillon

Apocynaceae

Dogbane family

Centers of Diversity: Native of Gabon, Republic of Congo, N.W. Zaire and Guinea.

Common/Vernacular Names: *English:* Iboga of Gabon people

Somatic Chromosome Numbers and Genome Constitution: 2n = 22

Description: A shrub to small tree attaining up to 2m in height and exuding a white, milky latex. Leaves opposite and glabrous; leaflets elliptical, 7.5-12.5 cm long. Flowers small, white with pink spots. Inflorescens smaller than leaves.

Lore, Legend and Romance: The plant is cultivated in Gabon. The root bark is the part of the plant used by the indigenous people in combination with other medicinal plants as a psychotomimetic for religious ceremony and as a medicine.

The roots contain several indol alkaloids. The most important is ibogaine, which is a stimulant, and in large doses, a hallucinogen. Roots of wild plants are collected; this over-exploitation has resulted in the extinction of this plant in several districts of Gabon.

There are seven species within the genus and all of them occur in Tropical Africa. Most of these contain a small amount of the active ingredient, ibogaine, but the most concentrated source is from the species TABER-NANTHE IBOGA.

Ibogaine ($C_{20}H_{26}N_2O$), the alkaloid isolated from the roots of **T. iboga**, has anti-depressant and euphoric properties, it is isometric with tabernanthine which has been shown effective as an analgesic with anti-serotonin properties.

In the past few years, this plant has gained a wide exposure because of its purported use as a cure for drug addiction. The extracted alkaloid has been administered to addicts of heroin with complete cures which, with one dosage, has lasted up to six months. It is claimed that this drug actually removes the desire for the drug heroin. These studies, however, have not been given the full test by the Food and Drug Administration, and has not been approved for use in this country.

Because this plant is near extinction, and holds so much promise for use in medicine in the Western world, cultivation is necessary on a large scale. To this end, THE NORTH SCALE INSTITUTE has initiated an ongoing research into all aspects of cultural practices related to the successful propagation and cultivation of this plant.

Normal methods of propagation of **T. iboga** is by seed or vegetative means using semi-mature wood cuttings. Air-layering methods of propagation have also been successfully attained. Studies are also being undertaken to determine the chemical potency of the indol alkaloids in the cultured plants which have been raised outside their natural habitat.

CORYNANTHE PACHYCERAS K. Schum.   Rubiaceae

Syn. Corynanthe paniculata Welw.   **Gardenia or Coffee family**

Centers of Diversity: Tropical West Africa

Common/Vernacular Names: *Africa:* Hwema, Pamprama (Ghana), Ako-igbon, Nikiba (Nigeria) Dyombe-wa (Cameroon).

Somatic Chromosome Numbers and Genome Constitution: 2n=

Description: A tree to 18.3 m in height and 2.1 m girth; crown dense, bark rather rough, dark green to reddish brown, branchlets glabrous. Flowers, July–Dec., very small, fragrant, whitish turning rusty brown on drying. Fruits, Mar.–June, Sept.–Dec., are red tinged, longitudinally furrowed into 2 lobes, many seeded.

Lore, Legend and Romance: The bark is used in Tropical Africa for *"strengthening fermented drinks."* The bark is a constituent of arrow poisons on the Ivory Coast. The bark is sometimes chewed as a cough rememdy. Bark decoction is used for leprosy. The bitter astringent bark and the bark infusion is used on the Ivory Coast for fever. It contains various crystalized alkaloids, the most important being corynanthine, corynantheine, corynanthidine, and corynantheidine, the chemical composition of which resembles that of yohimbine. Corynanthine has been used in medicine and has a marked sympatholitic action and a local anaesthetic action inferior to that of cocaine. The bark is used in Tropical Africa as an aphrodisiac.

OXYANTHUS UNILOCULARIS Hiern.   Rubiaceae

"Sacred Tree"   **Gardenia or Coffee family**

Centers of Diversity: West Tropical Africa; Sierra Leone to Zaire, Sudan and Uganda.

Common/Vernacular Names: *Africa:* Osuom Purom Pori, Supuya, Ahintuo (Ghana), Nkpo-azu (Nigeria), Bwirri (Sierra Leone)

Somatic Chromosome Numbers and Genome Constitution: 2n=????

Description: A shrub to small tree up to 3.7 m high and 30.5 cm girth; short brown-hairy branchlets angular, hollow; leaves crinkled, 30.5 x 2.5 cm, ovate-elliptic, light green, hairy on lateral nerves below, 12–14 pairs; stipules leafy, pointed; flowers slender, greenish-white, fragrant, in dense cymes, corolla-tube 10–15 cm, 2.2 cm long, ovoid (April, Aug., Oct.).

Lore, Legend and Romance: This is a sacred tree in Akwapin and Ashanti regions of Ghana. The Ashantis smoke the leaves. The bark and the leaves are used medicinally in Sierra Leone and Ghana.

PAUSINYSTALIA LANE-POOLEI (Hutch.) Hutch. ex Lane-Poole   Rubiaceae

Gardenia or Coffee family

Centers of Diversity: Sierra Leone to Ghana.

Common/Vernacular Names: *English:* Yohimbe; *Africa:* Pamprama (Ghana), Igbepo, Idagbon (Nigeria)

Somatic Chromosome Numbers and Genome Constitution: 2n=????

Description: A tree up to 30.5 m in height and 0.9 m in diameter. Leaves glabrous, oblong-elliptic, acuminate, entire, lateral nerves 10–14 pairs. Flowers yellow-white, turning purple-pink, small, profuse, of striking appearance in dense axillary panicles or compound cymes; Dec.

Lore, Legend and Romance: The pulverized bark is used in Liberia as a dressing for yaws and ground itch. From the bark of another species, **Pausinystalia yohimbe,** two active principles, yohimbinine and yohimbine are extracted, the latter being tonic and aphrodisiac, though also poisonous.

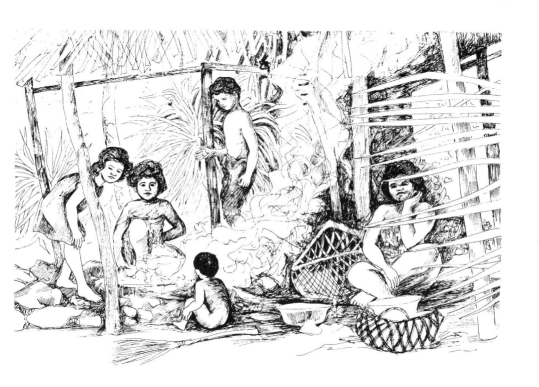

South Sea Island (Samoa)
Pen drawing of legend and landscape

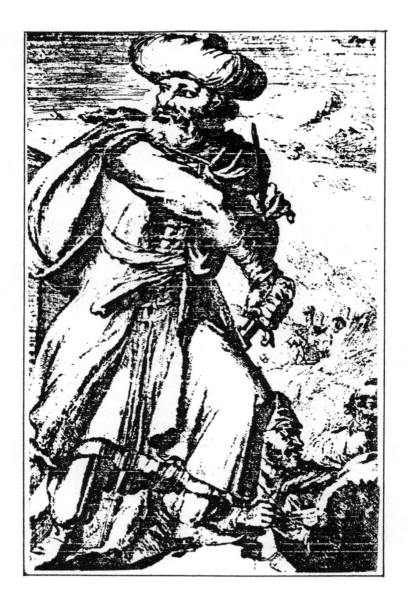

Mohammed, prophet of Islam, was a spice trader and camel driver.

KIGELIA AFRICANA (Lam.) Benth.   **Bignoniaceae**

Bignonia family

Centers of Diversity: Native to Tropical Africa. Cultivated for medicine and magic.

Common/Vernacular Names: *English:* Sausage tree; *Africa:* Nufuten, Nyakpe (Ghana), Pandoro, Nonon-giwa (Nigeria)

Somatic Chromosome Numbers and Genome Constitution: 2n=40

Description: A small to medium-sized tree up to 15 m high; leaves pinnate, glabrous, elliptic, or oblong-elliptic, leathery, apex round, generally entire, base unequal-sized. The tree is leafless in the dry season. The fruits attain a length of well over 30 cm, phallic shaped, but are not edible. The flowers, which open before the leaves, are very large, dark red and hang in racemes from the outermost branches, where they are pollinated by bats. Flowers in lax panicles, spikes pendulous (Jan.–Mar., May –July), seeds are numerous.

Lore, Legend and Romance: This tree is used medicinally in Ghana for piles, being boiled and drunk or used as an enema. The root decoction is drunk for constipation and for tapeworms. The bark and leaves alone, or with **Clerodendron capitatum, Carapa procera,** and **Xylopia aethiopica** (seed) are used on the Ivory Coast for dysentery and stomach and kidney troubles. The bark is used in Ghana as a remedy for rheumatism and dysentery.

    In Northern Nigeria, the somewhat bitter bark is boiled with red natron and Guinea-corn flour, or prepared as an infusion with other herbs and Guinea-grains and is used for syphilis and gonorrhea. The fruit is used sympatically in Ivory Coast in fertility rites.

    The fruits are sold in local medicine markets in West Africa as a purgative and for dysentery. The fruits, cut up and boiled with peppers, are used for constipation while the bark and fruit heal sores and restore taste.

    In Central Africa, another distinct species, **Kigelia pinnata** DC. is regarded with reverence, and religious meetings are held in its shade. Charms are often cut from this tree. The Zulus use an infusion of the fruit in the pre-battle preparation of the warriors.

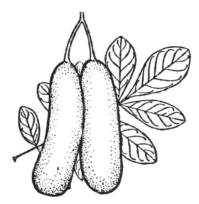

Kigelia pinnata

NEWBOULDIA LAEVIS Seem.   **Bignoniaceae**

"Around Sacred Groves"   **Bignonia family**

Centers of Diversity: Senegal to Zaire.

Common/Vernacular Names: *Africa:* Sasanemasa, Avia (Ghana), Akoko, Okurimi (Nigeria)

Somatic Chromosome Numbers and Genome Constitution: 2n=????

Description: A glabrous, erect shrub or tree up to 15.2 m high; leaves pinnate, leaflets 7–13, subsessile, oblanceolate to broadly elliptic, 20 x 10 cm. Flowers are pinkish-purple and white, tubular, spotted inside; corolla over 5 cm long, in dense terminal racemes or panicles.

Lore, Legend and Romance: This is a distinctly decorative tree, with shiny dark green leaves and purple tubular flowers. It is a common boundary tree around sacred groves and shrines. The tree is widely used in West African medicine, and it is esteemed as a sacred plant in parts of Nigeria.

   A decoction of the roots and leaves is drunk as an aphrodisiac, and is used in Senegal and Gambia for dysentery. It is also applied locally to rheumatic swellings.

STEREOSPERMUM XYLOCARPUM Cham.   **Bignoniaceae**

                                                                 Bignonia family

Centers of Diversity: Native of South India.

Common/Vernacular Names: *English:* Padri tree of India

Somatic Chromosome Numbers and Genome Constitution: 2n = 40

Description: A large spreading tree with small pinnate leaves, deciduous for a short period in the dry season. It bares a profusion of white, bell-shaped flowers for 2–3 weeks.

Lore, Legend and Romance: Padri Tree is considered a sacred tree in India and neighboring countries. Devout religious worshipers of various sects sit under the tree, which affords a good shade to meditate.

   There are some 24 species of **Stereospermums** on a world wide basis, all of them occurring in Tropical Africa and Asia.

   Mention might be made of **Stereospermum kunthianum** Cham., an indigenous tree of Tropical Africa, occurring from Senegambia to Zaire Basin, Malawi, Ethiopia and south to Zimbabwe. In Ghana, the plant is called *"Tunturei"* while it is known in Nigeria as *"Ajade."* The fruit pods are eaten with salt in Zimbabwe for coughs. Young African girls chew the bark like Cola to stain lips reddish-brown. A bark decoction, with natron, is used for venereal diseases, or in Sokoto, the bark with white Guinea-corn to which red natron is added while decoction is boiling, and is used for gonorrhea.

Bignoniaceae

Bignonia family

Centers of Diversity: Endemic to the warmer parts of the Andes mountains; occurring specifically in Brazil, Northern Argentina, Paraguay and Bolivia.

Common/Vernacular Names: *English:* Taheebo; *Spanish:* Lapacho colorado, Lapacho morado

Somatic Chromosome Numbers and Genome Constitution: $2n = 40$

Description: A medium-sized tree of the Andes forests, with light, hard wood. Flowers hermaphrodite.

Lore, Legend and Romance: The efficacies of this medicinal plant have been known and used by the Callaway tribe, descendants of the Inca medicine men, long before the advent of the Spanish and Portuguese in the New World. It has been reported that **Tabebuia altissima,** with its exceedingly hard wood, has a root system so deep and well anchored in the soil that not even the worst winter storms can blow it down. It is called *"taheebo"* by the Indians. That word is spelled *"tajibo"* by the Spanish populace, which also called the tree *"labacho morado"* (purple lapacho) because of the color of its flowers.

The purple flowers and the inner bark, including the sap, form the basis of the preparation of potions that effect thaumaturgies (miracle cures) for a host of diseases that are still officially deemed to be *"incurable."*

In recent years, the healing properties of the **Tabebuia altissima** has gained the attention of contemporary physicians in South America and the United States of America, where bark extracts have been successfully used to cure leukemia. Dr. Theodoro Meyer of the Universidad Nacional of Tucuman, a province of the Argentine Andes and Dr. Prats Ruiz, a general practitioner in Concepcion, a city in Tucuman province, have done an extensive work in the plant's chemical composition. These two modern medical practitioners isolated the species' active principles and found in it xyloidin, an antibiotic with virucidal properties. No other antibiotic capable of killing viruses had ever been mentioned in any scientific literature. Dr. Meyer learned of the taheebo from the Callawayas. He promptly used it on his patients and reported complete cures from five leukemia victims. These cures spurred further research in Brazil, a study funded by the United States government. Their findings also confirmed the compounds isolated from the plant, which was called *"quechua,"* and found it to be a powerful antibiotic with virus-killing properties. American herbal medicine experts Dr. James Duke, of the National Insitute of Health, and Dr. Norman Farnsworth, of the University of Illinois, confirmed the claims that: *"Taheebo undoubtedly contains a substance found to be highly effective against cancer."* However, the substance was found to be too toxic to be given to humans. For this reason, the National Cancer Institute lost interest.

The plant, however, is no more toxic than many drugs currently used to treat cancer in the United States. Again, it should be remembered that, despite American fears, Taheebo appears to be no more toxic than excessive aspirin or caffeine. Ample clinical data has been compiled by Professor Carlos Hugo

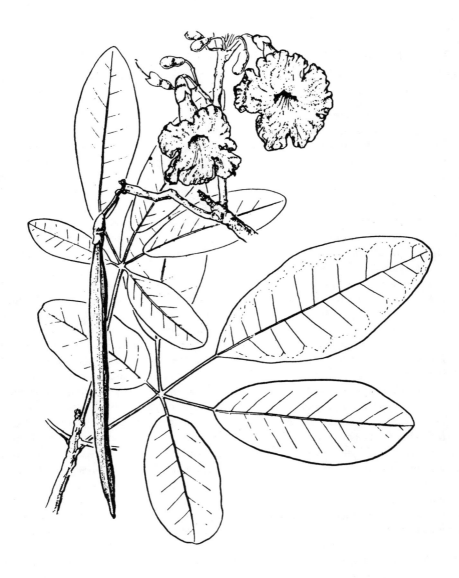

Tabebuia sp.

Burstaller in his book on the medicinal flora of Paraguay and Argentina (*"La Vueha a los Vegetales, Buenos Aires,"* 1968).

As the clinical data on the use of Taheebo in medicine has accumulated, this item of the Callawaya pharmacopoeia emerges as a veritable *"treasure of the Incas."* Within 30 days of the commencement of using the taheebo, most patients no longer showed symptoms of the dread diseases which follow: Anemia, arteriosclerosis, asthma, bronchitis, cancer of all types, colitis, cystitis, diabetes, eczema, external sores of any kind, even old sores, gastritis, gonorrhea and hemorrhages. Also, Hodgkin's disease, inflammations of the genital system, leukemia, leukorrhea, lupus, osteomyelitis, paralysis of the eyelids, Parkinson's disease, polyps (intestinal and vesical), prostatitis and psoriasis. Also, rheumatism, ringworm, scabies, skin diseases in general, syphilis and sequela, ulcerations of the intestines and varicose ulcers.

The malignant microbes that cause all those diseases cannot withstand the antibiotics this mighty tree secretes. Taheebo may, in the end, prove to be the greatest treasure the Incas have left us.

The native practitioners use herbal remedies collected on the slopes of the Andes, in the desert and on the seashore, plus ashes, volcanic mucks, waters and incantations to *"Pachacamac,"* the God of the Universe.

Since the early 1960's the bark has been used regularly at the Municipal Hospital of Santo Andre, on the outskirts of Sao Paulo. Taheebo has been used in leukemia as well as numerous diseases where viruses were suspected as the cause. Both the herb stores and the *"legitimate"* pharmacies in Brazil now carry this bark.

It should be pointed out that another species, **Tabebuia avellana,** occurring in the same eco-niche as **Tabebuia altissima** has been used interchangeably to cure the various ailments. **Tabebuia avellana** contains chemical alkaloids similar to those of **Tabebuia altissima**; the natives do not distinguish between the two.

"Ipe" and *"pau d'arco"* are the names used to denote a great number of trees of the genus **Tecoma** (or **Tabebuia**, according to some recent authorities) of the family **Bignoniaceae.** The wood of the trees is of great value, as it is beautiful, of very good quality, and practically indestructible.

Among the principal species may be mentioned the yellow ipes, *"ipes amarelos,"* **Tabebuia eximia** Mig. and **Tabebuia rigida** Dutra.; *"ipe do compo,"* **Tabebuia chrysotricha** Mart.; *"ipe pardo,"* the brown ipe, **Tabebuia ochracea** Cham.; *"ipe preto or una,"* the black ipe, **Tabebuia impetiginosa** Mart,; and the *"ipe-tabaco,"* **Tabebuia longiflora** Bur. & K. Sch. It should be emphasized that these common/vernacular names refer to the respective woods, as the same species are known by other names when used as ornamental plants.

Ipe wood exists in various shades of brown with fine yellow specks which contain a yellow dye, lapachol. This, a naphthoquinone derivative, turns red when wetted with alkali. The wood is very heavy, hard, and infinitely durable. It is employed widely for ship building and railway ties, floors and barrels. Another species, **Tabebuia cassinoides,** commonly called **Tabebuia** or **Tamanqueira** in South America, has a white or pale pink wood which turns a dirty white with time. Due to its lightness and softness it is used in pencils, toys, wooden shoes, chests and musical instruments. The wood of **Tabebuia obtusifolia** Bur. is similar and is employed as above mentioned.

NYCTANTHES ARBOR-TRISTIS L.

Verbenaceae

Vervain family

Centers of Diversity: Native of India; planted near temples and cultivated as an ornamental.

Common/Vernacular Names: *English:* Tree of sadness, Night-flowering jasmine; *Asia:* Nai-hua, Hung-mo-li (China), Hursinghar (India)

Somatic Chromosome Numbers and Genome Constitution: 2n=44

Description: A small shrub to 3 m high. Leaf yields a yellow dye. The aromatic oil is used in perfumery.

Lore, Legend and Romance: This is the *"night-blooming jasmine"* or musk flower of Eastern India. It is called *"Hursinghar"* in India, and in both India and China, it is used as a saffron dye and as an ornamental. It is not distinguished in the Pen ts'ao from **Jasminum sambac.** According to Chinese medicine, all evening flowers are good for heart troubles.

The leaf juice is stimulant, febrifuge and anthelmintic, and is taken in chronic biliary derangement, bilious, phlegmatic and remittent fever, for constipation and intestinal worms. Commonly used in India as a leaf brew for rheumatism, gout, sciatica, and backache. Bark is febrifuge and expectorant. Powdered seed rubbed on the scalp removes dandruff.

Many people easily confuse **Nyctanthes arbor-tristis** L., the true night-flowering jasmine, with **Cestrum nocturnum** L. which incidentally is also commonly called night-blooming jasmine, poison berry or Lady of the night. This plant is native to the Caribbean Basin. **Nyctanthes arbor-tristis** belongs to the family **Verbenaceae,** quite a distinct family from **Solanaceae** to which **Cestrum nocturnum** belongs. The flowers are used in Hindu worship as votive offerings. On a world-wide basis, this is among the various species of plants which furnishes scented flowers.

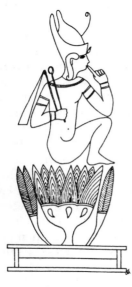

Egyptian god, Horus, seated on a lotus flower

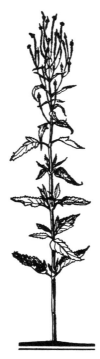

Verbena hastata

STACHYTARPHETA INDICA Vahl.   **Verbenaceae**

Syn. Stachytarpheta jamaicensis Gardn.   **Vervain family**
Syn. Verbena folio
Syn. Verbena jamaicensis

Centers of Diversity: Widely distributed in tropical Africa, Asia and America.

Common/Vernacular Names: *English:* Bastard vervain of Jamaica; *Africa:* Iru-ala-ngba, Iru amurin, Payun payun, Atitipa (Nigeria), Crete-dinde (Guinea), Cachinde ca menha (Angola), Herbe queue de Rat (Seychelles), Nsunsu, Abontennua (Ghana)

Somatic Chromosome Numbers and Genome Constitution: 2n = c112

Description: A shrubby plant, 1–2 m high, variously described as an annual, biennial or triennial. Cultivated from seed or cuttings. A common weed in waste places.

Lore, Legend and Romance: This plant is regarded as a valuable remedy for dysentery. It is used as *"tea."* It is also used for digestive disorders and sterility. It is a good febrifuge in cases of virus infections, and the fruits have been found to be valuable in the treatment of diseases of vitamin deficiencies particularly that of rickets.

NELUMBIUM SPECIOSUM Willd.   Nelumbonaceae

Syn. Nelumbium nucifera Gaertn.   **Waterlily family**

Centers of Diversity: Asia, India, Tibet and China.

Common/Vernacular Names: *English:* Lotus lily, Sacred lotus, Nelumbo; *Africa:* Osipata, Bado (Nigeria); *China:* Ho, Fu-ch'u

Somatic Chromosome Numbers and Genome Constitution: $2n = 16$

Description: A beautiful aquatic plant with a large, handsome peltate, circular petioles, erect; flowers large, bright pink or white, scented on stout stalks. Leaves incapable of being wetted, owing apparently to waxy surface, but really due to closely minute hairs. Seeds and root-stock edible.

Lore, Legend and Romance: This plant has been held sacred by the Egyptians from time immemorial, and is also venerated in parts of India, Burma, Sri-Lanka and China. This is the Sacred Lotus, the Egyptian National Floral Emblem, which is now rare in the Nile. This aquatic lily has a tuberous root which is taken in indigestion, diarrhea and for dysentery. Oral use of leaf juice is a good remedy for hemoptysis (hemostatic), and for digestive disorders. Stamens are used for bleeding piles and in parturition.

In China, this exceedingly popular and very useful plant has a distinct name for its every part. The stem is called *"Ch'ieh"*; the rootlets on the lower part of the stem or the top of the rhizome is called *"Mi."* Leaves are called *"Hsia"*; flowers are called *"Han-t'ao"*; fruit known as *"Lien"*; roots are known as *"Ou"* and the seed is called *"Ti."* This plant is used as a refreshing preventitive of fluxes, promotes the circulation and stregthens the virility. They are recommended for leucorrhea and gonorrhea. The prolonged use of this plant is reported to drive away old age and give a fine complexion.

It is well to mention here that the length of the dormant period in fruits and seeds not only varies as between different species, but also as between individual seeds of the same species. Because of the longevity of the viable seeds of the Sacred Lotus it is probably a *"Signature"* which has influenced the Chinese to believe that the use of this plant prolongs life.

As example of the germination period for plants: if a number of clover seeds are placed under favorable conditions, some will germinate quickly, others more slowly, so that seedlings appear at intervals over a long period. This variation may be of biological advantage since it was that the chance of some of the seedlings developing under optimum conditions is thereby increased.

During the period of dormancy just described, the embryo remains alive and capable of eventual growth. Such seeds which retain their ability to germinate are said to be viable.

The seeds of willows retain their viability for only a day or so. The seeds of coconut (**Cocos nucifera**) also retain their viability for only a relatively short time. Wheat and barley grains will give full germination after storage for ten years. Many seeds of **Leguminosae,** characterized by the possession of very hard seed coats, will germinate after a much longer period. Becquerel found that the seeds of a species of **Cassia** were capable of germination after being stored in the Paris Natural History Museum for 115 years.

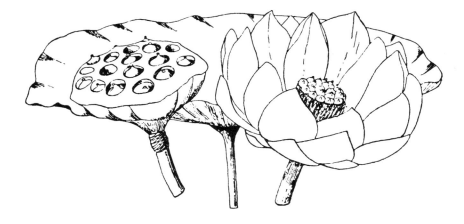

Nelumbo lutea

Another interesting example is afforded by the Sacred Lotus. Robert Brown (1850) was able to germinate some seeds of this plant after they had remained dry in Sir Hans Sloan's collection 120 years old. Reports that wheat grains from Egyptian tombs, for example, that of Tutankamen, are still capable of germination are, however, entirely unfounded.

In 1933, some seeds of the Sacred Lotus were supplied to the Royal Botanic Gardens, Kew, by a Japanese botanist who had found them in peat of a long dried-up Manchurian lake. They were tested and found to be still viable. In 1951, seeds having the same origin were germinated in Washington. The longevity of the seeds was then examined by Professor R.W. Chancey of the University of Chicago. From their investigations it seems that these still viable **Nelumbium speciosum** seeds were at least 1040 years old.

The Sacred Lotus has many symbolic meanings; for some it represents human fertility and for others it is symbolic of the world. It typifies Lower Egypt as the Papyrus plant does Upper Egypt.

It is sacred in India. Brahma alighted on the lotus when he sprang from the navel of the god Vishnu. The Orientals use the lotus plant to signify the growth of man through the three periods of human consciousness—ignorance, endeavor and understanding. The *"lotus eaters"* are those who become so addicted to eating the lotus that they live only where it grows and care for nothing and no one else. The fragrant flowers are used in perfumery. The tubers are poisonous, but when prepared properly, are edible.

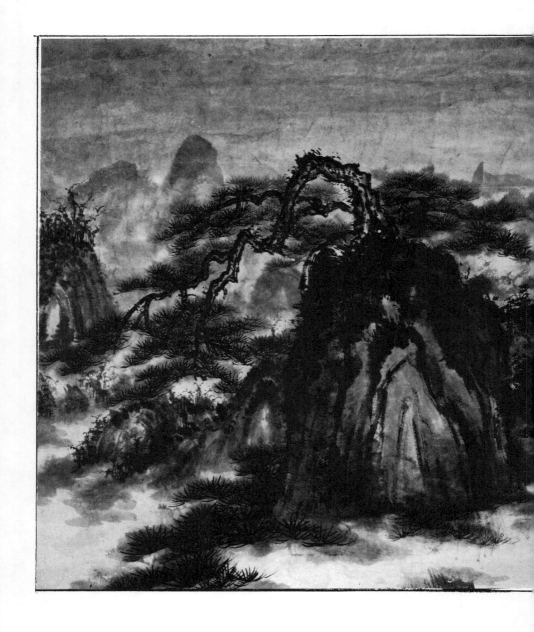

Painting by Dr. Andrew Tseng

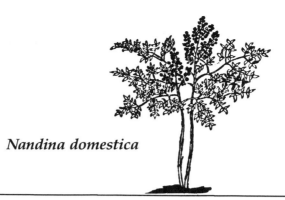

Nandina domestica

NANDINA DOMESTICA Thunb.   Nandinaceae

Heavenly Bamboo family

Centers of Diversity: Native to South China, and much esteemed in that country as well as in Japan. It is used around temples. Now, it is grown in most parts of the world as an aesthetic plant. Some horticultural varieties, particularly **Nandina domestica** *"Wood's Dwarf"* makes an excellent rock-garden material as well as Bonsai material when it shows its autumn colors.

Common/Vernacular Names: *English:* Nandin, Sacred Bamboo of China; *China:* Nan-chu, Nan-tien-chu, T'ien-chu-huang

Somatic Chromosome Numbers and Genome Constitution: $2n = 20$

Description: An erect evergreen or semi-deciduous shrub with bipinnate leaves and numerous bamboo-like stems, producing panicles of creamy flowers followed by beautiful red berries. Heavenly Bamboo can attain a height of 2.5 m in its slow to moderate growth habit. It loses its leaves when the temperature is below freezing; killed to the grown at temperatures of –10 degrees C but usually recover fast.

Lore, Legend and Romance: According to the *"Chinese Medicinal Herbs"* compiled by Li Shih-Chen, translated and researched by F. Porter Smith, M.D. and G.A. Stuart, M.D., the generic name is taken from the sound of the first two characters in the second name given above (China). Fortune, from the error of supposing that the last character in the Chinese name was *"Chu,"* translated the supposed name *"t'ien-chu"* into *"Heavenly bamboo,"* a name which the plant still retains among foreigners. The berries are called *"Hou-shu,"* *"Monkey beans,"* by the common people, and the plant also goes by the name of *"Wu-fan-ts'ao,"* because the leaves are used in preparing a kind of rice dish called *"Wu-fan"* or *"Ch'ing-ching-fan."*

    In China, the branches and leaves are reputed to check discharges, drive away sleepiness, strengthen the tendons, benefit the breath, prolong life, prevent hunger and keep off old age.

    The plant being a dicotyledon, is not a bamboo (monocotyledon) as its common vernacular name alludes; it is only reminiscent of bamboo in its lightly branched, cane-like stems and delicate, fine-textured foliage.

    This is the only genus in the family; an isolated type, probably related to **Berberidaceae** and **Podophyllaceae** also exists.

PIPER NIGRUM L.   Piperaceae

Pepper family

Centers of Diversity: Native to the slopes of mountains in the Ghats and in damp jungles of the Malabar Coast of Southwestern India at an altitude between 150–2400 m, but now widely cultivated in the tropics of both hemispheres. Cayenne, red, green and sweet peppers are **Capsicum** spp. of the family **Solanaceae.**

Common/Vernacular Names: *English:* Pepper, Black pepper; *Spanish:* Pimienta; *Africa:* Iwere (Nigeria), Mpilipili manga, Pilipili manga (Swahili); *China:* Huchiao

Somatic Chromosome Numbers and Genome Constitution: 2n=48, 52, 104, 128

Description: A woody perennial, glabrous, evergreen climbing vine to 10 m in height. The world's most important and oldest spice is prepared from the small round berries produced by the plant. Leaves simple and alternate, petiole 2–5 cm long, grooved above. Flowers unisexual (monoecious or dioecious) or hermaphrodite. Fruit, sessile, globose drupe, 4–6 mm in diameter, with pulpy mesocarp, exocarp turning red when ripe, drying black.

Lore, Legend and Romance: This is the true pepper and should not be confused with the three wholly different spices which are often erroneously called peppers. I am referring specifically to the **Capsicum** group which includes paprika, cayenne pepper, chili pepper, red pepper, bell pepper and other pod-like fruits of the Nightshade family. Also included in this group is the Jamaican pepper, known as pimento or allspice, and botanically called **Pimenta dioica;** and Melegueta pepper, or *"grains of paradise"* called **Amomum melegueta** Roscoe, an indigenous species of West Africa.

    Five centuries ago, *"grains of paradise"* were popular in Europe as a substitute for true pepper, but today the demand for the seeds is limited almost entirely to Ghana and Nigeria, whose inhabitants use them as a seasoning. The section of West Africa once known as the *"Grain Coast"* owed its name to the spice.

    Over 3,000 years ago references to pepper were made in India, in ancient Sanskrit medical literature. Most names for pepper are derived from the Sanskrit, *"pippali."*

    Pepper contains the alkaloids piperin and piperidine, the latter in much smaller quantity. Freedom from adulteration in ground pepper is ascertained by the percentage of piperine. The pungency of pepper is due to the resin chavioine, which is most abundant in the mesocarp; consequently, white pepper is not as pungent as black pepper.

    I should mention also that another important **Piper** species, **Piper methysticum** Forst., is an indigenous plant of the Polynesian, Melanesian and Hawaiian Islands (once called the Sandwich Islands and related Oceanic regions, collectively known as the South Sea Islands or Pacific Islands). It is also found in some areas of South New Guinea known as Maclay coast. In Fiji, the plant, the root and the beverage prepared from the rhizome (rootstock) are called *"Yaqona"* pronounced *"yanggona."* In English it is called Kava kava.

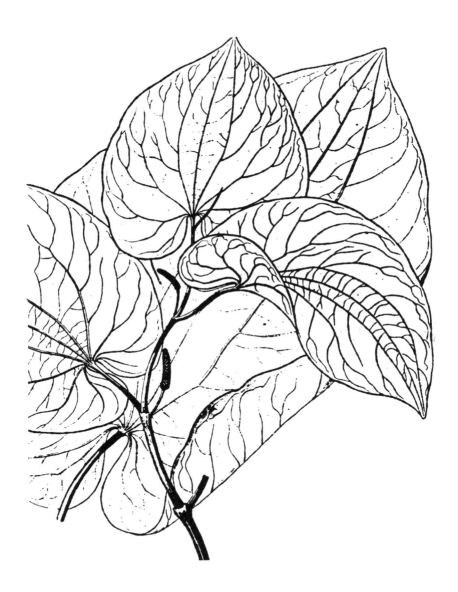

Piper methysticum

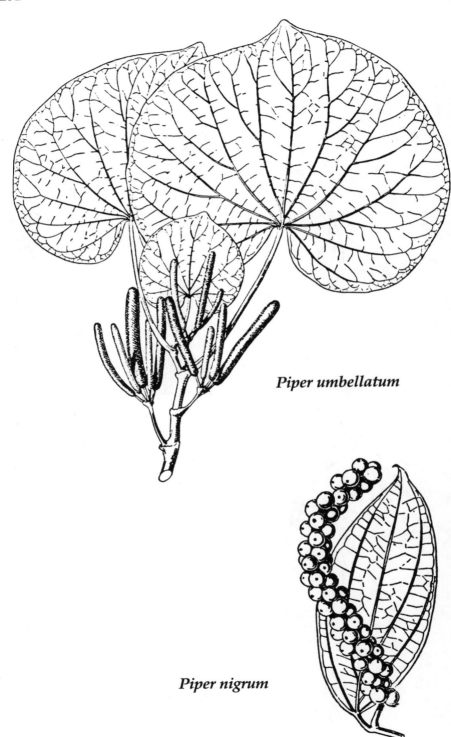

Piper umbellatum

Piper nigrum

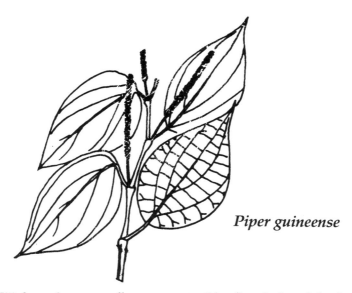

Piper guineense

In Fiji, kava kava usually represents "the first fruits of the land" and is presented as a mark of homage to the high chief, or as a mark of welcome to honored visitors. Captain James Cook, the so-called *"discoverer"* of the islands, was the first European whose attention was drawn to the custom of kava drinking; the peculiar method of ceremonial preparation and the effect of the beverage received his special attention. Daniel Carl Solander, a Swedish botanist and pupil of Linnaeus, and Sydney Parkinson, an artist with the task to make drawings of newly discovered plants, accompanied Captain Cook on his voyage with the *"H.M.S. Endeavour"* (1768–1771). The Forsters (father and son) accompanied Cook on his second voyage (1772–1775). No doubt Solander and Parkinson were the first white men who saw and described the kava plant, but the notes of Johann George Forster were published first. The beverage forms a national drink, widely used as a token of respect and goodwill, and is a ritual drink at magico-religious and ceremonial occasions. For a white man to ignore the etiquette followed at kava parties would be considered the height of ill-breeding.

Kava, which was once condemned by Christian missionaries as devil worship, is now being promoted by the government of the state of Vanuata, the former Anglo-French colony of New Hebrides, as a significant export crop. In 1933 the British biologist and explorer, Tom Harrison, saw the kava drink as a soothing alternative to alcohol. Harrison stated that the effect of the drink was most pleasant on the head which left the person feeling friendly, while not bringing on the feelings of sentimentality or aggressive behavior as does alcohol. Kava drink also does not leave a person with headache or hangover as does alcohol.

The root and rhizome preparation taken in small quantities is a stimulant, but in large doses it is a narcotic. It is also used in such ailments as hypertension, bronchitis, diarrhea, gout, rheumatism, nephritic colic, dropsy, vaginitis, gonorrhea, urethritis, metritis, salpingitis, enteritis and nocturnal incontinence of urine due to muscular weakness. It is antibacterial, antiseptic, fungicidal, anesthetic, soporific and diuretic.

PETIVERIA ALLIACEA L.	Phytolaccaceae

Pokeweed family

Centers of Diversity: Grows wild in moist woods and disused in areas in Southern Texas, Southern Florida, including most of the Caribbean Basin countries, and throughout mild temperate and tropical Mexico, including Central and South America. The plant is now naturalized and established in some parts of tropical Asia and Africa.

Common/Vernacular Names: *English:* Conga root, Garlic weed, Guinea hen weed, Gully root, John Doctor, Kojo root, Obean bush, Pipi root, Skunkweed, Strong man's weed, *Spanish:* Anamu, Ave, Avette, Chasser vermine, Feuilles ave, Herbe aux poules, Huevo de gato, Malpouri, Hierba de toro, Verbajo de ajo, Zorillo

Somatic Chromosome Numbers and Genome Constitution: $2n = 72$

Description: A perennial herb or sub-shrub to 1.5 m high, with a deep, thick, somewhat twisted taproot and tough, slender, erect stems. The whole plant, including the roots, is strongly garlic-scented. Leaves are alternate, short-petioled, elliptic, oblong or obovate, pointed at the apex, 3-15 cm long, 2-6 cm wide, sometimes slightly hairy, thin, prominently veined. Flowers are whitish, greenish or pinkish, star-like, tiny in slender axillary or terminal spikes. Fruit, 8-10 cm long, triangular, with 1-6 recurved spines, which cling to clothing and also penetrate human and animal skin.

Lore, Legend and Romance: This is a widely acclaimed folk remedy plant. The plant is very much used in the Santeria religion, where it is employed in spiritual work in South Florida. In Panama, the decoction of leafy stems are taken as diuretic and also helps calm the nerves. In Guatemala, it is drunk to stop diarrhea. The plant decoction is taken as an emmenagogue, and in Puerto Rico, the decoction of the leafy stems, boiled with leaves of **Guaicum officinale**, is taken as an abortifacient. It is likewise used by the Cuban and Barbadians as an abortifacient. In Jamaica, the plant is boiled with **Eryngium foetidum** and the *"tea"* is drunk to dispel fever and headache. Fresh leaves are bound around the head to dispel headache. The plant decoction is valued as a remedy for nervous spasms, paralysis, hysteria, asthma and whooping cough in Argentina and Mexico. Cubans take a combined decoction of this and **Rosmarinus officinalis** to overcome hoarseness. In Jamaica, it has been taken to relieve heart trouble. In Trinidad, the root infusion is a remedy for influenza, cystitis, veneral diseases and menstrual dysfunctions, womb inflammation and is also used as an abortifacient.

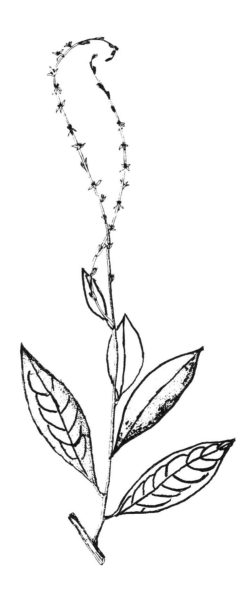

Petiveria alliacea

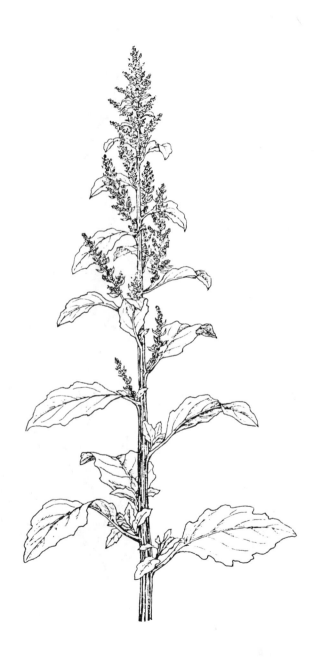

Chenopodium ambrosioides

CHENOPODIUM AMBROSIOIDES L.

Chenopodiaceae

Syn. Ambrina ambrosioides Spach.   Goosefoot family
Syn. Chenopodium ambrosioides var. anthelminticum Gray
Syn. Chenopodium suffructicosum Willd.
Syn. Onthosporum anthelminticum R.Br.

Centers of Diversity: Widespread in tropical and sub-tropical American countries, in sandy fields and disused places; also introduced in North America and naturalized in other parts of the tropics. Probably indigenous to Southern Europe.

Common/Vernacular Names: *English:* Bitter weed, Hedge mustard, Mexican tea, Semicontract, Spanish tea, Jerusalem tea, Jesuit tea, Ambrosia; Jerusalem oak, Goosefoot, American wormseed, Stink-weed; *China:* T'u Ching-Chieh; *Africa:* Dungurachirombo, Bigicana (Zimbabwe)

Somatic Chromosome Numbers and Genome Constitution: $2n = 16, 32, 36, 64$

Description: A bushy taprooted annual or perennial herb up to 3 m high, aromatic of garlic scent and the roots strongly pungent; lower leaves sinuate-toothed, 5-8 cm long, 1-2 cm broad oblong in shape; flowers minute in axillary clusters; stamens yellow or white; fruit subglobose. Flowers and fruits, Dec.-July.

Lore, Legend and Romance: This plant has been used as a tonic and antispasmodic, for nervous afflictions, as an injection for mucous membrane of the lungs, cholera in infants, for lumbrici in children. It is narcotic, acrid, poison affecting the brain, spinal cord and stomach. It is used as an anthelmintic, in ammenorrhea, for painful and profuse menstruation. The herb is said to be nervine and emmenagogue; the seeds and oil are vermifuge, diaphoretic, diuretic and expectorant. It contains a volatile oil and chenopodin, which has the effect of a narcotic. The entire plant is employed in Santeria works.

OENOTHERA BIENNIS L.   **Onagraceae**

Syn. Onagra biennis Scop.   **Evening Primrose family**

Centers of Diversity: North America to Mexico. Occurs in moist fields, meadows and disused areas throughout the United States and gregarious over a large part of the world. Cultivated as a fodder crop.

Common/Vernacular Names: *English:* Evening Primrose, Scabish, Cure-all, Tree Primrose, Common Evening Primrose, King's cure-all.

Somatic Chromosome Numbers and Genome Constitution: $2n=14$

Description: A biennial plant attaining 0.91 m in height with large yellow flowers; commonly encountered as a weed on railway embankments, road escarpments, quarries and similar habitats. It was introduced into gardens in the 18th century as a fleshy root-vegetable (yellow lamb's lettuce) and as an ornamental. The behavior of the species is such that, in the first year, it forms a rosette of leaves lying quite flat on the ground. The tall stem is not formed until the second year and as it grows, it keeps producing one or two new flowers every few weeks on end. They wither away during the next day. Leaves lanceolate, 5 cm–12 cm with a width of 2.5 cm–5 cm.

Lore, Legend and Romance: The rapid rise to fame of the evening primrose is intimately linked to the discovery of a family of hormone-like substances known as prostaglandins. These compounds hold great promise to millions of people for the relief of such diverse ailments as high blood pressure, ulcers, asthma, allergies, migraine, headaches, arthritis, glaucoma, menstrual cramps and possibly some types of cancer. Prostaglandins is actually a family of compounds closely related to essential fatty acids, similar to essential amino acids in that they cannot be manufactured by the body and need to be provided in the diet.

Medicinally, evening primrose is astringent, mucilaginous and sedative. It is useful in gastrointestinal and hepatic ailments, useful for coughs and mental depression. In recent times, the profusion of the tiny seeds produced by the plant has been of immense interest to research scientists around the globe. The oil from the seeds has made the plant one of the modern day "wonder plants." Among its notable efficacies are the ability to lower serum cholesterol levels, reduce blood pressure, inhibit thrombosis, control arthritis and other forms of inflammation, treat eczema, decrease hyperactivity in children, and benefit those suffering problems from alcoholism to obesity to cancer.

Mention might be made of the "Primrose League" which arose in England. This was a political society of English women founded for the furtherance of conservative opinions in England, and named after the favorite flower of Earl Beaconsfield, one year after his death, April 19, 1881. This anniversary is observed by wearing of the primrose flower at the annual meetings in each great center of population.

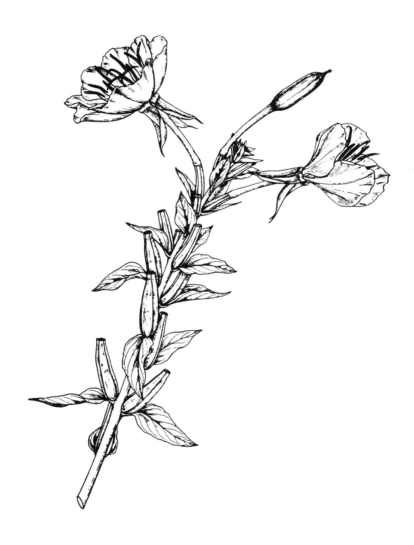

Oenothera biennis

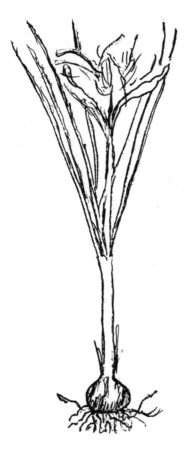

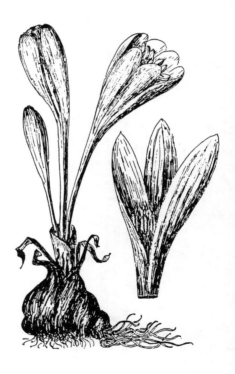

Crocus sativus
(Saffron)

Colchicum autumnale
(*meadow saffron*)

(See page 20)

PIMPINELLA ANISUM L.   **Umbelliferae**

Syn. Anisum vulgare Gaertn.   **Parsley or Carrot family**
Syn. Anisum officinarum Moench.

Centers of Diversity: Indigenous to Asia Minor, the Greek islands and Egypt.

Common/Vernacular Names: *English:* Anise seed; *Spanish:* Anis; *China:* Heui-Hsiang, Pa-Yueh-chi

Somatic Chromosome Numbers and Genome Constitution: 2n=18, 20

Description: A graceful pubsecent annual herb up to 1 m high with feathery leaves, the source of one of the oldest known aromatic seed-like fruits. The bulk of the world's supply of anise, also known as aniseed, is produced in Mexico, Spain, Germany, Turkey and Italy but it is widely cultivated in most temperate and warm climates, including India and South and Central America. Leaves compound-pinnate. Flowers yellowish, small, in compound umbels. Fruits ovate, ribbed.

Lore, Legend and Romance: Throughout Latin America, anise-flavored "aguardiente" (distilled from sugar cane) is one of the most universally popular alcoholic drinks. Anise oil is distilled in medicine for its carminative and expectorant properties and is a masking agent for flavoring otherwise evil-smelling and bitter-tasting drugs; it has been used also as an antiseptic.

In 1305 anise was listed by King Edward I among the commodities liable to taxation and was sufficiently popular that such fees helped produce the funds to repair London Bridge.

This plant was well known to the ancient Egyptians, Hebrews, Greeks and Romans, and in the Middle Ages it was highly valued as a medicine.

AMBROSIA PERUVIANMA Willd.   **Asteraceae (Compositae)**

Syn. Ambrosia paniculata Michx.   **Composite or Sunflower family**

Centers of Diversity: Florida, Bahamas, Cuba, Dominican Republic

Common/Vernacular Names: *English:* Wild tansy, wormwood

Somatic Chromosome Numbers and Genome Constitution: 2n=18, 36

Description: A shrubby herb 0.6 to 1.2 m high; leaves peltate to narrowly ovate in outline, thinly pubescent, slightly aromatic. Common in disused areas and pasture margins. Flowers and fruits Dec.–Aug. Adams states that the taxonomic affinities of Jamaican plants are not clear; the variations and relationships of local populations require further study.

Lore, Legend and Romance: This is a highly esteemed plant of the Santeria religion. In combination with other herbs, it forms an ingredient of the holy bath.

And the Lord said unto Moses, *"Take unto thee sweet spices, stacte, and onycha and galbanum, these sweet spices with pure frankincense: of each shall there be a like weight: And thou shalt make it a perfume, a confection after the art of the apothecary, tempered together, pure and holy."*

Exodus 30:34-36

"Moreover the Lord spake unto Moses, saying, 'Take thou also unto thee principal spices, of pure myrrh five hundred shekels, and of sweet cinammon half so much, even two hundred and fifty shekels, and of sweet calamus two hundred and fifty shekels, and of cassia five hundred shekels. After the shekel of the sanctuary, and of oil olive an hin: And thou shalt make it an oil of holy ointment, an ointment compounded after the art of the apothecary: it shall be a holy anointing oil.'"

Exodus 30:22-25

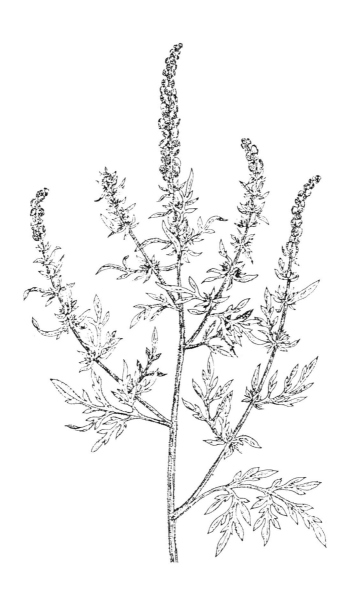

Ambrosia maritima

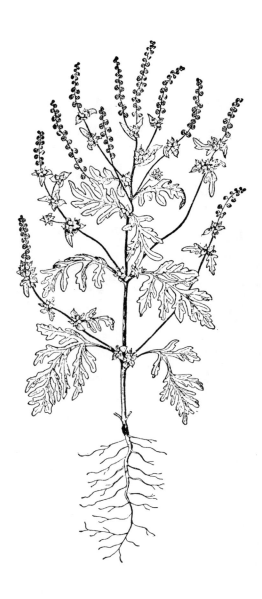

Ambrosia artemisiifolia

ARTEMISIA ABSINTHIUM L.   Asteraceae (Compositae)

Syn. Artemisia officinalis Lam.   Composite or Sunflower family
Syn. Artemisia vulgare Park

Centers of Diversity: Native to Central and Southern Europe, Southern Siberia, Kashmir and Mediterranean region. Now cultivated and naturalized throughout the world, both in temperate and sub-tropical ecosystems, including many localities in the Southern United States.

Common/Vernacular Names: *English:* Bitter artemisia, Wormwood, Absinthium, Common wormwood Maderwort, Mingwort, Old-woman, Mugwort; *Spanish:* Ajenjo, Ajenjo mayor, Absinthe batarde de Plaine, Ajorizo, Fueilles ameres; *China:* Ta-feng Ai, Yun Chen Ho

Somatic Chromosome Numbers and Genome Constitution: $2n=18$

Description: A perennial shrubby herb, to 3 m high, entirely coated with fine, silvery, silky hairs; the slender stems are much branched. Leaves are alternate, 5–7 cm long, divided into triangular segments, each subdivided into narrow, indented or toothed lobes. Flowers yellowish, minute, in profuse globose heads 4–6 mm in diameter.

Lore, Legend and Romance: The plant is ascribed to the Greek goddess Artemis and it comes under the rulership of the Moon. Artemisia's record goes back to 600 B.C. In the Bibical times, wormwood was employed as a symbol of bitterness, for of all plants it possesses that bitter characteristic. On the last night in Egypt, Moses had the escaping children of Israel flavor their paschal lamb with bitter herbs; later, no matter how much they yearned for the cucumbers, melons, leek, onions and garlic that they had left behind, wise Moses kept the cleansing bitterness in their diet with his strict health and food laws which even today have been shown to be relevant.

From the book of Exodus to the final Apocalypse runs mention of the wormwood, or reference to it as the bitter symbol of futility and the purge of repentance.

With rare unanimity, authorities state that the artemesia of historic record was either **Artemisia pontica**, called Roman wormwood, or **Artemisia absinthium**, the common wormwood, or both. **Artemisia pontica** is found on the shores of the Mediterranean Sea and Southern Europe; it is indigenous to the Black Sea region, and has proven a difficult plant to keep in bounds. **Artemisia absinthium**, on the other hand, occurs practically all over Europe. In the second century A.D., Dioscorides declared it to be a remedy against intoxication; Gerard in the 16th century used it as a vermifuge and pharmacists recommended it for its tonic properties, employing it as a stomachic.

Its virtues have been known since ancient times; Galen advocated it as a powerful tonic; the Salernitan school recommended it as a preventive medicine against seasickness, adding that it soothes the stomach and the nerves, expels worms, mitigates the effects of any poison that might have been drunk and, mixed with ox-gall, is a miraculous treatment for buzzing in the ears.

218

In the Yoruba Pantheon, the plant is claimed by Yemaya, the goddess who controls the seas and the water elements; thus, Moses' intent when ordering the use of wormwood before crossing the Red Sea was probably to employ the protection of the good spirits of the water. Moses, as we know, was a high ranking priest and magician in the "Egyptians Mysteries," and was highly trained in the use of herbs as medicine, in religious ceremonies and in magic.

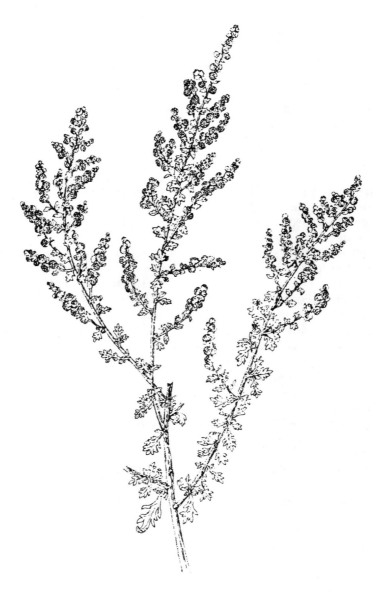

Artemisia judaica

VERNONIA AMYGDALINA Delile   Asteraceae (Compositae)

Composite or Sunflower family

Centers of Diversity: Widely distributed in West Tropical Africa, extending to Zaire and Ethiopia. Occasionally cultivated. This species is often confused with **Vernonia colorata** Drake (Syn. **Vernonia senegalensis** Less.). Both species have the same vernacular names.

Common/Vernacular Names: *English:* Bitter leaf of Sierra Leone, Libo (St. Thomas); *Africa:* Glabra (Ethiopia), Ewuro, Olubo (Nigeria), Mpon asere ("concubine laughs"), Akpa, Gboti (Ghana); Waatsa (Swahili); Sika-vakadzi (Zimbabwe)

Somatic Chromosome Numbers and Genome Constitution: $2n = 18$

Description: A shrub to small tree up to 5 m high; branchlets striped, pubsecent, becoming glabrous; leaves simple, 15 x 5 cm, obovate oblanceolate, entire or minutely toothed, finely glandular below. Flowers white, fragrant, bee infested, about 60 mm broad, in copious corymbose panicles; pappi white.

Lore, Legend and Romance: An esteemed utility plant, it is used as a shade tree for young coffee plants in Kenya. The Yorubas and Ugandans use the twigs as a "chewstick." It is much used as a tooth cleaner and is often chewed as a stomachic, tonic and appetizer. It is mixed with red natron by the Hausas of Northern Nigeria for gastro-intestinal troubles. The slightly bitter and scented leaves are eaten by the Creoles of Sierra Leone, where plants are especially cultivated for this purpose.

On the Ivory Coast a root decoction, with that of **Rauwolfia vomitoria** is taken several times a day for gonorrhea. Like other very bitter plants such as *"quinquina"* **Cinchona, Khaya senegalensis** and certain **Rubiaceae** such as **Morinda, Mitragyna** and others, these plants tend to be used as febrifuges. A leaf decoction is used as a cough medicine in Ghana and Tanzania. The marcerated leaves, strained through a cloth with peppers or spices, are used for purgative enema.

According to Irvine, 1961, Professor Paris, in his unpublished work, demonstrated the presence of a bitter principle, vernonine, which was poisonous to mice. When adminstered simultaneously—10 g. per kg of body weight—proved a 100% fatal dose. It also has a hypotensive action on dogs. These plants are said to be harmful to goats, hence the Ewe name *"gboti"* (*"goat tree"*), and the Timne name (Sierra Leone) *"edifioire"* meaning *"it kills goats."*

CAPSICUM ANNUUM L.   Solanaceae

Nightshade family

Centers of Diversity: Indigenous to Mexico, Central America, the West Indies and much of South America. Prehistoric Capsicum peppers are known from burial sites at Ancon and Huaca Prieta in Peru and were widely spread throughout the New World tropics in pre-Colombian times. Secondary center is Asia. It should not be confused with black or white pepper which is the product of **Piper nigrum**.

Common/Vernacular Names: *English:* Paprika, Cayenne pepper, Chili pepper; *Spanish:* Chile, pimentao; *Africa:* Mpilipili (Swahili); *China:* Hsiung-ya-li-chiao; La-chiao

Somatic Chromosome Numbers and Genome Constitution: 2n=24

Description: A variable herbaceous plant or sub-shrub up to 1.5 m high and widely distributed and grown in gardens from sea level to 6000 ft. or more in the tropics. Leaves very variable in size, simple; lamina broadly lanceolate to ovate, entire, thin, subglabrous. Flowers usually borne singly, terminal; calyx campanulate, July–Aug. Fruit indehiscent, many seeded berry, pendulous or erect, borne singly at nodes, very variable in size, shape and color and degree of pungency.

Lore, Legend and Romance: The Spaniards came to the New World looking for the black pepper of Asian origin that they had known in Europe. Instead, they accidentally came upon an even more pungent spice in the multi-colored, variformed pods of **Capsicum** peppers, already cultivated for many centuries by the native Indians in tropical America.

Long before the arrival of the Spaniards, the Mayan Indians of Northern Guatemala used **Capsicum** peppers medicinally, calling them *"ic,"* and taking them internally to cure cramps and diarrhea. Columbus took back fruits to Spain on his first voyage to the New World. The long viability of the seeds and the ease with which they can be transported assisted in the rapid spread in the tropics and subtropics throughout the world after 1492.

By 1650 the cultivation and use of the **Capsicum** peppers as a condiment had spread throughout Europe as well as to the Asian and African tropics. It should be pointed out here that, in the different soils and climates, the **Capsicum** fruits took on modified characteristics—probably through selection by man. After a long period of cultivation in many different environments, much hybridization has taken place. Considerable variation exists among **Capsicums** in growth habit, size, color, shape, flavor pungency, and even in their botanical classification. Linnaeus (1707–1778) described two species of **Capsicum** in 1753, and in 1776 he added two more. By 1832, no less than 25 different spp. of **Capsicum** had been described. Currently some 90 species are known to exist. however, only five distinct and recognizable pure lines of **Capsicum** is cultivated: **Capsicum annuum, Capsicum frutescens, Capsicum chinensis, Capsicum pendulum, Capsicum pubescens.**

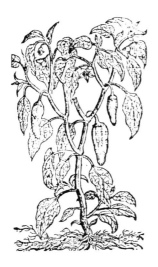

Capsicum annuum

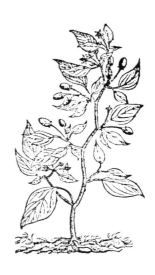

Capsicum chinensis

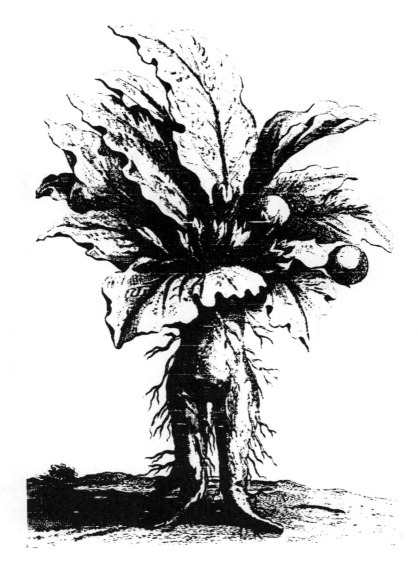

Mandragora officinarum vernalis—Mandrake

DATURA FASTUOSA L.   Solanaceae

Nightshade family

Centers of Diversity: Cosmopolitan in the tropics; the variety alba is recorded from the West Coast of Africa.

Common/Vernacular Names: *English:* Black Datura; *Spanish:* Estramonio; *Africa:* Jila-Andundo (Ghana), Mutumbella (Angola)

Somatic Chromosome Numbers and Genome Constitution: 2n=24

Description: An erect annual plant 1–1.6 m high, with large handsome flowers, white inside, violet outside in the type, all white in the variety alba, less foetid than the leaves. Flowers and fruits in June and July.

Lore, Legend and Romance: In Mexico, **Datura** species were known as *"Ololiuqui,"* an important plant in magico-religious rites, and is still widely used as a divinatory hallucinogen. There was much confusion over the use of this plant as the Indians tried to keep it from the conquistadors, the invading Spaniards.

Another plant indigenous to Mexico and gregarious in Oaxaca, which is worth mentioning in this regard, is **Rivea corymbosa** belonging to the family **Convulvulaceae**. It has also been variously described as *"Ololiuqui."* The seeds of this plant are highly hallucinogénic and it is reported to induce apathy and anergia, together with heightened visual perception and increased hypnogogic phenomena; it promotes an acute awareness combined with alteration of time perception, followed a few hours later by a period of calm, alert euphoria. Hernandez observed that through *"Ololiuqui,* Aztec priests *communed with their gods...to receive a message from them, eating the seeds to induce a delirium when a thousand visions and Satanic hallucinations appeared to them."* Interestingly, the seeds of this plant contain alkaloids allied to the synthetic LSD, lysergic acid diethylamid, some of them identical with the hallucinogenic alkaloids isolated from ergot, a comparatively primitive fungus. Ergot was the fungus from which LSD was first synthesized.

A lot has been written about the magic-religious significance of the **Datura** as a group of higher plants. I would like to quote from William E. Safford's paper on *"Daturas of the Old World and New "* which was presented by S. Henry Wassén, Gothenburg Ethnographical Museum, Sweden, at the 1968 Botanical Museum of the Harvard University-sponsored symposium on **Plants in the Development of Modern Medicine.** *"I have come to get you, but not without a purpose. You were placed as medicine, and it is for medicine that I seek you. Be not humiliated, oh powerful one."*

The above quotation explains how Luiseño Indians in gathering **Datura metaloides** for ceremonial or medicinal purposes were treating the plant *"with great deference."* Before plants are dug up or parts taken from them, the medicine man had to address it in the way they quoted. Such an apologetic preliminary is the universal custom of all medicine men from all cultures the world over. Similar incantations are made by certain Mexican tribes in gathering the narcotic *"peyote,"* and the African witch doctor or medicine man in gathering his herbals; also, these apologies were offered by the European herb gatherers of the Middle Ages in connection with the dreaded *"mandragora."*

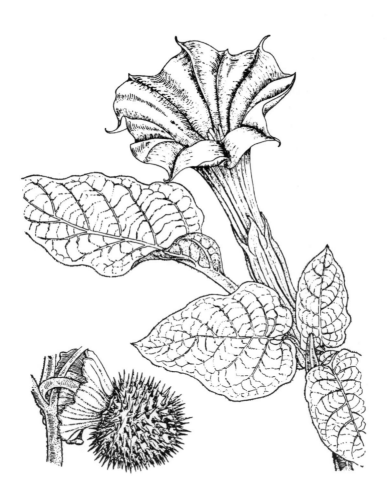

Datura metel

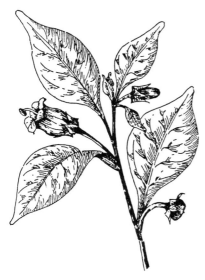

Atropa belladonna

In the Blue Ridge Mountains of North Carolina, I encountered **Datura tatula** L., commonly called Purple Jamestown weed or Purple thorn apple. It was gregarious in disused places and flowering between July and September. The seeds were said to be very poisonous. A decoction was at one time used in leprosy. The leaves and seeds contain atropine, hyoscyamine and hyoscine.

DATURA METEL L. Solanaceae

Nightshade family

Centers of Diversity: Indigenous to India. Cosmopolitan in the Tropics; also in the United States from New England to Florida and westward and in the lower districts of North Carolina and South Carolina.

Common/Vernacular Names: *English:* Guayaquil thorn apple, Downy thorn apple, Egyptian henbane, Hindu datura; *Spanish:* Chamico blanco; *Africa:* Mnanaha, Mranaa (Swahili); *China:* Man-t'o-lo

Somatic Chromosome Numbers and Genome Constitution: 2n=24

Description: A herbaceous plant, stem erect 60–120 cm high, found growing near villages, apparently wild, and on waste grounds by rivers. Cultivated throughout Mexico.

Lore, Legend and Romance: A poison. The seeds and leaves have been found to contain 0.25% and the capsules 0.12% of the total alkaloid in cultivated plants. This medicinal plant is now introduced and naturalized in many parts of the globe. It is often cultivated as an ornamental plant.

CORDIA MILLENII Bak. **Boraginaceae**

Syn. Cordia irvingii Bak. **Borage family**
"Sacred Tree"

Centers of Diversity: Native to Tropical Africa; Ghana to Angola, Congo, Sudan, Uganda and Kenya.

Common/Vernacular Names: *English:* Drum tree; *Africa:* Kyenedua (i.e., *"drum tree"* (Ghana); Omo, Kilbo-eki (Nigeria); Mkamasi, Mkoria (Swahili)

Somatic Chromosome Numbers and Genome Constitution: 2n = 48

Description: A fine spreading tree up to 18 m high; buttressed, foliage dense. Leaves 30 x 25 cm, base rounded to deeply cordate, entire or crenulate; flowers, male and female separate, yellowish, fragrant, Mar.–Aug. Fruits, a drupe, strongly scented, 4 x 2.5 cm, narrowly ellipsoid, in an enlarged, hardened, cup-shaped calyx, Sept.

Lore, Legend and Romance: This plant is employed as a shade tree in African villages and is often regarded as a sacred tree. The close-grained, yellow lustrous wood with brownish heart wood, makes durable household utensils and accessories. It is much used to make drums, including the Ashanti *"talking drums"* and other domestic utensils. The leaves are boiled and the liquid bottled and administered two spoonsful morning and evening for roundworms. A leaf decoction, or the dried leaves are smoked as tobacco, and used in Nigeria for asthma, colds and cough.

Some botanical authorities still continue to use the families **Boraginaceae** and **Ehretiaceae** interchangeably. Zeven and Ahukovsky, 1975, gives **Cordia dodecandra** D.C. as belonging to the family **Ehretiaceae**. This, of course, is the Copte tree of Mexico, a tall tree cultivated for its fruits.

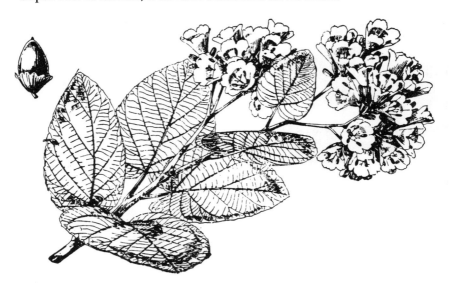

Cordia abyssinica

OCIMUM SANCTUM L. — Labiatae

Mint family

Centers of Diversity: Native to Arabia and Australia. Cultivated throughout India where it is regarded as sacred. Introduced into the Caribbean Basin and Tropical America. In Trinidad, it is often planted in home gardens of people of Indian ancestry. It is an abundant weed in moist areas of Puerto Rico, especially in cultivated fields. It is listed among plants of the world that furnish scented flowers.

Common/Vernacular Names: *English:* Sacred basil, Sweet basil, holy basil; *Spanish:* Albahaca cimarrona, Hole anis, Jerba hole blanco, Yerba hole; *Asia:* Tulsi (Hindi), Manjari, Krishna tulsi (Sanskrit); *Africa:* Mrihani wa kiunguja (Swahili)

Somatic Chromosome Numbers and Genome Constitution: 2n=64

Description: A herbaceous perennial plant 60–90 cm high, much branched, softly hairy. Leaves elliptic-oblong, lanceolate or ovate, pointed or blunt at the apex, downy on both surfaces. Flowers lavender, purple or crimson, 3 mm long in whorls of 3–8, closely set in slender, spike-like racemes 5–14 cm long, sometimes branched. Strongly aromatic.

Lore, Legend and Romance: Known as the mosquito plant, it is so highly esteemed by Indians that every Hindu keeps a plant on his house premises or religious sanctuary. In Hindu tradition this plant is so important that its precious sanctity is regarded as assuring entrance into heaven; and homes where they are grown are reputed to be guarded by the protective spirit of this herb.

Ancient authors proclaim or denounce the virtues of this herb. The very earliest reference, according to the American Herb Society, is where Chrysippus, about 250 B.C. declares that *"Ocimum exists only to drive men insane."*

This plant is so important in infantile ailments that one in India cannot do without it. Leaf juice relieves cold, cough, catarrh, bronchitis, fever, indigestion, grippe, bilious derangement and choked throat, especially among children. Pasted twigs are taken in gonorrhea. Leaf and root brew arrests malarial and other fevers, and increase sexual appetite (aphrodisiac).

This is one of the very popular folk-remedy herbs of Curacao. A leaf decoction with cinnamon is drunk to ease delivery. A decoction, with or without cloves, is a remedy for colds. It is sometimes used as a substitute for betel.

OCIMUM VIRIDE Willd.   Labiatae

"Drive away evil ghosts"   **Mint family**

Centers of Diversity: Senegal to Angola, Zaire and East Africa.

Common/Vernacular Names: *English:* Tea bush, Fever plant of Sierra Leone; *Africa:* Onumum, Suru, Bebusui (Ghana); Efinrin (Nigeria); Arachia (Swahili)

Somatic Chromosome Numbers and Genome Constitution: 2n=40, 48, 64

Description: An erect shrub attaining 2 m with nearly glabrous stems. Leaves ovate or obovate, acuminate, base cuneate or unequal-sided, margins toothed. Flowers paniculate racemes, creamy-white or yellowish, July.

Lore, Legend and Romance: This plant is much used in West African medicine and is often especially grown in compounds and sold in markets as a well-known febrifuge. In many parts of West Africa, it is reputed to drive out evil spirits and demons. It is used in Ashanti for fumigation at birth and to drive away evil spirits. The whole plant may be used as a poultice for rheumatism and lumbago. It is called "mosquito plant" and since it is reputed to keep away mosquitoes, the leaves are sometimes hung around beds for this purpose.

A hot leaf infusion is commonly used, also by some Europeans as a familiar febrifuge and diaphoretic, being taken like tea, with milk and sugar. Sometimes a leaf decoction is drunk, or used in baths, against fever and coughs. The leaves boiled with peppers are drunk in Ghana for fevers. The leaves also have stomachic properties, and is used as such in most African countries where the plant grows.

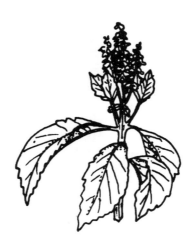

Ocimum viride

ANNONA SENEGALENSIS Pers.   Annonaceae

Syn. Annona chrysophilla Boj.   **Custard-apple family**

Centers of Diversity: Cape Verde Islands to Northern Nigeria and then to South Central Africa.

Common/Vernacular Names: *English:* Wild custard-apple; *Africa:* Saa-borofere, Batanga (Ghana), Abo, Gwandar-daji (Nigeria), Mkonokono mwitu (Swahili), Mense/Chingwa (Zimbabwe)

Somatic Chromosome Numbers and Genome Constitution: $2n = 14$

Description: A prostrating shrub to small tree up to 6 m in height, coppicing readily. Branchlets usually tomentellous; leaves up to 12.5 x 7.5 cm, fragrant, lighter below, closely reticulate, broadly elliptic, glabrous, pubescent when young. Flowers axillary, green turning yellow, generally softly pubescent outside, falling easily, Feb.–April. Fruits almost 5 cm diameter, globose, smooth, yellow when ripe, with outline of carpels on the surface.

Lore, Legend and Romance: The family **Annonaceae**, to which **Annona senegalensis** belongs, is a very large one comprising 120 genera with more than 2000 species, mainly tropical. All are woody plants, mostly trees and shrubs, but some are climbers as well. Roughly half the total number of species is found in Asia, Australia, and Polynesia; one-third is found in America, the rest in tropical Africa. Only two genera are common to both the Old and New Worlds; one of them is **Annona** which lent its name to the entire family, and which, in its turn, is so called after Anon, the Haitian name for *"custard-apple"*— the tasty fruit of **Annona reticulata**. In his endeavor to eliminate *"barbaric"* names, Linnaeus changed anon to the Latin annona, meaning *"fruit of the year."* The custard apple (or Bullock's heart), which is now cultivated in all tropical countries, is the size and shape of a large apple, but tastes of pears and cinnamon. The aromatic and prickly fruit of another West Indian species, **Annona muricata**, known as sour sop, is in great demand.

As with all fruits of **Annona** species, **Annona senegalensis** is edible. The Nankanis of Northern Ghana use the fresh sepals in making soup. The flowers are used elsewhere to flavor local foods. The leaves and roots are sold in Hausa medicine markets. The roots are used for venereal disease and, when powdered, for intestinal disorders and as tonic for horses. The root and bark serve as vermifuge and as an ingredient in a sleeping sickness remedy in Northern Nigeria; it is also used for dysentery and diarrhea in Senegal. In Central Africa the root-bark is used as an antidote to snake-bite. The Tonga tribe of Zambia regards the plant as a good *"war"* medicine, and they administer the root to a suckling child to wean it from its mother's breast, as the plant is supposed to cause forgetfulness. The Shangana have a similar use for the **Annona** root. It is said that it is the duty of the first wife of the chief of a Tonga clan to keep a perpetual fire burning in the sacred hut where the great talisman is housed. This fire is considered a great sacred monument. If by mischance it should die out, the fire has to be relit with the aid of two

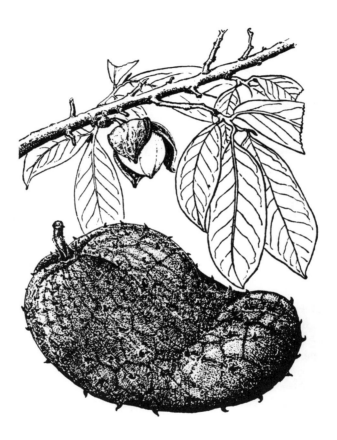

Annona muricata

friction sticks of the **Annona** plant. These are not used for lighting ordinary fires.

The Bemba tribe, also of Zambia, tie amulets of the wood around the neck of their hunting dogs as a charm to protect them from being gored by warthogs.

SECHIUM EDULE (Jacq.) Sw.   Cucurbitaceae

Syn. Chayota edulis Jacq.   **Gourd family**

Centers of Diversity: Indigenous to Central America, Mexico, Venezuela and the West Indies.

Common/Vernacular Names: *Spanish:* Chayote, Chou-chou, Cocombre, Meliton, Tayota, Guisquil, Christophine

Somatic Chromosome Numbers and Genome Constitution: $2n=24$

Description: A quick growing climber attaining 10 m in height, naturalized and extensively cultivated in many warmer parts of the world. Fruit large, green or cream-colored according to the variety, and covered with soft prickles.

Lore, Legend and Romance: This plant comes under the rulership of Venus, the planet of love, beauty, art, music and wealth. In the Santeria religion where the whole plant is used in their initiation, the plant is claimed by the deity, Oshun and it corresponds with Netzach of the Qabalistic Tree of Life.

The plant was common among the Aztecs prior to the conquest. It then spread throughout the tropics.

The fruit is a most wholesome vegetable cooked like squash or pumpkin; it can also be made into tarts with lime. It is sometimes added to soup, or soup made with it, or is eaten boiled, and mashed with oil and pepper; the prickly skin being first removed. In San Francisco, California, the Mexican nationals like to eat the fruit; these are sold in supermarkets in the South City frequented by them.

The Gourd family comprises some 850 species in 100 genera. By far the largest number is found in the tropics and sub-tropics—only a few extend into the temperate zone.

Some genera of the family of tropical African origin must have reached southern Asia a very long time ago. It was known to the ancient Greeks and Romans, and is mentioned in Charlemagne's *"Capitulare de villis"* (A.D. 800), by St. Hildegard (c. 1150) and Albertus Magnus (c. 1250).

Lagenaria siceraria (Molina) Standl. with a synonym of **Lagenaria vulgaris** Ser., also a member of the family **Cucurbitaceae** is an interesting species worth mentioning. The plant was known in antiquity as *"kolokynthis"* by the Greeks and as *"cucurbita"* by the Romans. It has a white flower with petals that are free right down to the base. The fruits may be spherical, elongated, and pear or bottle shaped. The woody shell is used throughout the tropics as a water bottle; the small bottle-shaped types can, moreover, be cut in half and are often fashioned into spoons.

The bottle gourd with a chromosome constitution of $2n=22$, grows wild not only in the Old World but also in the New. It was formerly thought that it was introduced to America by Europeans, but recent various vessels and tools made of bottle gourds have been discovered among pre-Inca remains in Peru going back to the fourth millenium B.C. and also among later remains (second and first millenium B.C.) in Mexico and southern North America. In other words, the bottle gourd was known in America long before the arrival of Columbus. All the same, it is likely to have originated in the Old World since in Africa, it grows wild in places far from any human habitation past or present.

American botanists, who floated a bottle gourd in sea water for 224 days under normal oceanic conditions, found that germinating power of its seeds remained unimpaired. This suggests that the fruits may have reached America across the Atlantic without any human assistance.

It should be pointed out that a number of species indigenous to Africa have also been found growing in the Americas on the same latitude. The author has encountered numerous such species, the chief two West African species that come to mind are the **Abrus precatorius** and **Caesalpinia bunduc** complex of Southern Florida.

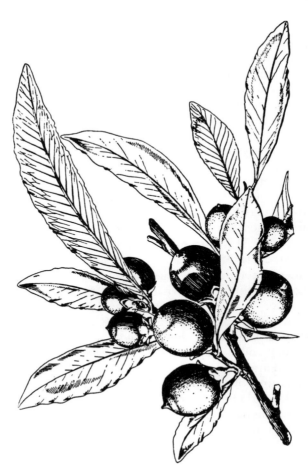

Diospyros mespiliformis

DIOSPYROS MONBUTTENSIS Gurke   Ebenaceae

Ebony family

Centers of Diversity: Ivory Coast to Cameroons and then to Zaire and Sudan.

Common/Vernacular Names: *English:* Ebony, Yoruba Ebony, Walking-stick ebony; *Africa:* Akyirinian, Ada piri (Ghana), Ogan-pupa, Okahimi, Okpu-ocha (Nigeria), Mpingo (Swahili)

Somatic Chromosome Numbers and Genome Constitution: $2n = 30$

Description: A small tree reaching 9 m in height and 60 cm in girth, rarely growing straight. Leaves obovate 15 x 7.5 cm, base long-cuneate, with 6–8 pairs of lateral nerves. Flowers greenish-yellow or creamy white, fragrant, calyx cynlindrical, March. Fruits, 3.7 x 1.2 cm, ovoid, calyx persistent, 8-seeded, velvety on both sides, June–Sept.

Lore, Legend and Romance: Diospyros spp. yields the famous brown-black, striped and jet black timber with the characteristic hard, dark black heart wood. The wood is much sought after the world over for its uses in carvings, the type **Diospyros sanzamanika** commanding high market prices.

The timber of **Diospyros monbuttensis** is yellowish-white, hard, dense and durable, and used for both household and light industrial purposes. The wood is also famous in the making of walking sticks.

A decoction of the bark and leaf-tips, with those of **Cassia occidentalis** and **Lippia adoensis** is drunk and used in bathing as an Ivory Coast leprosy remedy (Kerharo and Bouquet). The fruits are used medicinally in Nigeria.

In the Caribbean basin, where **Cassia occidentalis** forms the basic ingredient of the sacred *"Omiero"* of the Santeria religion, **Diospyros monbuttensis** is a highly sought plant where it is mixed with at least six of the *"Twenty-one Sacred Plants,"* is used in spiritual baths and is said to calm a tormented spirit.

Another interesting bit of legend about the ebony was their uses in the New World. The Africans who were brought to the Eastern Seaboard of the United States settling around Virginia and the Carolinas found a native species of the ebony, **Diospyros virginiana** L. which they recognized as a substitute for the African species, **Diospyros monbuttensis** Gurke. This American species, commonly called persimmon, played an important role in the food and medicine of the slaves. Because of the presence of tannins in the bark, it was used for diarrhea, dysentery, uterine hemorrhages and as a bitter tonic. The inner bark being very astringent, it was useful in sore throats and fevers. The Africans used to chew on the sticks of the bark, which enabled them to work in the fields for long periods of time without water.

The fruits were an important nutrient for the people. The ripe fruits were eaten and were used in the preparation of beer and brandy; these preparations were subastringent and nutrient, antiseptic and anthelmintic. The unripe fruit with alum was used for ulcerated sore throat.

234

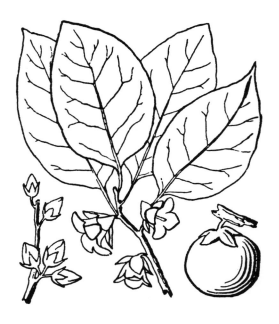

Diospyros virginiana

It is also interesting to note that the largest Black publishing company in the United States today, the Johnson Publishing Company of Chicago, Illinois, has named its two major publications after this family of trees; *"Ebony,"* a monthly magazine, is perhaps the largest circulated magazine in the world which originates in Black America. Another publication, *"Jet,"* is most important to the Black communities in America, for it gives a weekly digest of news of interest to the community, news which is ignored or adulterated by the major press syndicate, but which provides a significant link within the Black population of the United States. The word *"jet"* describes the heart wood of the ebony, deep black, or jet black. The native **Diospyros** of the United States, like these magazines, played an important role in the lives of the captive Africans, as do these publications which are sometimes *"life-savers"* for the present population of African descendants in America.

Tree of Life as depicted by several ancient religions

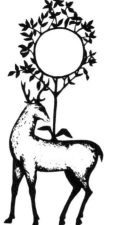

Japanese "Tree of Life" (circa 700 A.D.) from the Kusuga Mandara in Nara

Chinese version of the *"The Tree of Life."*

Han dynasty, circa 200 B.C.

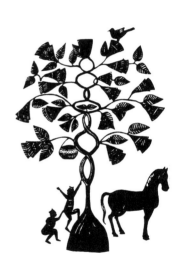

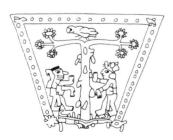

Aztec *"Tree of Life"* from a stone relief, Mexico

"And he shewed me a pure river of water of life, clear as crystal, proceeding out of the throne of God and of the Lamb. In the midst of the street of it, and on either side of the river, was there the TREE OF LIFE, which bare twelve manner of fruits, and yielded her fruit every month: and the leaves of the tree were for the healing of the nations. And there shall be no more curse: but the throne of God and of the Lamb shall be in it; and his servants shall serve him."

REVELATION 22: 1–4

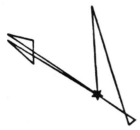

THE NORTH SCALE INSTITUTE
Education and Research Group

2205 TARAVAL   SAN FRANCISCO, CA 94116   (415) 759-9491

The North Scale Institute is dedicated to the preserva ion of the knowledge and wisdom of the ancient cultures throughout the world. In particular, this education and research group is concerned with two aspects of this ancient wisdom — Ethno-botany and Traditional Medicine.

ETHNO-BOTANY — This is a branch of plant science which studies the relationship between a people of a particular culture and the use these people make of the plants and herbs which grow around them. Not only does this study include the exact science of botany, it also embraces the anthropology, astronomy, history, lore, legend, romance, medicinal and spiritual practices of these peoples. These beliefs and practices have survived till today as a subconscious memory, even in the most advanced technological societies.

TRADITIONAL MEDICINE —The art and science of healing the sick has been an important part of all civilizations as long as mankind has walked the face of the earth. The "medicine men" have always held an esteemed position in all cultures. They have been the most important human factor in the survival of the people, as they have provided a cure for the diseases of the body, mind and spirit of their constituents. The "medicine man" of the American Indians, the "witch doctors" of Africa, the "shaman" of the indigenous people of the Americas, the "aryvedic doctors" of India, the "barefoot doctors" of China, the "herbalists" of Europe have preserved the ancient secrets of healing for thousands of years. All the independent thinkers of the world know deep within their hearts that this knowledge and wisdom is a precious truth. THE NORTH SCALE INSTITUTE IS DEDICATED TO THE PRESERVATION OF THIS TRUTH.

PRACTICAL WORK SHEET FOR PLANT STUDY II

MONOCOTYLEDON	DICOTYLEDON
1.	1.
2.	2.
3.	3.
4.	4.
5.	5.

PRACTICAL WORK SHEET FOR PLANT STUDY III
DISTINGUISHING FEATURES BETWEEN PLANTS & ANIMALS

1.	1.
2.	2.
3.	3.
4.	4.
5.	5.

PRACTICAL WORK SHEET IV
CLASSIFICATION OF PLANTS

DIVISION

I. Thallophyta

1. _____ _____

2. _____ _____

3. _____ _____

II. Bryophyta

1. _____ _____

2. _____ _____

III. Pteridophyta

1. _____ _____

2. _____ _____

3. _____ _____

IV. Gymnosperms

1. _____ _____

2. _____ _____

3. _____ _____

4. _____ _____

V. Angiosperms

1. _____ _____

2. _____ _____

PRACTICAL WORK SHEET FOR PLANT STUDY V

Botanical Name	Common/ Vernacular Name	Family	Origin/ Habit	Locality	Uses	Culture	Date
1.							
2.							
3.							
4.							
5.							
6.							
7.							
8.							
9.							
10.							
11.							
12.							
13.							
14.							
15.							
16.							
17.							
18.							
19.							
20.							
21.							
22.							
23.							
24.							
25.							

LEGEND: Trees (T)   Shrubs (S)   Herbs (H)   Climbers (C)

U.S. Measure and Metric Measure Conversion Chart
Formulas for Exact Measures

Length

Symbol:	When You Know:	Multiply by:	To Find:	Rounded Measures for Quick Reference:
in.	inches	2.54	centimeters	⅜ in. = 1 cm
ft	feet	30.48	centimeters	1 in. = 2.5 cm
yd	yards	0.9144	meters	2 in. = 5 cm
mi	miles	1.609	kilometers	2½ in. = 6.5 cm
km	kilometers	0.621	miles	12 in. (1 ft.) = 30 cm
m	meters	1.094	yards	1 yd. = 90 cm
cm	centimeters	0.39	inches	100 ft = 30 m
				1 mi = 1.6 km

Botanical Illustrations
Glossaries
Index

Botanical Illustrations

[After Lloyd, 1949]

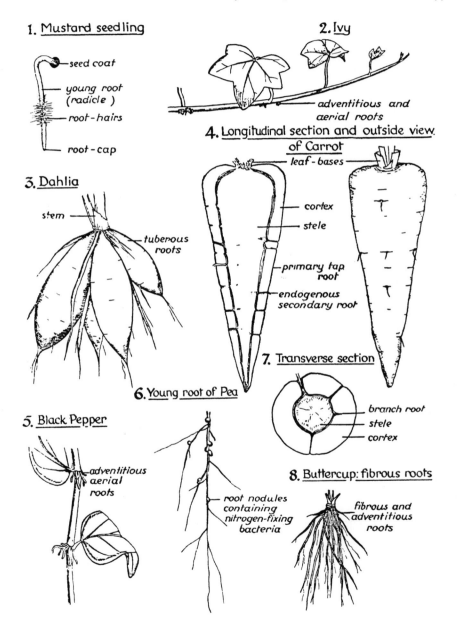

1. Mustard seedling
- seed coat
- young root (radicle)
- root-hairs
- root-cap

2. Ivy
adventitious and aerial roots

3. Dahlia
stem
tuberous roots

4. Longitudinal section and outside view of Carrot
- leaf-bases
- cortex
- stele
- primary tap root
- endogenous secondary root

5. Black Pepper
adventitious aerial roots

6. Young root of Pea
root nodules containing nitrogen-fixing bacteria

7. Transverse section
- branch root
- stele
- cortex

8. Buttercup: fibrous roots
fibrous and adventitious roots

ROOTS

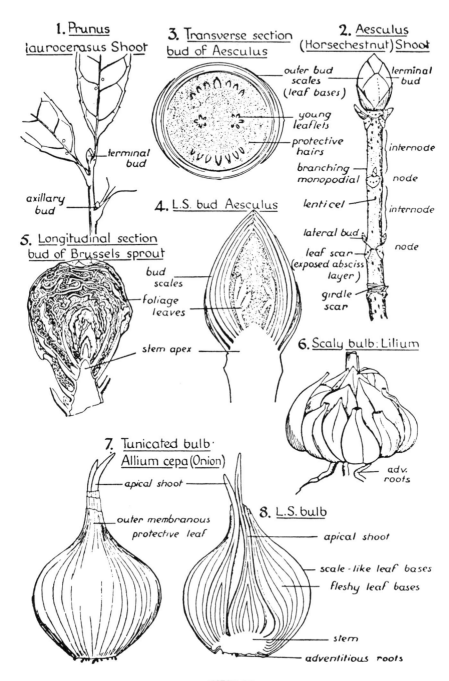

1. Prunus laurocerasus Shoot
terminal bud
axillary bud

3. Transverse section bud of Aesculus
outer bud scales (leaf bases)
young leaflets
protective hairs

2. Aesculus (Horsechestnut) Shoot
terminal bud
internode
branching monopodial
node
lenticel
internode
lateral bud
leaf scar (exposed absciss layer)
node
girdle scar

4. L.S. bud Aesculus

5. Longitudinal section bud of Brussels sprout
bud scales
foliage leaves
stem apex

6. Scaly bulb: Lilium
adv. roots

7. Tunicated bulb. Allium cepa (Onion)
apical shoot
outer membranous protective leaf

8. L.S. bulb
apical shoot
scale-like leaf bases
fleshy leaf bases
stem
adventitious roots

STEMS

Botanical Illustrations

[After Lloyd, 1949]

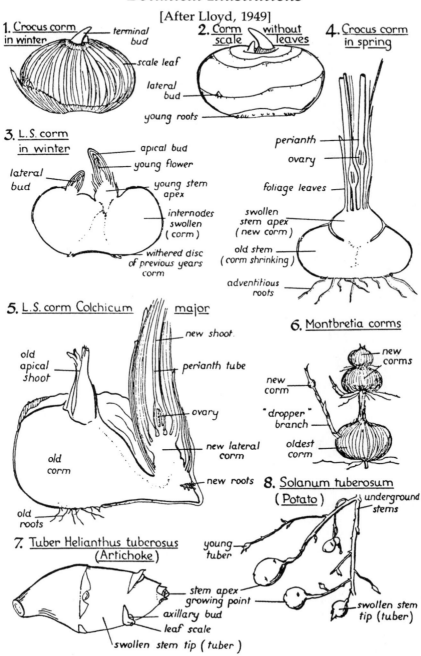

1. Crocus corm in winter — terminal bud, scale leaf, lateral bud, young roots

2. Corm scale without leaves

4. Crocus corm in spring — perianth, ovary, foliage leaves, swollen stem apex (new corm), old stem (corm shrinking), adventitious roots

3. L.S. corm in winter — apical bud, young flower, lateral bud, young stem apex, internodes swollen (corm), withered disc of previous years corm

5. L.S. corm Colchicum major — new shoot, old apical shoot, perianth tube, ovary, new lateral corm, old corm, new roots, old roots

6. Montbretia corms — new corms, new corm, "dropper" branch, oldest corm

7. Tuber Helianthus tuberosus (Artichoke) — stem apex growing point, axillary bud, leaf scale, swollen stem tip (tuber)

8. Solanum tuberosum (Potato) — underground stems, young tuber, swollen stem tip (tuber)

STEMS—Continued

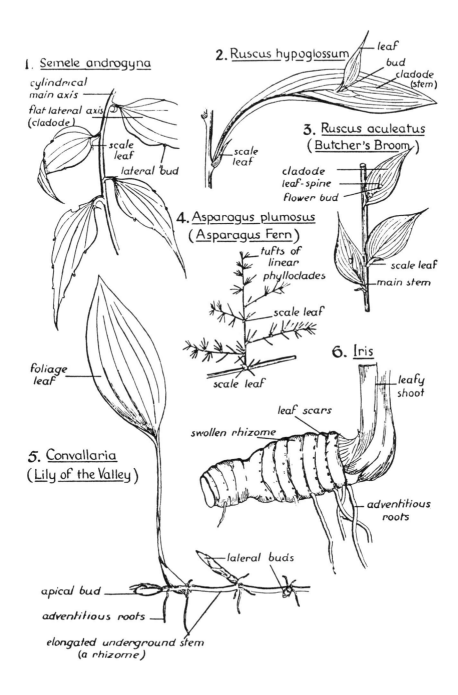

1. Semele androgyna
- cylindrical main axis
- flat lateral axis (cladode)
- scale leaf
- lateral bud
- foliage leaf

2. Ruscus hypoglossum
- leaf
- bud
- cladode (stem)
- scale leaf

3. Ruscus aculeatus (Butcher's Broom)
- cladode
- leaf-spine
- flower bud
- scale leaf
- main stem

4. Asparagus plumosus (Asparagus Fern)
- tufts of linear phylloclades
- scale leaf
- scale leaf

5. Convallaria (Lily of the Valley)
- foliage leaf
- lateral buds
- apical bud
- adventitious roots
- elongated underground stem (a rhizome)

6. Iris
- leafy shoot
- leaf scars
- swollen rhizome
- adventitious roots

STEMS—Continued

Botanical Illustrations

[After Lloyd, 1949]

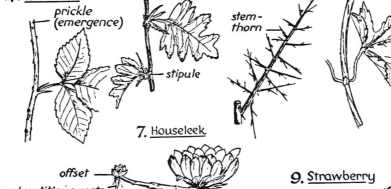

1. Passiflora

2. Virginian Creeper

3. Hop

stipules
tendril

twining stem

5. Hawthorn

suction disc

stem-thorn

6. Whin (Gorse.)

4. Bramble

prickle
(emergence)

stem-
thorn

stipule

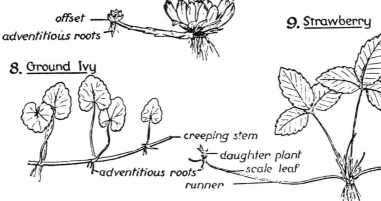

7. Houseleek

offset
adventitious roots

9. Strawberry

8. Ground Ivy

creeping stem

daughter plant
scale leaf

adventitious roots
runner

STEMS—Continued

1. <u>Diagram showing tissue arrangement as seen in transverse section</u>
<u>Vanilla planifolia (climber)</u>

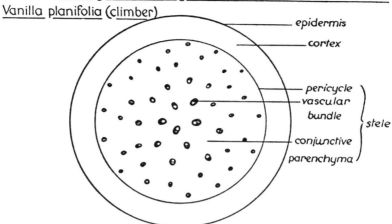

- epidermis
- cortex
- pericycle ⎫
- vascular bundle ⎬ stele
- conjunctive parenchyma ⎭

2. <u>T.S. single V.B</u>
$\frac{1}{60}$ mm.

0·1   0·2   0·3   0·4   0·5   mm.

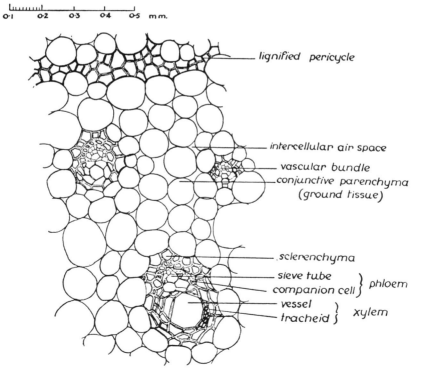

- lignified pericycle

- intercellular air space

- vascular bundle
- conjunctive parenchyma (ground tissue)

- sclerenchyma
- sieve tube ⎫ phloem
- companion cell ⎬
- vessel ⎫ xylem
- tracheid ⎬

MONOCOTYLEDONOUS STEM : VANILLA

248

Botanical Illustrations

[After Lloyd, 1949]

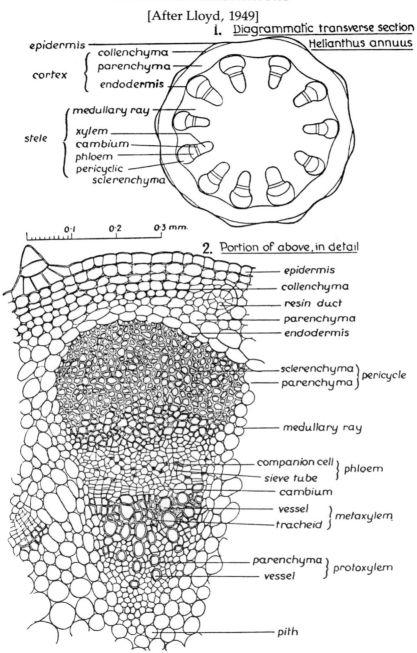

1. Diagrammatic transverse section
Helianthus annuus

epidermis
cortex {
collenchyma
parenchyma
endodermis
}

stele {
medullary ray
xylem
cambium
phloem
pericyclic
sclerenchyma
}

0·1   0·2   0·3 mm.

2. Portion of above, in detail

epidermis
collenchyma
resin duct
parenchyma
endodermis

sclerenchyma } pericycle
parenchyma }

medullary ray

companion cell } phloem
sieve tube }
cambium
vessel } metaxylem
tracheid }

parenchyma } protoxylem
vessel }

pith

YOUNG DICOTYLEDONOUS STEM: HELIANTHUS

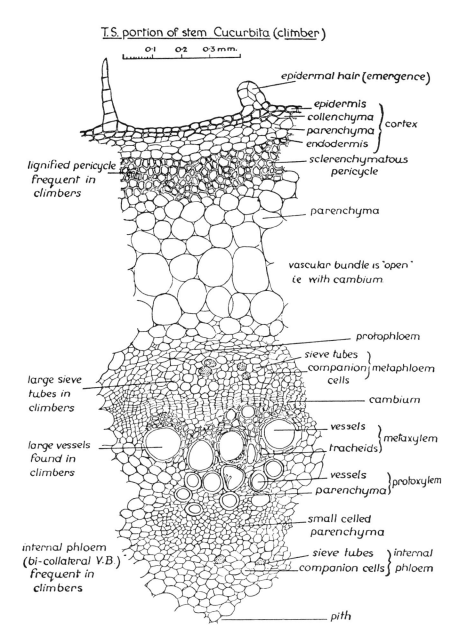

T.S. portion of stem Cucurbita (climber)

0·1   0·2   0·3 mm.

epidermal hair (emergence)

epidermis
collenchyma
parenchyma } cortex
endodermis

lignified pericycle
frequent in
climbers

sclerenchymatous
pericycle

parenchyma

vascular bundle is "open"
ie with cambium.

protophloem

sieve tubes
companion | metaphloem
cells

large sieve
tubes in
climbers

cambium

large vessels
found in
climbers

vessels
tracheids } metaxylem

vessels
parenchyma } protoxylem

small celled
parenchyma

internal phloem
(bi-collateral V.B.)
frequent in
climbers

sieve tubes
companion cells } internal
phloem

pith

CLIMBING STEM : CUCURBITA

Botanical Illustrations

[After Lloyd, 1949]

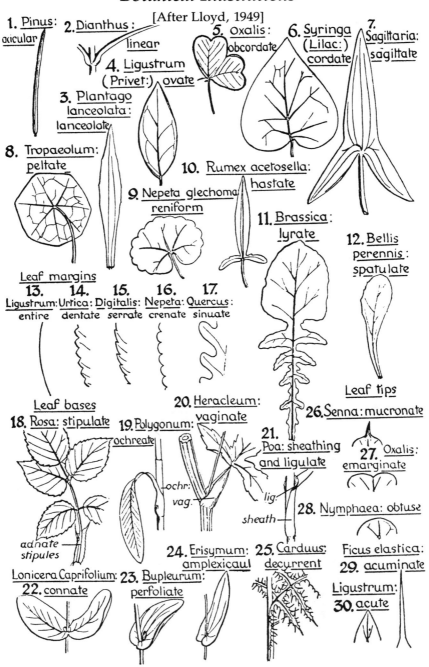

1. Pinus: acicular
2. Dianthus: linear
3. Plantago lanceolata: lanceolate
4. Ligustrum (Privet:) ovate
5. Oxalis: obcordate
6. Syringa (Lilac:) cordate
7. Sagittaria: sagittate
8. Tropaeolum: peltate
9. Nepeta glechoma: reniform
10. Rumex acetosella: hastate
11. Brassica: lyrate
12. Bellis perennis: spatulate

Leaf margins

13. Ligustrum: entire
14. Urtica: dentate
15. Digitalis: serrate
16. Nepeta: crenate
17. Quercus: sinuate

Leaf bases

18. Rosa: stipulate — adnate stipules
19. Polygonum: ochreate — ochr:
20. Heracleum: vaginate
21. Poa: sheathing and ligulate — vag. lig. sheath
22. Lonicera Caprifolium: connate
23. Bupleurum: perfoliate
24. Erisymum: amplexicaul
25. Carduus: decurrent

Leaf tips

26. Senna: mucronate
27. Oxalis: emarginate
28. Nymphaea: obtuse
29. Ficus elastica: acuminate
30. Ligustrum: acute

LEAVES

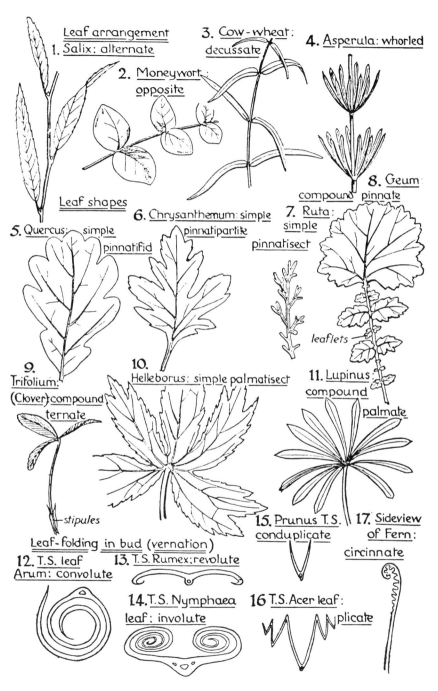

Leaf arrangement
1. Salix: alternate
2. Moneywort: opposite
3. Cow-wheat: decussate
4. Asperula: whorled

Leaf shapes
5. Quercus: simple pinnatifid
6. Chrysanthemum: simple pinnatipartite
7. Ruta: simple pinnatisect
8. Geum: compound pinnate

leaflets

9. Trifolium: (Clover) compound ternate
10. Helleborus: simple palmatisect
11. Lupinus: compound palmate

stipules

Leaf-folding in bud (vernation)
12. T.S. leaf Arum: convolute
13. T.S. Rumex: revolute
14. T.S. Nymphaea leaf: involute
15. Prunus T.S. conduplicate
16. T.S. Acer leaf: plicate
17. Sideview of Fern: circinnate

LEAVES—Continued

Botanical Illustrations

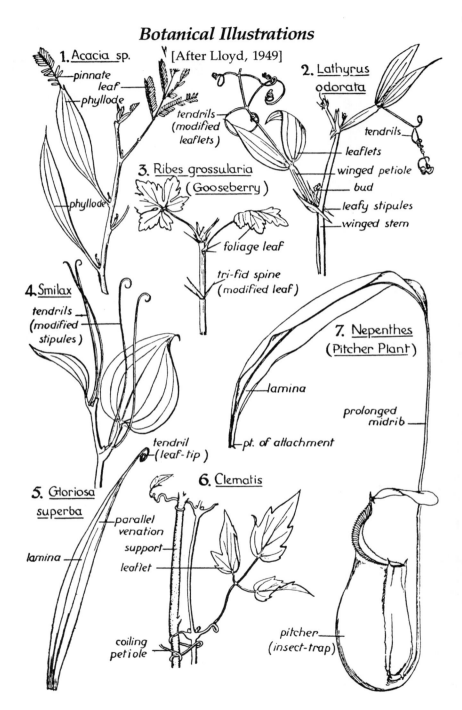

[After Lloyd, 1949]

1. Acacia sp.
pinnate leaf
phyllode
phyllode
phyllode

tendrils (modified leaflets)

2. Lathyrus odorata
tendrils
leaflets
winged petiole
bud
leafy stipules
winged stem

3. Ribes grossularia (Gooseberry)
foliage leaf
tri-fid spine (modified leaf)

4. Smilax
tendrils (modified stipules)

7. Nepenthes (Pitcher Plant)
lamina
prolonged midrib
pt. of attachment

tendril (leaf-tip)

5. Gloriosa superba
parallel venation
support
leaflet
lamina

6. Clematis

coiling petiole

pitcher (insect-trap)

LEAVES—Continued

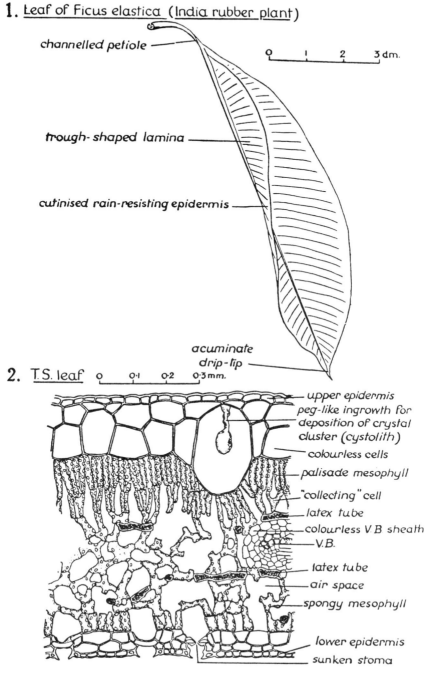

1. Leaf of Ficus elastica (India rubber plant)

channelled petiole

0   1   2   3 dm.

trough-shaped lamina

cutinised rain-resisting epidermis

acuminate
drip-tip

2. T.S. leaf   0   0·1   0·2   0·3 mm.

upper epidermis
peg-like ingrowth for
deposition of crystal
cluster (cystolith)
colourless cells
palisade mesophyll
"collecting" cell
latex tube
colourless V.B sheath
V.B.
latex tube
air space
spongy mesophyll
lower epidermis
sunken stoma

DICOTYLEDONOUS LEAF : FICUS

Botanical Illustrations
[After Lloyd, 1949]

1. <u>Diagrammatic T.S. Iris leaf</u>

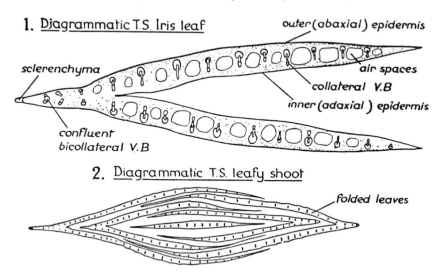

2. <u>Diagrammatic T.S. leafy shoot</u>

3. <u>V.S. leaf through V.B.</u>

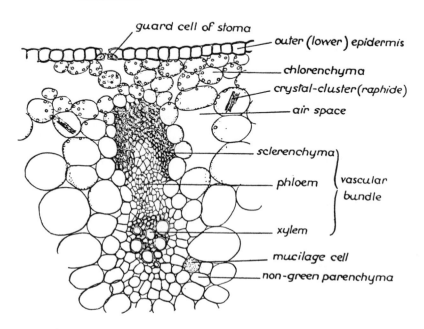

MONOCOTYLEDONOUS LEAF : IRIS

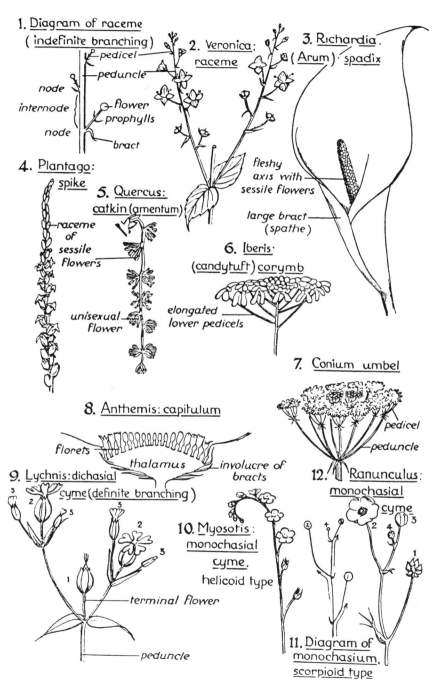

1. Diagram of raceme
   (indefinite branching)
   ̲pedicel̲
   ̲peduncle̲
   node
   internode
   ̲flower̲
   ̲prophylls̲
   node
   ̲bract̲

2. Veronica:
   raceme

3. Richardia.
   (Arum)· spadix

fleshy
axis with
sessile flowers

large bract
   (spathe)

4. Plantago:
   spike

5. Quercus:
   catkin(amentum)

̲raceme̲
of
sessile
flowers

unisexual
flower

6. Iberis·
   (candytuft) corymb

elongated
lower pedicels

7. Conium umbel

pedicel
peduncle

8. Anthemis: capitulum

florets
thalamus
involucre of
bracts

9. Lychnis: dichasial
   cyme (definite branching)

12. Ranunculus:
    monochasial
    cyme

10. Myosotis:
    monochasial
    cyme.
    helicoid type

terminal flower

peduncle

11. Diagram of
    monochasium.
    scorpioid type

INFLORESCENCES

Botanical Illustrations

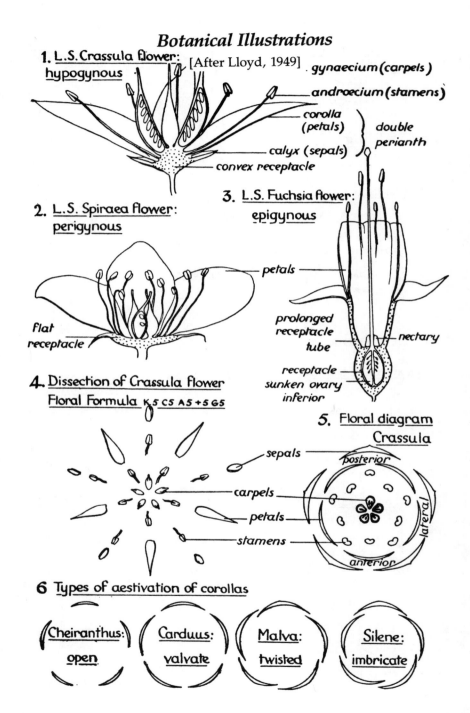

1. L.S. Crassula flower: hypogynous · [After Lloyd, 1949] · gynaecium (carpels)

androecium (stamens)

corolla (petals)

double perianth

calyx (sepals)

convex receptacle

2. L.S. Spiraea flower: perigynous

3. L.S. Fuchsia flower: epigynous

petals

flat receptacle

prolonged receptacle tube

nectary

receptacle

sunken ovary inferior

4. Dissection of Crassula flower

Floral Formula K 5 C5 A5 +5 G5

5. Floral diagram Crassula

sepals

carpels

petals

stamens

posterior

lateral

anterior

6 Types of aestivation of corollas

Cheiranthus: open

Carduus: valvate

Malva: twisted

Silene: imbricate

THE FLOWER

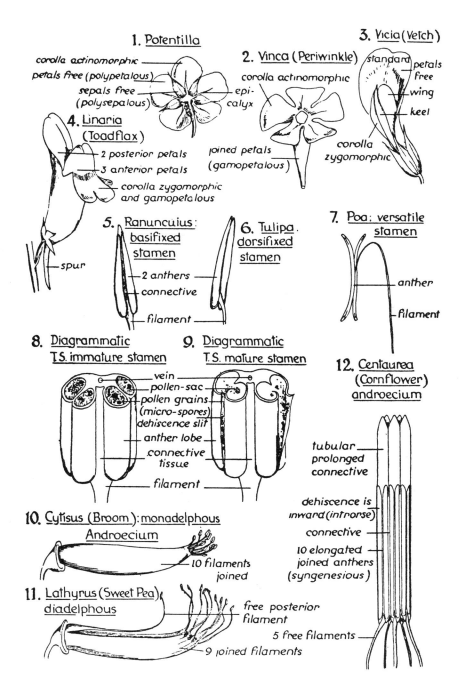

1. Potentilla
corolla actinomorphic
petals free (polypetalous)
sepals free (polysepalous)
epi-calyx

2. Vinca (Periwinkle)
corolla actinomorphic
joined petals (gamopetalous)

3. Vicia (Vetch)
standard
petals free
wing
keel
corolla zygomorphic

4. Linaria (Toadflax)
2 posterior petals
3 anterior petals
corolla zygomorphic and gamopetalous
spur

5. Ranunculus: basifixed stamen
2 anthers
connective
filament

6. Tulipa. dorsifixed stamen

7. Poa: versatile stamen
anther
filament

8. Diagrammatic T.S. immature stamen

9. Diagrammatic T.S. mature stamen
vein
pollen-sac
pollen grains (micro-spores)
dehiscence slit
anther lobe
connective tissue
filament

10. Cytisus (Broom): monadelphous Androecium
10 filaments joined

11. Lathyrus (Sweet Pea) diadelphous
free posterior filament
5 free filaments
9 joined filaments

12. Centaurea (Cornflower) androecium
tubular prolonged connective
dehiscence is inward (introrse)
connective
10 elongated joined anthers (syngenesious)

PERIANTH AND ANDRŒCIUM

Botanical Illustrations

[After Lloyd, 1949]

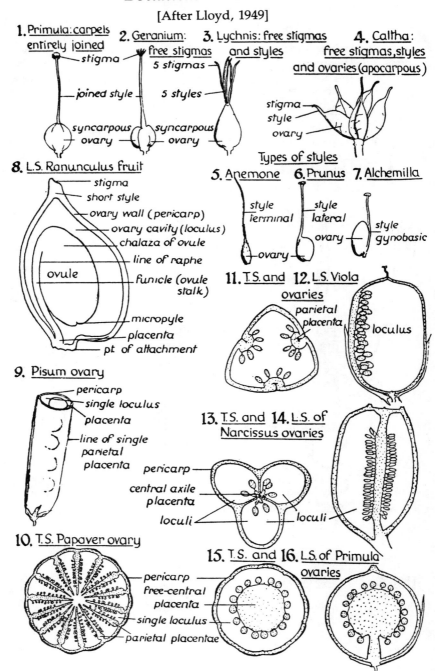

1. Primula: carpels entirely joined
   - stigma
   - joined style
   - syncarpous ovary

2. Geranium: free stigmas
   - 5 stigmas
   - 5 styles
   - syncarpous ovary

3. Lychnis: free stigmas and styles

4. Caltha: free stigmas, styles and ovaries (apocarpous)
   - stigma
   - style
   - ovary

Types of styles

8. L.S. Ranunculus fruit
   - stigma
   - short style
   - ovary wall (pericarp)
   - ovary cavity (loculus)
   - chalaza of ovule
   - line of raphe
   - ovule
   - funicle (ovule stalk)
   - micropyle
   - placenta
   - pt. of attachment

5. Anemone
   - style terminal
   - ovary

6. Prunus
   - style lateral
   - ovary

7. Alchemilla
   - style gynobasic

11. T.S. and 12. L.S. Viola ovaries
   - parietal placenta
   - loculus

9. Pisum ovary
   - pericarp
   - single loculus
   - placenta
   - line of single parietal placenta

13. T.S. and 14. L.S. of Narcissus ovaries
   - pericarp
   - central axile placenta
   - loculi

10. T.S. Papaver ovary
   - pericarp
   - free-central placenta
   - single loculus
   - parietal placentae

15. T.S. and 16. L.S. of Primula ovaries

GYNÆCIUM

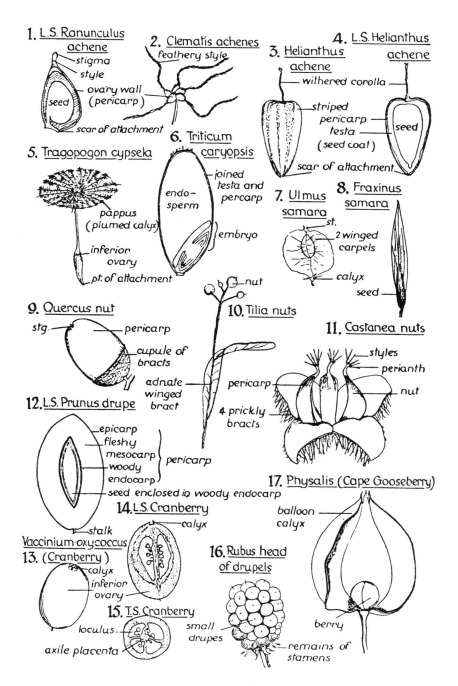

1. L.S. Ranunculus achene
- stigma
- style
- ovary wall (pericarp)
- seed
- scar of attachment

2. Clematis achenes
feathery style

3. Helianthus achene
- withered corolla
- striped pericarp
- testa (seed coat)
- scar of attachment

4. L.S. Helianthus achene
- seed

5. Tragopogon cypsela
- pappus (plumed calyx)
- inferior ovary
- pt. of attachment

6. Triticum caryopsis
- joined testa and percarp
- endosperm
- embryo

7. Ulmus samara
- st.
- 2 winged carpels
- calyx

8. Fraxinus samara
- seed

9. Quercus nut
- stg.
- pericarp
- cupule of bracts

10. Tilia nuts
- nut
- adnate winged bract
- pericarp
- 4 prickly bracts

11. Castanea nuts
- styles
- perianth
- nut

12. L.S. Prunus drupe
- epicarp
- fleshy mesocarp
- woody endocarp
- pericarp
- seed enclosed in woody endocarp
- stalk

Vaccinium oxycoccus
13. (Cranberry)
- calyx
- inferior ovary

14. L.S. Cranberry
- calyx

15. T.S. Cranberry
- loculus
- axile placenta

16. Rubus head of drupels
- small drupes

17. Physalis (Cape Gooseberry)
- balloon calyx
- berry
- remains of stamens

FRUITS

Botanical Illustrations

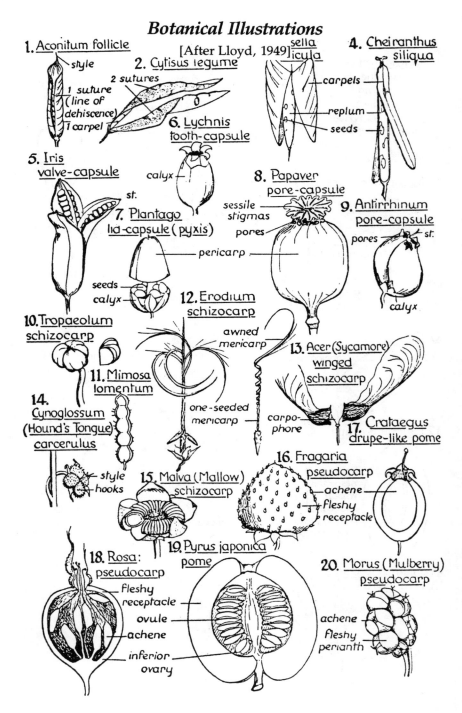

[After Lloyd, 1949]

1. Aconitum follicle
   - style
   - 1 suture (line of dehiscence)
   - 1 carpel

2. Cytisus legume
   - 2 sutures

4. Cheiranthus siliqua
   - sella icula
   - carpels
   - replum
   - seeds

6. Lychnis tooth-capsule
   - calyx

5. Iris valve-capsule
   - st.

8. Papaver pore-capsule
   - sessile stigmas
   - pores

9. Antirrhinum pore-capsule
   - pores
   - st.
   - calyx

7. Plantago lid-capsule (pyxis)
   - pericarp
   - seeds
   - calyx

12. Erodium schizocarp
   - awned mericarp

10. Tropaeolum schizocarp
   - one-seeded mericarp

13. Acer (Sycamore) winged schizocarp
   - carpo-phore

11. Mimosa lomentum

14. Cynoglossum (Hound's Tongue) carcerulus
   - style
   - hooks

15. Malva (Mallow) schizocarp

17. Crataegus drupe-like pome

16. Fragaria pseudocarp
   - achene
   - fleshy receptacle

18. Rosa: pseudocarp
   - fleshy receptacle
   - ovule
   - achene
   - inferior ovary

19. Pyrus japonica pome

20. Morus (Mulberry) pseudocarp
   - achene
   - fleshy perianth

FRUITS—Continued

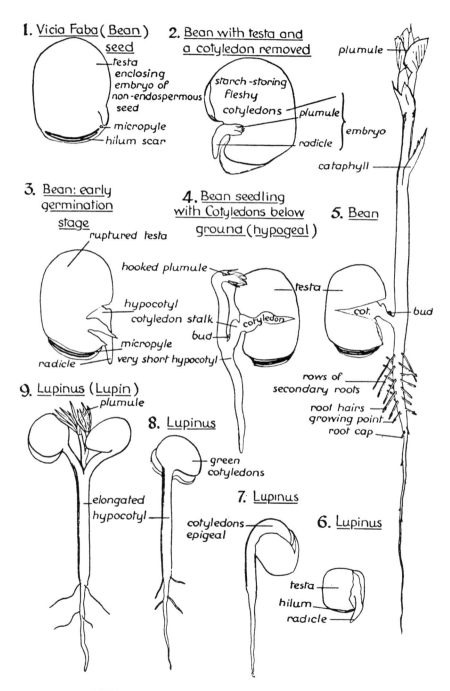

1. <u>Vicia Faba (Bean)</u>
   <u>seed</u>
   — testa
   enclosing
   embryo of
   non-endospermous
   seed
   — micropyle
   — hilum scar

2. <u>Bean with testa and</u>
   <u>a cotyledon removed</u>
   starch-storing
   fleshy
   cotyledons
   plumule
   radicle
   } embryo

plumule
cataphyll

3. <u>Bean: early</u>
   <u>germination</u>
   <u>stage</u>
   ruptured testa
   hypocotyl
   cotyledon stalk
   micropyle
   radicle
   very short hypocotyl

4. <u>Bean seedling</u>
   <u>with Cotyledons below</u>
   <u>ground (hypogeal)</u>
   hooked plumule
   testa
   cotyledon
   bud

5. <u>Bean</u>
   cot.
   bud

rows of
secondary roots
root hairs
growing point
root cap

9. <u>Lupinus (Lupin)</u>
   plumule
   elongated
   hypocotyl

8. <u>Lupinus</u>
   green
   cotyledons

7. <u>Lupinus</u>
   cotyledons
   epigeal

6. <u>Lupinus</u>
   testa
   hilum
   radicle

SEEDS AND SEEDLINGS—Continued

Botanical Illustrations

[After Lloyd, 1949]

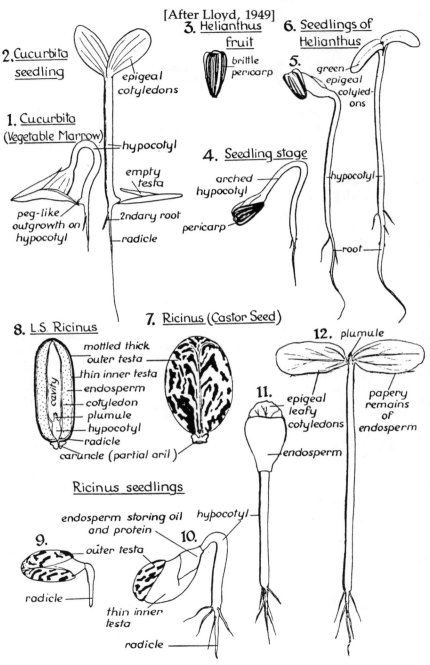

2. Cucurbita seedling

epigeal cotyledons

1. Cucurbita (Vegetable Marrow)

hypocotyl

empty testa

peg-like outgrowth on hypocotyl

2ndary root

radicle

3. Helianthus fruit

brittle pericarp

4. Seedling stage

arched hypocotyl

pericarp

6. Seedlings of Helianthus

5.

green epigeal cotyledons

hypocotyl

root

8. L.S. Ricinus

mottled thick outer testa

thin inner testa

endosperm

cotyledon

plumule

hypocotyl

radicle

caruncle (partial aril)

cavity

7. Ricinus (Castor Seed)

12. plumule

11.

epigeal leafy cotyledons

endosperm

papery remains of endosperm

Ricinus seedlings

endosperm storing oil and protein

hypocotyl

9.

outer testa

radicle

10.

thin inner testa

radicle

SEEDS AND SEEDLINGS—*Continued*

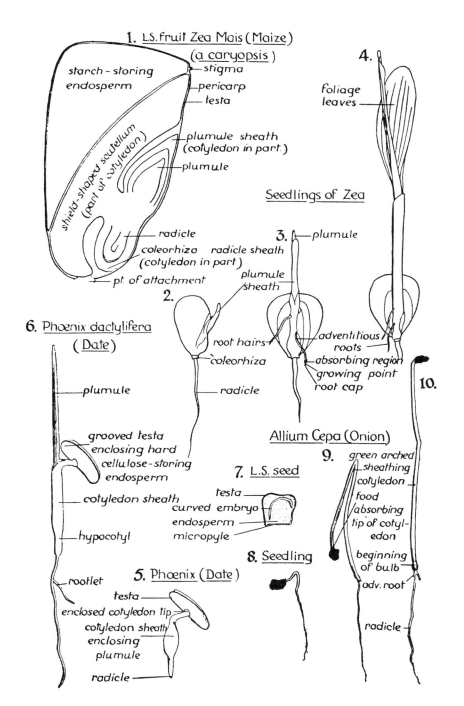

1. L.S. fruit Zea Mais (Maize)
(a caryopsis)

starch-storing endosperm

— stigma
— pericarp
— testa

shield-shaped scutellum (part of cotyledon)

— plumule sheath (cotyledon in part)
— plumule

— radicle
coleorhiza
radicle sheath (cotyledon in part)

pt. of attachment

4.

foliage leaves —

Seedlings of Zea

3. — plumule

plumule sheath

2.

root hairs

coleorhiza

radicle

adventitious roots
absorbing region
growing point
root cap

10.

6. Phoenix dactylifera (Date)

plumule

grooved testa enclosing hard cellulose-storing endosperm

cotyledon sheath

hypocotyl

rootlet

Allium Cepa (Onion)

9. green arched sheathing cotyledon
food absorbing tip of cotyledon

7. L.S. seed

testa
curved embryo
endosperm
micropyle

8. Seedling

beginning of bulb
adv. root

5. Phoenix (Date)

testa
enclosed cotyledon tip
cotyledon sheath enclosing plumule
radicle

radicle

SEEDS AND SEEDLINGS—Continued

Botanical Illustrations

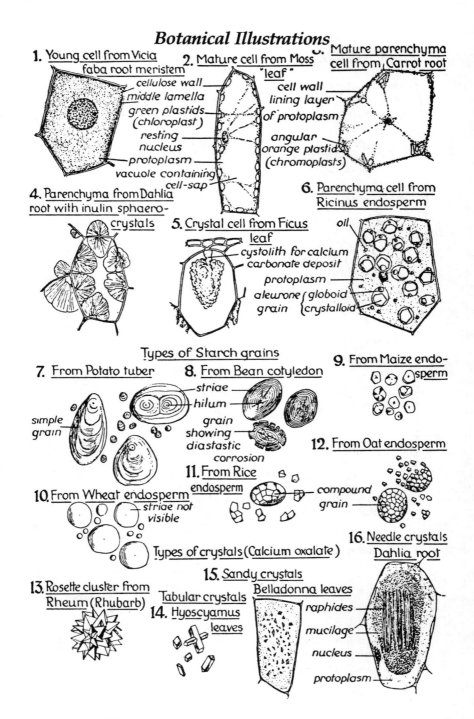

1. Young cell from Vicia faba root meristem
— cellulose wall
— middle lamella
— green plastids (chloroplast)
— resting nucleus
— protoplasm
— vacuole containing cell-sap

2. Mature cell from Moss "leaf"
— cell wall
— lining layer of protoplasm
— angular orange plastids (chromoplasts)

3. Mature parenchyma cell from Carrot root

4. Parenchyma from Dahlia root with inulin sphaero-crystals

5. Crystal cell from Ficus leaf
— cystolith for calcium carbonate deposit
— protoplasm

6. Parenchyma cell from Ricinus endosperm
oil
aleurone { globoid grain { crystalloid

Types of Starch grains

7. From Potato tuber
simple grain

8. From Bean cotyledon
— striae
— hilum
— grain showing diastastic corrosion

9. From Maize endosperm

10. From Wheat endosperm
— striae not visible

11. From Rice endosperm

12. From Oat endosperm
compound grain

Types of crystals (Calcium oxalate)

13. Rosette cluster from Rheum (Rhubarb)

14. Hyoscyamus leaves
Tabular crystals

15. Sandy crystals
Belladonna leaves

16. Needle crystals
Dahlia root
— raphides
— mucilage
— nucleus
— protoplasm

CELLS AND CELL CONTENTS

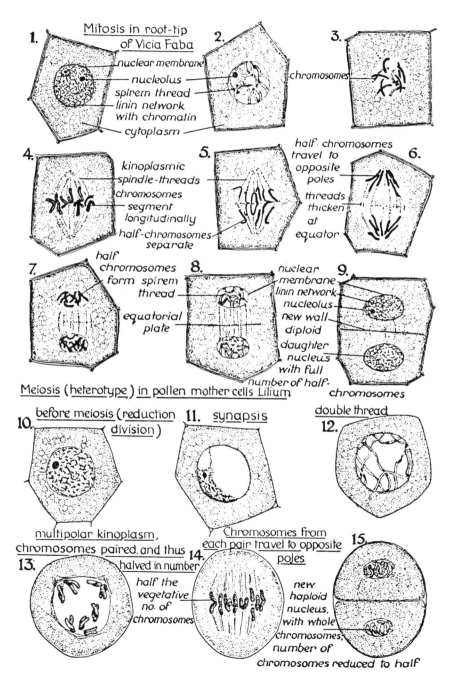

Mitosis in root-tip of Vicia Faba

1. nuclear membrane
   nucleolus
   spirem thread
   linin network with chromatin
   cytoplasm

2. chromosomes

3. chromosomes

4. kinoplasmic spindle-threads
   chromosomes
   segment longitudinally
   half-chromosomes separate

5. half chromosomes travel to opposite poles

6. threads thicken at equator

7. half chromosomes form spirem thread

8. nuclear membrane
   linin network
   nucleolus
   new wall
   diploid daughter nucleus with full number of half-chromosomes
   equatorial plate

9. chromosomes

Meiosis (heterotype) in pollen mother cells Lilium

10. before meiosis (reduction division)

11. synapsis

12. double thread

13. multipolar kinoplasm, chromosomes paired, and thus halved in number
    half the vegetative no. of chromosomes

14. Chromosomes from each pair travel to opposite poles

15. new haploid nucleus, with whole chromosomes; number of chromosomes reduced to half

NUCLEAR DIVISION : KARYOKINESIS

Botanical Illustrations

[After Lloyd, 1949]

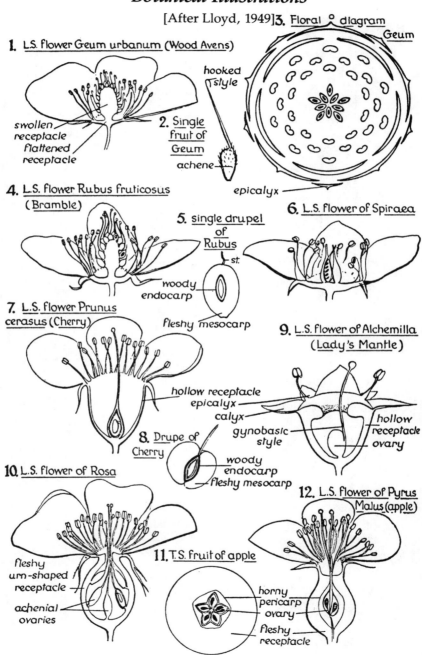

3. Floral ♀ diagram Geum

1. L.S. flower Geum urbanum (Wood Avens)

hooked style

swollen receptacle flattened receptacle

2. Single fruit of Geum

achene

epicalyx

4. L.S. flower Rubus fruticosus (Bramble)

5. single drupel of Rubus

st.

woody endocarp

fleshy mesocarp

6. L.S. flower of Spiraea

7. L.S. flower Prunus cerasus (Cherry)

9. L.S. flower of Alchemilla (Lady's Mantle)

hollow receptacle
epicalyx
calyx
gynobasic style

hollow receptacle
ovary

8. Drupe of Cherry

woody endocarp
fleshy mesocarp

10. L.S. flower of Rosa

fleshy urn-shaped receptacle

achenial ovaries

11. T.S. fruit of apple

horny pericarp
ovary
fleshy receptacle

12. L.S. flower of Pyrus Malus (apple)

ROSACEÆ

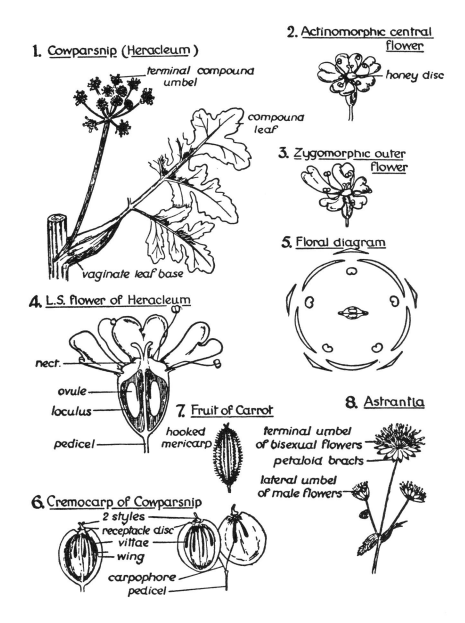

1. Cowparsnip (Heracleum)

terminal compound umbel

compound leaf

vaginate leaf base

2. Actinomorphic central flower

honey disc

3. Zygomorphic outer flower

5. Floral diagram

4. L.S. flower of Heracleum

nect.

ovule

loculus

pedicel

7. Fruit of Carrot

hooked mericarp

8. Astrantia

terminal umbel of bisexual flowers

petaloid bracts

lateral umbel of male flowers

6. Cremocarp of Cowparsnip

2 styles

receptacle disc

vittae

wing

carpophore

pedicel

UMBELLIFERÆ

Botanical Illustrations

[After Lloyd, 1949]

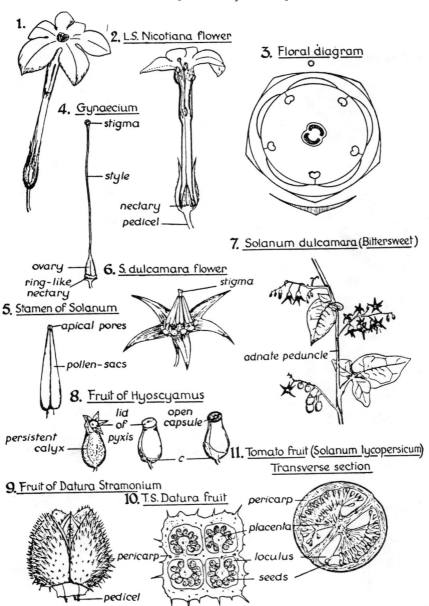

1.

2. L.S. Nicotiana flower

3. Floral diagram

4. Gynaecium
- stigma
- style
- nectary
- pedicel

ovary
ring-like
nectary

5. Stamen of Solanum
- apical pores
- pollen-sacs

6. S. dulcamara flower
- stigma

7. Solanum dulcamara (Bittersweet)

adnate peduncle

8. Fruit of Hyoscyamus
lid of pyxis
open capsule
persistent calyx
c

11. Tomato fruit (Solanum lycopersicum)
Transverse section

9. Fruit of Datura Stramonium
10. T.S. Datura fruit
- pericarp
- pericarp
- placenta
- pedicel
- loculus
- seeds

SOLANACEÆ

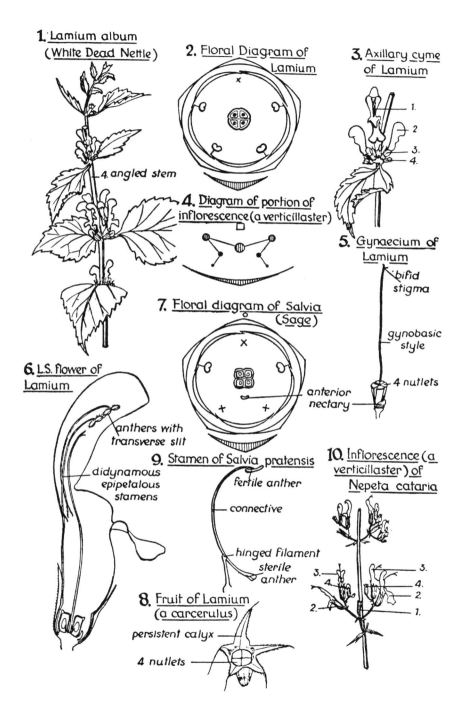

1. Lamium album
(White Dead Nettle)

4. angled stem

2. Floral Diagram of
Lamium

3. Axillary cyme
of Lamium

1.
2.
3.
4.

4. Diagram of portion of
inflorescence (a verticillaster)

5. Gynaecium of
Lamium

bifid
stigma

gynobasic
style

4 nutlets

7. Floral diagram of Salvia
(Sage)

anterior
nectary

6. L.S. flower of
Lamium

anthers with
transverse slit

didynamous
epipetalous
stamens

9. Stamen of Salvia pratensis

fertile anther

connective

hinged filament
sterile
anther

10. Inflorescence (a
verticillaster) of
Nepeta cataria

3.
3.
4.
4.
2.
2.
1.

8. Fruit of Lamium
(a carcerulus)

persistent calyx

4 nutlets

LABIATÆ

Botanical Illustrations

[After Lloyd, 1949]

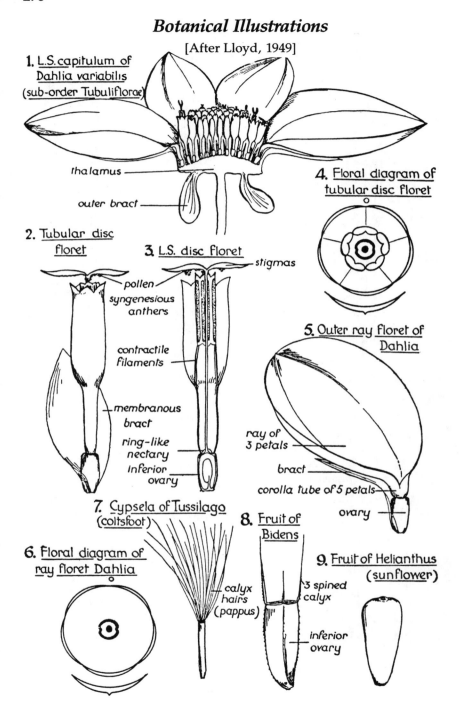

1. L.S. capitulum of Dahlia variabilis (sub-order Tubuliflorae)

thalamus

outer bract

4. Floral diagram of tubular disc floret

2. Tubular disc floret

3. L.S. disc floret

stigmas

pollen

syngenesious anthers

contractile filaments

membranous bract

ring-like nectary

inferior ovary

5. Outer ray floret of Dahlia

ray of 3 petals

bract

corolla tube of 5 petals

ovary

7. Cypsela of Tussilago (coltsfoot)

8. Fruit of Bidens

9. Fruit of Helianthus (sunflower)

6. Floral diagram of ray floret Dahlia

calyx hairs (pappus)

3 spined calyx

inferior ovary

COMPOSITÆ

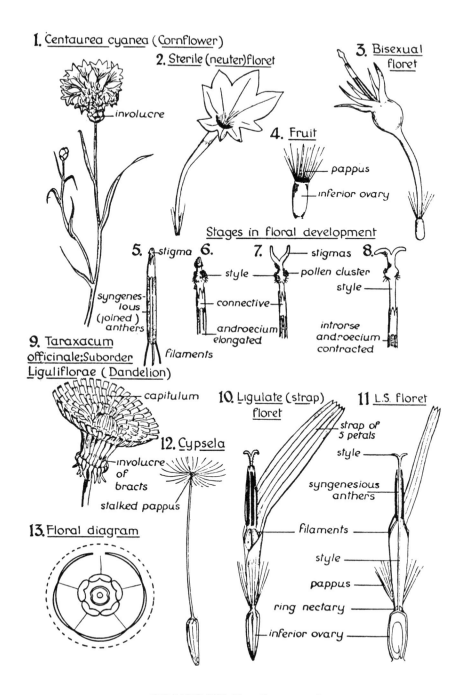

1. Centaurea cyanea (Cornflower)

2. Sterile (neuter) floret

3. Bisexual floret

involucre

4. Fruit

pappus

inferior ovary

Stages in floral development

5. stigma 6. 7. stigmas 8.

style pollen cluster

style

syngenes-
ious
(joined)
anthers

connective

androecium
elongated

introrse
androecium
contracted

filaments

9. Taraxacum
officinale: Suborder
Liguliflorae (Dandelion)

capitulum

10. Ligulate (strap)
floret

11. L.S. floret

strap of
5 petals

style

involucre
of
bracts

12. Cypsela

syngenesious
anthers

stalked pappus

filaments

style

13. Floral diagram

pappus

ring nectary

inferior ovary

COMPOSITÆ—Continued

Botanical Illustrations

[After Lloyd, 1949]

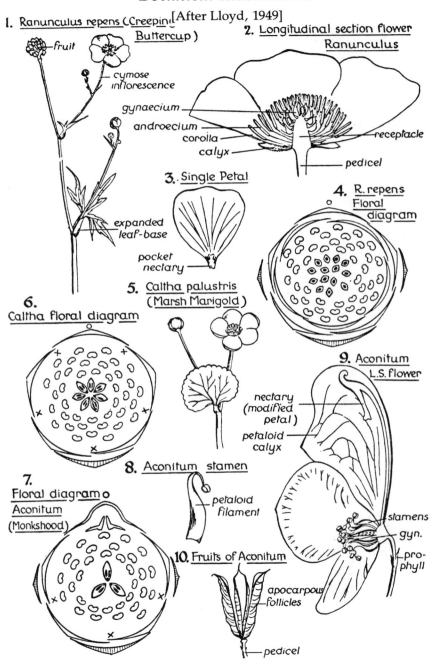

1. Ranunculus repens (Creeping Buttercup)
   — fruit
   — cymose inflorescence
   — expanded leaf-base

2. Longitudinal section flower Ranunculus
   gynaecium
   androecium
   corolla
   calyx
   — receptacle
   — pedicel

3. Single Petal
   pocket nectary

4. R. repens Floral diagram

5. Caltha palustris (Marsh Marigold)

6. Caltha floral diagram

7. Floral diagram Aconitum (Monkshood)

8. Aconitum stamen
   — petaloid filament

9. Aconitum L.S. flower
   nectary (modified petal)
   petaloid calyx
   — stamens
   — gyn.
   — pro-phyll

10. Fruits of Aconitum
    apocarpous follicles
    — pedicel

RANUNCULACEÆ

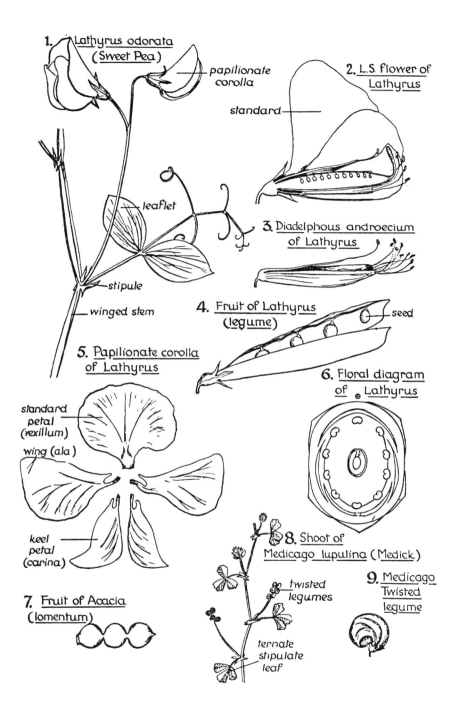

1. Lathyrus odorata (Sweet Pea)

papilionate corolla

standard

leaflet

stipule

winged stem

2. L.S. flower of Lathyrus

standard

3. Diadelphous androecium of Lathyrus

4. Fruit of Lathyrus (legume)

seed

5. Papilionate corolla of Lathyrus

standard petal (vexillum)

wing (ala)

keel petal (carina)

6. Floral diagram of Lathyrus

7. Fruit of Acacia (lomentum)

8. Shoot of Medicago lupulina (Medick)

twisted legumes

ternate stipulate leaf

9. Medicago Twisted legume

LEGUMINOSÆ

Botanical Illustrations

[After Lloyd, 1949]

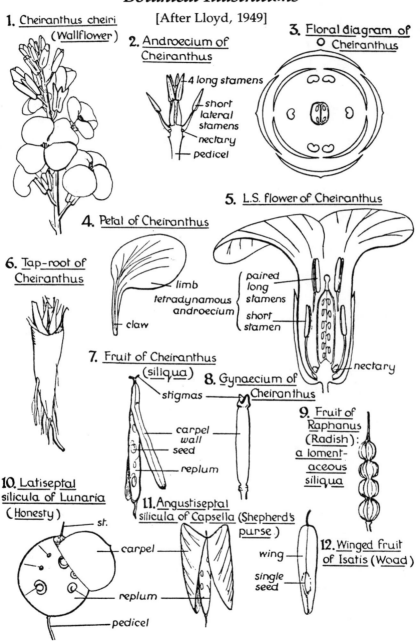

1. Cheiranthus cheiri (Wallflower)

2. Androecium of Cheiranthus
- 4 long stamens
- short lateral stamens
- nectary
- pedicel

3. Floral diagram of ♂ Cheiranthus

4. Petal of Cheiranthus
- limb
- tetradynamous androecium
- claw

5. L.S. flower of Cheiranthus
- paired long stamens
- short stamen
- nectary

6. Tap-root of Cheiranthus

7. Fruit of Cheiranthus (siliqua)
- stigmas
- carpel wall
- seed
- replum

8. Gynaecium of Cheiranthus

9. Fruit of Raphanus (Radish): a loment-aceous siliqua

10. Latiseptal silicula of Lunaria (Honesty)
- st.
- carpel
- replum
- pedicel

11. Angustiseptal silicula of Capsella (Shepherd's purse)

12. Winged fruit of Isatis (Woad)
- wing
- single seed

CRUCIFERÆ

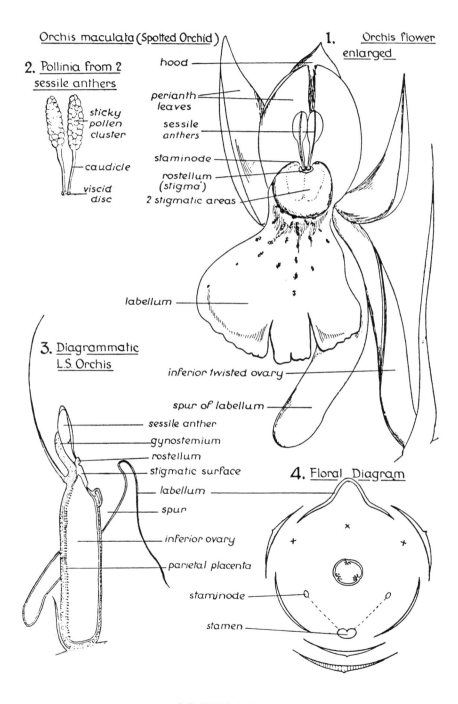

Orchis maculata (Spotted Orchid)

1. Orchis flower enlarged

2. Pollinia from 2 sessile anthers

sticky pollen cluster

caudicle

viscid disc

hood

perianth leaves

sessile anthers

staminode

rostellum (stigma)

2 stigmatic areas

labellum

inferior twisted ovary

spur of labellum

3. Diagrammatic L.S. Orchis

sessile anther

gynostemium

rostellum

stigmatic surface

labellum

spur

inferior ovary

parietal placenta

4. Floral Diagram

staminode

stamen

ORCHIDACEÆ

Botanical Illustrations

[After Lloyd, 1949]

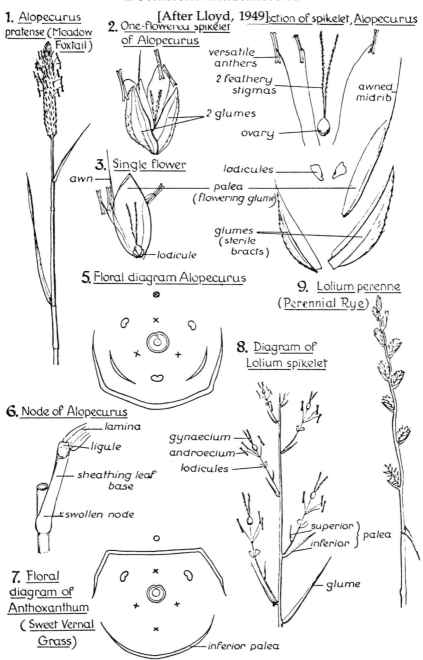

1. Alopecurus pratense (Meadow Foxtail)

2. One-flowered spikelet of Alopecurus

...ction of spikelet, Alopecurus

versatile anthers

2 feathery stigmas

2 glumes

ovary

awned midrib

3. Single flower

awn

lodicule

lodicules

palea (flowering glume)

glumes (sterile bracts)

5. Floral diagram Alopecurus

9. Lolium perenne (Perennial Rye)

8. Diagram of Lolium spikelet

6. Node of Alopecurus

lamina

ligule

sheathing leaf base

swollen node

gynaecium

androecium

lodicules

superior
inferior
} palea

glume

7. Floral diagram of Anthoxanthum (Sweet Vernal Grass)

inferior palea

GRAMINEÆ

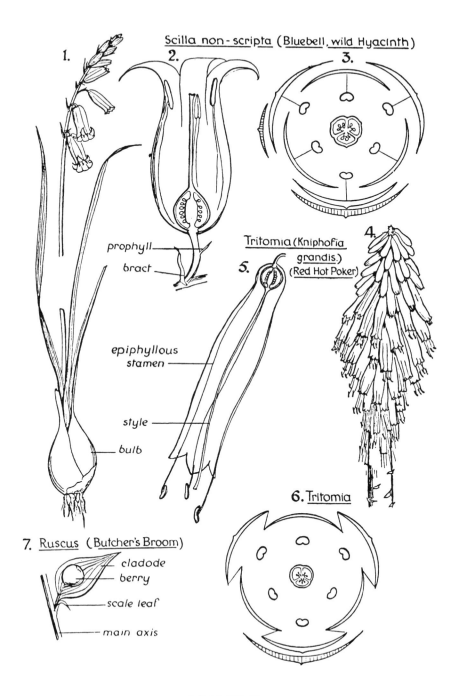

1.

Scilla non-scripta (<u>Bluebell, wild Hyacinth</u>)

2.

3.

prophyll

bract

Tritomia (Kniphofia grandis.) (Red Hot Poker)

5.

4.

epiphyllous
stamen

style

bulb

6. <u>Tritomia</u>

7. <u>Ruscus</u> (<u>Butcher's Broom</u>)

cladode

berry

scale leaf

main axis

LILIACEÆ

Botanical Illustrations

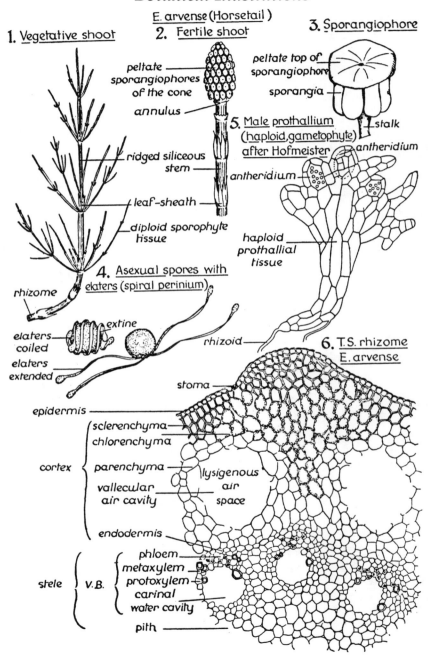

E. arvense (Horsetail)

1. Vegetative shoot

2. Fertile shoot

3. Sporangiophore

peltate sporangiophores of the cone

annulus

ridged siliceous stem

leaf-sheath

diploid sporophyte tissue

rhizome

peltate top of sporangiophore

sporangia

stalk

5. Male prothallium (haploid, gametophyte) after Hofmeister

antheridium

antheridium

haploid prothallial tissue

4. Asexual spores with elaters (spiral perinium)

extine

elaters coiled

elaters extended

rhizoid

6. T.S. rhizome E. arvense

stoma

epidermis

sclerenchyma

chlorenchyma

cortex

parenchyma

lysigenous air space

vallecular air cavity

endodermis

phloem

metaxylem

protoxylem

carinal water cavity

pith

stele

V.B.

EQUISETALES : EQUISETUM

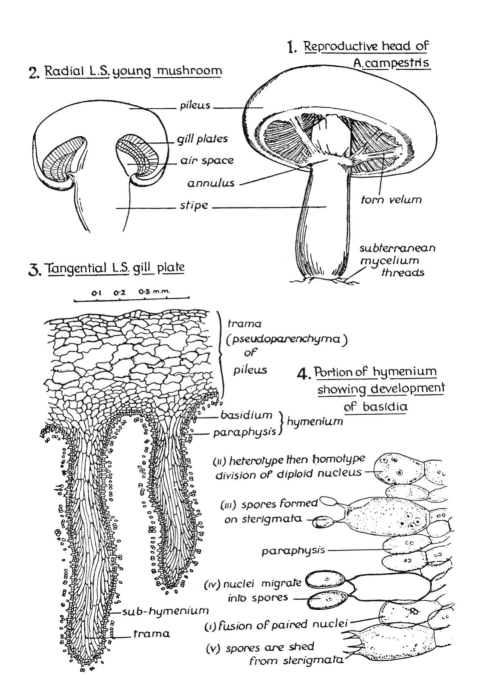

2. Radial L.S. young mushroom

1. Reproductive head of A.campestris

pileus

gill plates

air space

annulus

stipe

torn velum

subterranean mycelium threads

3. Tangential L.S. gill plate

0·1   0·2   0·3 m.m.

trama (pseudoparenchyma) of pileus

4. Portion of hymenium showing development of basidia

basidium ⎱ hymenium
paraphysis ⎰

(II) heterotype then homotype division of diploid nucleus

(III) spores formed on sterigmata

paraphysis

(IV) nuclei migrate into spores

sub-hymenium

trama

(I) fusion of paired nuclei

(V) spores are shed from sterigmata

FUNGI : AGARICUS

ACHENE a small dry indehiscent fruit, strictly of one free carpel.

ACICLE a very slender prickle or stoutish bristle.

ACTINOMORPHIC having flowers of a regular star pattern, capable of bisection in two or more planes into similar halves.

ACUTE sharply pointed but not drawn out.

ALLELE Genes situated at corresponding positions in a pair of chromosomes.

ALTERNATE arranged successively on opposite sides of a stem.

AMPLEXICAUL clasping the stem with their base.

ANGLE(D)(S) the meeting of two planes to form an edge

ANNUAL a plant completing its life cycle from germination to death within one year.

ANTHER the terminal portion of a stamen containing the pollen grains.

APEX the growing point of a stem; the tip of an organ.

APICULATE furnished with a small broad point at the apex.

APPRESSED lying flat along the whole length of an organ.

AQUATIC living in water.

ARCUATE bent like a bow.

ARIL the exterior covering of the seed in certain plants; e.g., Taxus baccata, developed from the stalk or base of the ovule.

ARISTATE awned.

ATTENUATE gradually tapering to a point.

AURICLES small ear-like appendages at the base of a leaf.

AWN a brittle-like part.

AXIL the upper angle formed by the union of the stem and the leaf.

AXILLARY growing in an axil.

AXIS the central part of a plant, around which the organs are developed.

BEAK a pointed projection.

BEARD awn.

BICONVEX having a more or less rounded surface on both sides.

BIENNIAL a plant requiring two years to complete its life cycle, growing in the first year, and flowering and fruiting in the second.

BIFID divided halfway down into two parts.

BINOMIAL the use of a generic and specific name to connote a given organism.

BIPINNATE when the divisions of a pinnate leaf are themselves pinnate.

BISERRATE doubly serrate.

BLUNT ending in a rounded form, neither tapering to a point, nor truncate.

BOLE the trunk of a tree.

BRACT(S)dmodified leaves intermediate between the calyx and the normal leaves.

BRACTEATE having bracts.

BRACTEOLES minute bracts.

BULB an underground organ which is really a modified plant bud with fleshy scales, yielding stem and roots.

BULBILS Small bulbs or tubers usually arising in the axils of the leaves or amongst the florets of an inflorescence, but sometimes found on the root.

CALYX the outermost of the floral envelopes.

CAMPANULATE bell-shaped.

CAPILLARY hair-like.

CAPITATE growing in heads; pin-headed.

CAPITULUM a close cluster of sessile flowers.

CAPSULE a dry, dehiscent fruit.

282

GLOSSARY OF TAXONOMICAL TERMS

CARPEL a modified leaf of one, or several, of which the pistil is formed.

CARPOPHORE the continuation of the stalk between the carpels.

CAULINE borne on the stem, not radical.

CERNUOUS nodding.

CHROMOSOME fibrillar bodies of definite number formed during nuclear division, dividing by fission into new groups, and contributing to form the daughter nuclei; a structure in the nucleus containing a linear thread of DNA which transmits genetic information.

CILIATE fringed with hairs.

CLADODE a leaf-like branch, as in Ruscus aculeatus.

CLASPING grasping.

CLAW the narrow base of a petal in certain genera, e.g. Dianthus.

CLEFT deeply cut, but not to the midrib.

COMMISSURE the faces by which two carpels adhere, particularly in Umbeliferae.

CONFLUENT united at some part.

CONNATE similar organs distinct in origin but eventually becoming united.

CONNIVENT making contact or converging.

CONTIGUOUS adjacent to each other; making contact at the edges.

CORDATE heart-shaped.

CORM bulb-like fleshy underground stem, as in Anemone, etc.

COROLLA the petals as a whole.

CORONA the circumference or margin of a radiated compound flower, particularly in Compositae.

COTYLEDON(S) the first leaf or leaves of the embryo.

CRENATE with rounded marginal teeth.

CRENULATE minutely crenate.

CRUCIFORM cross-shaped.

CRYPTOGAM a flowerless plant.

CULTIVAR an assemblage of cultivated individuals which is designated by any characters, morphological, physiological, chemical or others, significant for the purpose of agriculture, horticulture or forestry, and which, when produced sexually or asexually, retains its distinguishing features. A cultivar may be: (1) a clone which consists of individuals vegetatively propagated from a single plant and which are, therefore, of genetic uniformity, e.g. Theobroma cacao; (2) a line, which is an assemblage of sexually reproducing individuals of uniform appearance propagated by seeds, the stability of which is maintained by selection to a standard, e.g. Phaseolus vulgaris, Canadian wonder; (3) an assemblage of individuals, usually reproducing sexually and showing genetic differences, but having one or more characters by which it can be differentiated from other cultivars, e.g. watermelon "Dixie Queen;" (4) a uniform group which is a first generation hybrid reconstituted on each occasion by crossing two or more breeding stocks maintained either by inbreeding or as clones, e.g. maize "U.S. 13," a double-cross involving four inbred lines.

CUNEATE wedge-shaped.

CUSPIDATE spear-shaped at the tip.

CYME a flower-cluster of a broad and flattened type, as in Sambucus nigra.

CYTOLOGY the study of cells, their origin, structure, function and pathology.

DECIDUOUS dropping off; shedding its leaves in the autumn.

DECUMBENT lying on the ground but tending to rise at the end.

DECURRENT extending downwards, as when leaves are extended beyond their insertion and run down by a wing on the stem as in Carduus and Cirsium.

DEFLEXED bent sharply downwards.

DEHISCENT opening to shed its seeds.

DELTOID shaped like an equilateral triangle.

DENTATE toothed; notched.

DENTICULATE minutely toothed.

DEPRESSED when flattened vertically or at the top.

DICHOTOMOUS forked, parted by pairs from top to bottom.

DIFFUSE widely or loosely spreading.

DIGITATE a compound leaf divided into five leaflets, as in Aesculus hippocastanum.

DIOECIOUS having the sexes on different plants.

DISK the central part of a capitulum in Compositae as opposed to the ray florets; the expanded base of a style in Umbelliferae.

DOCTRINE OF SIGNATURES the theory stating that each plant bore a visible mark that revealed its intended use.

DRUPE a fleshy or leathery fruit containing a stone with a kernel.

ECOSYSTEMS an ecological community in relationship to the nonliving factors of its environment.

EDAPHIC the influence of the soil on the plants growing upon it; relating to soil, drainage and salinity

EFFICACY power to produce effects; as, the efficacy of a medince.

ELLIPTIC(AL) oval but acute at each end.

ELONGATE much lengthened.

EMARGINATE slightly notched at the edges.

ENDEMIC confined to a given region or geographical area.

ENDOCARP the inner layer of a pericarp.

ENTIRE with an even margin; not toothed or cut at the edges.

EPICALYX an involucre resembling an accessory calyx, as in Malva.

EPICHILE the terminal part of the labellum of an orchid when it is distinct from the basal portion.

ETHNO-BOTANY the interdisciplinary approach to the study of indigenous peoples and their use of plants in the environments; the basic disciplines involved have been botany, chemistry, and pharmacology, but anthropology, archaeology, linguistics, history, sociology, and comparative religion have contributed appreciably to this field.

EVERGREEN bearing green foliage all the year.

EXCURRENT where the stem remains central, the other parts being regularly placed around it.

EXOTIC said of a plant not native to the place where it is found.

EXSERTED protruding.

FAMILY a group of related genera.

FARINACEOUS of the nature of starch, containing starch.

FASCICLE(D) a cluster of bundle.

FASTIGIATE tapering to a point like a pyramid.

FILAMENT the stalk of an anther.

FILIFORM thread-like

FIMBRIATE with a fringed margin.

FLEXUOSE zigzag.

FLORET a small flower, one of a cluster.

FOLLICLE a dry dehiscent fruit formed of one carpel opening by a ventral suture to which the seeds are attached.

FRINGE with hair-like appendages on the margins.

GLOSSARY OF TAXONOMICAL TERMS

FROND the leaf-like part of a fern and other cryptogams.

FRUIT the ripe seeds and their surrounding structure.

GAMOPETALOUS having the petals united at the edges in the form of a tube.

GENE POOL

GENOME CONSTITUTION a description of the complete set of hereditary factors, as contained in the haploid assortment of chromosomes.

GENUS the smallest natural group containing related but distinct species.

GIBBOUS swollen on one side.

GLABROUS smooth, devoid of hair or other clothing.

GLAND a wart-like structure on the surface, embedded or protruding, from any part of a plant.

GLANDULAR having glands

GLAUCOUS covered with a bluish green bloom.

GLOBOSE round.

GLUME a small bract with a flower in the axil as in grasses.

GREGARIOUS growing in company, associated but not matted.

HABITAT the place where a plant grows naturally.

HAMMOCK tree islands on higher elevations characterized by tropical hardwoods.

HASTATE spear-shaped.

HERB any non-woody vascular plant.

HERBACEOUS having the texture of leaves.

HERMORPHRODITE having the characters of both sexes; the stamens and pistils in the same flower.

HIRSUTE hairy, with long, usually soft, hairs.

HISPID clothed with stiff hairs or bristles.

HOODED formed into a hood at the end.

HYALINE very thin and translucent.

HYBRID a plant produced by the fertilization of one species by another.

HYPOCHILE the basal portion of the labellum in an orchid.

INCUMBENT resting or leaning upon.

INDIGENOUS original to the country, not introduced.

INFERIOR below the ovary.

INFLORESCENCE the arrangement of the flowers on a stem or branch.

INTERCALARY inserted between or amongst others.

INTERNODE the space between two adjacent nodes.

INTRODUCED used of plants which have been brought from another country.

INVOLUCRE the whorl of bracts enclosing a number of flowers as in Compositae and Umbelliferae.

INVOLUTE having the margins rolled upwards.

KAROTYPE the chromosomal constitution of the nucleus of a cell.

KEEL(ED) the lower petal or petals when shaped like the keel of a boat as in Vicia, Lathyrus, etc.

LABELLUM the lower petal of certain flowers, particularly orchids.

LACINIATE jagged; deeply and irregularly divided into segments.

LANCEOLATE narrow, tapering at each end.

LATERAL fixed on, or near, the side of an organ.

LATEX the milky juice of such plants as spurge and lettuce.

LEAFLET a subdivision of a compound leaf.

LEMMA the flowering glume of a grass.

LENTICEL corky spots having the shape of a double-convex lens on young bark.

LIGULATE strap-shaped.

LIGULE a small thin projection from the top of the leaf-sheath in grasses; a strape-shaped petal, e.g. Compositae.

LIMB the border or exposed part of a calyx or corolla, as distinct from the tube or throat.

LINEAR slender.

LINEAR-LANCEOLATE

LOBED sets of leaves which are divided, but not into separate leaflets.

LUNATE shaped like the new moon.

MEMBRANOUS thin, dry and semitransparent.

METAPHASE the second stage of cell division (mitosis or meiosis), during which the contracted chromosomes, each consisting or two chromatids, are arranged in the equatorial plane of the spindle prior to separation.

MITOTIC pertaining to mitosis.

MONOECIOUS when the male and female flowers are separate, but borne on the same individual plant.

MORPHOLOGY the study of form and its development.

MUCRONATE abruptly tipped with a short, straight point.

MURICATE with sharp points or prickles.

NATIVE pertaining to plants indigenous to a geographical area.

NATRON native sodium carbonate; also soda and sodium hydroxide.

NECTARY the honey gland of a flower.

NERVE a vien or slender rib.

NODE a point in a stem where a leaf is borne.

NOTCH an indentation.

OB as a prefix means inversely or oppositely.

OBLONG longer than broad.

OBTUSE blunt.

OCHREA provided with a tubular membranous stipule.

OOLITIC soil of limestone composition.

OPPOSITE growing in pairs at the same level on opposite sides of a stem.

ORBICULAR nearly round and flat.

OSTIOLATE furnished with an opening or mouth.

OVAL broadly elliptic.

OVARY the vessel in which the seeds are formed.

OVATE egg-shaped.

OVATE-OBLONG egg-shaped, but much longer than broad.

OVOID of a solid object which is egg-shaped in outline.

PALEA the inner bract or glume of a grass; the chaffy scales on the receptacle in many Compositae.

LALMATE lobed or divided into more than three leaflets arising from a central point.

PANICLE a raceme with branching pedicels.

PAPILAE small elongated protuberances.

PAPILLOSE warty; having papillae.

PAPPUS the tufts of hair on achenes or fruits, particularly in Compositae.

PECTINATE resembling the teeth of a comb.

PEDICEL the stalk of a single flower.

PEDUNCLE the stalk supporting either a flower or a flower-cluster.

PELLUCID transparent.

PELTATE shield-shaped with the stalk in the center.

PEN TS'AO the Materia Medica published in China in 1578 by Li Shih-Chen comprising 1,892 species of drugs from animal, vegetable and mineral sources and includes 8,160 prescriptions; origin said to be before 2000 B.C.

PERENNIAL a plant that lives for more than two years and usually flowers annually.

PERFOLIATE with the leaf united round the stem, as in Montia perfoliate.

PERIANTH the floral envelopes, calyx or corolla, or both.

PERICARP a seed vessel, including the adhering calyx if present.

PETAL a flower leaf, often brightly colored, forming part of a corolla.

PETALOID resembling a petal.

GLOSSARY OF TAXONOMICAL TERMS

PETIOLE a leaf-stalk.

PETIOLATE having a petiole.

PHYLOGENY a tribe; the developmental history of a tribe or group.

PHYSIOLOGY the science which studies facts about the functions of organs, tissues, cells, etc. in living animals or plants.

PILOSE hairy, usually with long soft hairs.

PINNATE with leaflets arranged on opposite sides of a common stalk or rachis.

PINNATIFID deeply cut into segments nearly to the midrib.

PISTIL the female organ of a flower, consisting when complete of ovary, style and stigma.

POLLINIA a pollen mass composed of large numbers of cohering pollen grains.

POLYGAMOUS with hermaphrodite and unisexual flowers on the same, or on different individuals of the same species.

POLYPETALOUS having many separate petals.

POLYPLOID having more than two full sets of homologous chromosomes.

PORE a small aperture.

PROCUMBENT trailing; lying loosely on the ground.

PROLIFEROUS bearing progeny as offshoots.

PROSTRATE lying closely on the surface of the ground.

PRUINOSE covered with a whitish bloom.

PUBESCENT covered with fine short hairs.

PYRIFORM pear shaped.

RACEME an unbranched inflorescence with flowers borne on equal pedicels.

RACHIS the axis of an inflorescence, compound leaf or branch.

RADICAL growing from the root.

RAY the outer part of a compound radiate flower.

RECEPTACLE the uppermost part of the stem nearing the flowers.

RECURVED bent moderately backwards in a curve.

REFLEXED bent abruptly backwards.

RENIFORM kidney-shaped.

RETICULATE marked with a network of veins.

RETUSE terminating in a rounded end, the center of which is slightly indented.

REVOLUTE rolled or curved downwards.

RHACHIS the axis of an inflorescence or compound leaf or frond.

RHIZOMATOUS having the character of a rhizome.

RHIZOME an underground, creeping stem, producing roots and leafy shoots.

RHOMBOID(AL) similar in shape to a diamond in a pack of playing cards.

RIB(BED) a primary vein; furnished with ribs.

ROSETTE a cluster of leaves in circular form, as in Plantago major.

ROTATE (OF A COROLLA) wheel-shaped, circular and flat with a short tube.

RUDERAL said of a plant which thrives in the surroundings of cities.

RUGOSE wrinkled.

SACCART pouched.

SAGITTATE shaped like the barbed head of an arrow.

SAPROPHYTE a plant that lives on decaying vegetable matter.

SCABRID rough.

SCALE a thin scarious structure, often a degenerate leaf.

SCAPE a leafless flower-stalk rising from the root.

SCARIOUS very thin, dry and semi-transparent.

SECUND all turned to one side.

SEGMENT a division into which a plant organ, e.g. a leaf, may be cleft.

SEPAL a leaf of the calyx, the outer whorl of the perianth.

SEPTATE divided into partitions.

SERRATE toothed like a saw.

SESSILE without a stalk.

SETAE bristles.

SHRUB a woody perennial of smaller structure than a tree, lacking a bole.

SINUATE having a deep wavy outline.

SINUOUS undulating.

SINUS a depression between two teeth.

SPADIX a succulent spike with a fleshy axis, as in Arum maculatum.

SPATHE a large bract enclosing a flower cluster, usually a spadix.

SPATHULATE spatula-shaped.

SPIKE an inflorescence in which the flowers are sessile round at axis.

SPIKELET a small spike; the inflorescence of grasses.

SPINE a thorn.

SPUR a slender projection from the bas of a perianth segment, or of a corolla, as in Aquilegia vulgaris.

STAMEN one of the male reproductive organs of a plant.

STAMINODES infertile, often reduced stamens.

STANDARD the large, often erect posterior petal of a corolla in Papilionaceae.

STELLATE star-shaped.

STIGMA the part of the pistil or style which receives the pollen.

STIPULE a leaf-like appendage usually at the base of the petiole.

STIPULATE having stipules on it.

STOLON a creeping stem which roots at intervals.

STOLONIFEROUS having stolons.

STRIATE(IONS) marked with slender streaks or furrows.

STRICT narrow, upright and very straight.

STYLE the space between the ovary and the stigma.

SUB under or below.

SUBULATE awl-shaped.

SUCCULENT juicy.

TEETH small marginal lobes.

TERETE long and round, without ridges or grooves.

TERMINAL borne at the top of the stem.

TESTA the outer coat of the seed.

TOMENTOSE densely pubescent, with woolly entangled hairs.

TRIFID three-cleft but not to the base.

TRIFOLIATE having three leaflets.

TRIGONOUS of a solid body, three-angled, with plane faces.

TRIQUETROUS triangular and acutely angled.

TRUNCATE as though abruptly cut off at the end.

TUBE the united parts of a corolla or calyx.

TUBER a thickened part of an underground stem or root on one year's duration.

GLOSSARY OF TAXONOMICAL TERMS

TUBERCLE a small spherical or ovoid swelling.

UMBEL a type of inflorescence in which equal pedicels proceed from a common center.

UMBELLATE having partial or secondary umbels.

UNARMED without spines or prickles.

UNDULATE wavy.

UNISEXUAL of one sex only.

VALVATE when parts of a flower bud meet but do not overlap.

VALVE one of the pices into which a capsule naturally separates at maturity.

VASCULAR furnished with vessels.

VERNAL appearing in spring.

VILLOUS covered with shaggy hairs.

VISCID clammy or sticky.

VITTA(E) the aromatic oil tubes of the pericarp in many species of Umbelliferae.

VIVIPAROUS producing young plants instead of flowers.

WHORL(ED) a ring of leaves or flowers around a stem at the same level as each other.

WING(ED) the lateral petals in the flowers of Fumariaceae and Papilionaceae; the flat membranous appendages of some seeds.

GLOSSARY OF MEDICAL TERMS

ABORTIFACIENT—causing abortion.

ALLERGY—a hypersensitive state which causes reaction to a particular irritant.

ALTERNATIVE—gradually changing, or tending to change a morbid state of health.

ANAESTHETIC—producing a numbing or sedative effect.

ANTHELMINTIC—expels worms.

AMINO ACID—the building blocks of proteins.

ANTIFEBRIL—having the quality of reducing or curing fever.

ANTIPERIODIC—preventing the return of periodic spasms, as in intermittent fevers.

ANTIPHLEGMATIC—preventing excess of the supposed humor called phlegm.

ANTIPHLOGISTIC—tends to check inflammation.

ANTIPRURITIC—relieving itch.

ANTISCORBUTIC—counteracts scurvy.

ANTISPASMODIC—prevents or allays spasms or convulsions.

APERIENT—gently laxative.

APHRODISIAC—any drug that arouses the sexual instincts.

AROMATIC—stimulating.

ARTHRITIS—inflammation of the joints.

ASCITES—effusion and accumulation of serous fluid in the abdominal cavity.

ASTHMA—a condition characterized by recurrent attacks of spasmodic contractions of bronchi, accompanied by wheezing.

ASTRINGENT—quality of causing constriction of tissues.

CANCER—a cellular tumor, the natural course of which is fatal.

CARMINATIVE—relieves flatulence.

CHANCRE—a painless sore occurring at the site of the entry of infection.

CHOLAGOGIC—increases the flow of bile.

CHRONIC—persisting over a long period of time.

COLIC—acute abdominal pain.

COLITIS—inflammation of the colon.

DECOCTION—boiling down; a medicine prepared by boiling ingredients.

DEMULCENT—mucilaginous or oil substance soothing and protecting to inflamed membrane.

DENTAL CARIES—decayed teeth.

DIAPHORETIC—increases perspiration.

DIARRHEA—abnormal infrequency or liquidy discharge of fecal matter.

DIURETIC—promotes or increases the discharge of urine.

DYSMENORRHEA—difficult and painful menstruation.

DYSENTERY—a term given to several conditions marked by inflammation of the colon.

DYSPEPSIA—impairment of the power or function of digestion.

DYSURIA—difficult or painful discharge of urine.

EXZEMA—a superficial inflammation of the outer skin, characterized by redness, itching and the outbreak of lesions that become encrusted and scaly.

EDEMA—the presence of abnormal amounts of fluids in the intercellular tissue spaces of the body.

EMMENAGOGUE—promotes menstrual discharge.

EMOLLIENT—softening and soothing to inflamed parts.

ENEMA—a liquid injected into the rectum for cleansing the lower colon.

EPILEPSY—seizures which result from disturbances of brain function.

EPISTAXIS—nosebleed.

ESSENTIAL FATTY ACIDS—those oils or fats which must be a part of the dietary intake.

ESTROGEN—a generic term for estrus-producing compounds, the female sex hormones, including estradiol, estriol and estrone. In humans, the estrogens are formed in the ovary, adrenal cortex, testis, and fetoplacental unit, and are responsible for female secondary sex characteristic development, and during the menstrual cycle, act on the female genetalia to produce an environment suitable for fertilization, implantation of the early embryo. Estrogen is used as a palliate in post menopausal cancer of the breast and in prostatic cancer, as oral contraceptives and for relief of menopausal discomforts.

EXPECTORANT—promotes discharge of mucus from the lungs.

FEBRIFUGE—removes or mitigates fever.

FLATULENCE—having or causing excessive gas in the digestive tract.

FLUX—fluid discharge from bowels or other parts.

GANGRENE—death of a tissue in considerable mass which is followed by decay.

GASTROINTESTINAL—pertaining to the stomach and intestines.

GALACTOGOGUE—promotes the flow of milk.

GLAUCOMA—pathological changes in the optic disc which causes defects in vision.

GONORRHEA—infection due to Neisseria gonorrhea transmitted venerally or to neonatal children at birth.

HEMOPTYSIS—expectoration of blood from the lungs.

HEMATURIA—passage of blood mixed with urine.

HEPATIC—related diseases of the liver.

HERPATIC—medicine for skin or ringworms.

HEADACHE—pain in the head.

HORMONE—a chemical substance produced by an organ or certain cells of an organ and which has a certain regulatory effect on an organ.

HYDROPHOBIA—rabies.

HYPERACTIVITY—abnormal or increased activity.

HYPERTENSION—high blood pressure; abnormally high arterial blood pressure.

HYSTERIA—a psychoneurosis characterized by uncontrollable emotions or actions.

INFLUENZA—an acute viral infection of the respiratory tract and sometimes intestinal tract.

INFUSION—the process of steeping a drug in water to extract its medicinal properties.

JAUNDICE—a condition characterized by excess belirubinemia and deposits of bile pigment in the skin which causes yellowing appearance.

KIDNEY—either of the two organs of the lower back region which filter the blood and perform various regulatory functions of metabolism; also known as the renal gland.

LEUKORRHEA—a whitish, viscid discharge from the vaginal area.

MENSTRUAL CRAMPS—painful menstrual spasms.

MENTAL DEPRESSION—a psychiatric syndrome consisting of dejected mood and low spirit, often accompanied by physical symptoms such as weight loss and slowness of movement.

MIGRAINE—a sever headache, usually temporal and commonly associated with other symptoms.

MATURATING—bringing boils to a head.

MENORRHAGIA—profuse menstruation.

MUCILAGINOUS—soothing to inflamed parts.

NERVOUS SPASMS—involuntary jumping or movement of the nerves of certain parts of the body.

ORCHITIS—inflammation of the testis marked by pain, swelling and a feeling of weight.

OBESITY—excessive accumulation of fat on the skeleton.

OPTHALMIC—remedy for eye disease.

PALPITATIONS—unduly rapid action of the heart which is noted by the patient.

PARTURITION—the act or process of giving birth to a child; labor.

PLEURISY—inflammation of the pleura, the serous membrane which encloses the thoracic cavity.

PROGESTERONE—the steroid hormone produced by the corpus luteum, adrenal cortex and placenta which serves to prepare the uterus for reception and development of the fertilized ovum by inducing secretions in the proliferated glands. A synthetic preparation is used in the treatment of functional uterine bleeding, menstrual cycle abnormalities and threatened abortion.

PROSTAGLANDINS—a group of naturally occurring fatty acids that stimulate contractility of many smooth muscles and have an effect on hormones; they have the ability to lower blood pressure.

RHEUMATISM—inflammation and degeneration of various types of connective structures in the body.

SEDATIVE—allaying irritability and excitement.

SERUM CHOLESTEROL—free flowing cholesterol in the clear liquid portion of the blood.

SOPORIFIC—causing or inducing sound sleep.

SPERMATORRHEA—involuntary and abnormally frequent release of semen without copulation.

STYPTIC—producing contractions, stopping bleeding.

SUDORIFIC—promoting flow of sweat.

SYPHILIS—a contagious veneral disease caused by the spirochete *"Treponema pallidum"* and transmitted by intimate contact.

TAENICIDE—an agent that destroys tapeworms.

THAUMATURGIES—miracle cures.

THROMBOSIS—clotting of the blood in the heart or great vessels before death.

TOXIC—pertaining to, due to, or of the nature of poison.

TUSSIC—pertaining to cough.

ULCER—an inflammatory lesion on the skin or an internal mucous surface of the body.

VENEREAL DISEASE—diseases which are propagated by sexual contact.

VERMIFUGE—any agent which expels intestinal worms.

VULNERARY—useful in healing wounds.

WOMB INFLAMMATION—inflammation of the uterus.

Glossary of Terms & Deities
Used in Reference to the Santeria Religion

BABALAWO—Father of Mysteries.

CHANGO—god of thunder, lightning and fire; St. Barbara.

ELEGBA—one of the three aspects of God; raw cosmic energy.

ELLEGUÁ—messenger of the gods; he opens and closes all doors to opportunity; Holy Guardian Angel.

IFA—the word from the mouth of God; god of impossible things; the 16 great books containing the laws of civilization, moral and ethical code, handed down orally until the 19th century, containing 1680 ways of expression.

OBA—king among the Yorubas.

OBATALA—father of the gods; Our Lady of Mercy in the Santería religion.

OCHOSI—god of hunting of birds and wild animals.

ODDUDUA—wife of Obatala.

OGGUN—god of war and iron, strength and determination; St. Peter.

OLODUMARE—God.

OMIERO—the sacred elixer of the Santería religious ceremony.

ORISHA—Yoruba god or goddess.

ORUNLA or ORUNMILA—the holy prophet; first teacher; St. Francis of Assissi.

OSHUN—goddess of love; associated with material well being and the sensual sacred aspect of life; uninhibited love and creative propagation; Our Lady of La Caridad del Cobre.

SANTERO, SANTERA—a priest or priestess of the Santería religion.

YEMAYÁ—goddess of fertility; mother of mothers; goddess of fresh waters; Our Lady of Regla.

YORUBA—a West African nation of people located in Nigeria and Benin.

GENERAL INDEX

GENERAL INDEX

GENERAL INDEX

INDEX TO COMMON/VERNACULAR NAMES
(ENGLISH)

INDEX TO COMMON/VERNACULAR NAMES
(ENGLISH)

INDEX TO COMMON VERNACULAR NAMES (ENGLISH)

INDEX TO COMMON VERNACULAR NAMES (ENGLISH)

INDEX TO COMMON VERNACULAR NAMES (ENGLISH)

INDEX TO COMMON/VERNACULAR NAMES
(SPANISH)

INDEX TO COMMON/VERNACULAR NAMES
(SPANISH)

INDEX TO COMMON/VERNACULAR NAMES
(AFRICA)

INDEX TO COMMON/VERNACULAR NAMES
(AFRICA)

INDEX TO COMMON
VERNACULAR NAMES
ASIA (CHINA, INDIA)

INDEX TO COMMON VERNACULAR NAMES (ASIA)

INDEX TO PLANT FAMILIES

INDEX TO PLANT FAMILIES

INDEX TO BOTANICAL NAMES
[Synonyms in Italics]

INDEX TO BOTANICAL NAMES

INDEX TO BOTANICAL NAMES

314

INDEX TO BOTANICAL NAMES

INDEX TO BOTANICAL NAMES

ABBREVIATIONS OF AUTHORS' NAMES
FOR THE PLANT SPECIES
No dates given for living authors

A. DC – Alphonse deCandolle (1806-1893)
Airy Shaw – H.K. Airy Shaw (1902-   )
Ait. – W. Aiton (1731-1793)
Ait. f. – W.T. Aiton (son) (1766-1849)
Alef. – Fredrich Georg Christoph Alefed (1820-1872)
Alston – A.H.G. Alston (1902-1958)
Arn. – George A.W. Arnott (1799-1868)
Aubl. – Jean Baptiste Aublet (1720-1778)
C. Bailey – C. Bailey (1838-1924)
Baill. – Henri E. Baillon (1827-1895)
H.G. Bak. – H. G. Baker
Bakh. – Bakhuizen van der Brink (1881-1945)
Balf. – John Hutton Balfour (1808-1884)
Benth. – George Bentham (1800-1884)
Bertero – C.G. Bertero (1789-1831)
Birdw. –
Blume – Karl L. Blume (1796-1862)
Boenn. – C.M.F. von Boenninghausen (1785-1864)
Boj. – Wenzel Bojer (1797-1856)
R. Br. – Robert Brown (1773-1858)
Brand. – Dietrich Brandis (1824-1907)
Breyn –
Britton – Nathaniel L. Britton (1859-1934)
Beauv. – George Eugene Beauvisage (1852-1925)
Bur. – Edouard Bureau (1830-1918)
Camb. – Jacques Cambessedes (1799-1863)
Cham. – A.L. von Chamisso (1781-1838)
Chev. – F.F. Chevallier (1796-1840)
Choisy – Jacques Denis Choisy (1799-1859)
Clark – Charles B. Clarke (1832-1906)
Comm. – P. Commersom (1727-1773)
Crantz – H.J.N. von Crantz (1722-1797)
Dam –
Dalz. – Alexander Nicolas Dalzell (1817-1878)
DC – Augustin deCandolle (1778-1841)
Del – A.R. Delile (1778-1850)
DeWild – Emile de Wildeman (1866-1947)
Diels – Friedrich L.E. Diels (1874-1945)
Dilile – Alire Raffeneau (1778-1850)
G. Don – George Don (1798-1856)
Drake – Emmanuel Drake del Castillo (1885-1904)
Dutra – João Dutra (1862-1939)
Edmonst – T. Edmonston (1825-1846)
Ehrh. – J.F. Ehrhart (1742-1795)
Engl. – Heinrich G.A. Engler (1844-1930)
Forst. – Johann R. Forster (1729-1798)
Gaertn. – Joseph Gaertner (1732-1791)
Gaertn. f. – Carl Friedrich von Gaertner (son) (1754-1825)

Gaudich – C. Gaudiehoud-Beaupre (1789-1854)
Gilib. – J.E. Gilibert (1741-1814)
Gmel. – Johanmn Georg Gmelin (1709-1755)
Graebn. – Karl Otto R.P.P. Graebner (1871-1933)
Gray – S.F. Gray (1766-1836)
Griseb. – August H.R. Grisebach (1814-1879)
Guill. – Andre Guillaumin (1885-1952)
H.B. & K. – Alexander von Humbold (1769-1859), Aime Bonpland (1773-1858), Karl S. Kunth (1788-1850)
Hassk. – Justus C. Hasskarl (1811-1894)
Hayek. – A.E. von Hayek (1871-1928)
Hepper – F.N. Hepper (1929-   )
Hitchc. – Charles Leo Hitchcock (1902-   )
Hiern. – William P. Hiern (1839-1925)
Hook. f. – Joseph D. Hooker (1817-1911)
Hua – Henri Hua (1861-1919)
Hutch. – John B. Hutchinson (1884-1972)
Ilj. – Alexei Iljinsky (1888-1945)
Jacq. – Nicolaus J. von Jacquin (1727-1817)
Juss. – Antoine L. de Jussieu (1748-1836)
Kotschy – Carl. G.T. Kotschy (1813-1866)
Kunth – Karl S. Kunth (1788-1850)
Kuntz. – Karl E. O. Kuntze (1843-1907)

L. – Carolus Linnaeus (C. Linne) (1707-1778)
L. f. – Carl von Linne (son) (1741-1783)
Lam. – J.B.A.P. de Lamarck (1744-1829)
Lem. – Charles Antoine Lemaire (1801-1871)
Less. – Christian F. Lessing (1809-1862)
Link – Johann H.F. Link (1767-1851)
Lodd. – Conrad Loddige (1732-1826)
Lour. – A. Lourteig (1913-   )
Mart. – Carl F. P. von Martius (1794-1868)
Maxim. – Karl J. Maximowicz (1827-1891)
Meissen. – C.F. Meissner (1800-1874
Merat – F.V. Merat (1780-1851)
Mill. – P. Miller (1691-1771)
Millsp. – Charles F. Millspaugh (1854-1923)
Milne-Redhead – Edgar Milne-Redhead (1906-   )
Miquel – Friedrich Miquel (1811-1871)
Moench – Konrad Moench (1744-1805)
Molina – Juan L. Molina (1740 [1737]-1829)
Moon – Alexander Moon (?-1825)
Moore, J.W. – John William Moore (1901-   )
Nees. – Christian G.D. Neese von Esenbeck (1776-1858)
Oken – Lorenz Oken (1779-1851)
Oliv. – Daniel Oliver (1830-1916)

ABBREVIATIONS OF AUTHORS' NAMES
FOR THE PLANT SPECIES

Park – Mungo Park (1771-1805)
Parkin – John Parkin (1873-1964)
Pav. – Jose Pavon (1750-1844)
Perr. – Claude Perrault
Pers. – C.H. Persoon (1762-1836)
Poir. – Jean Louis M. Poiret (1755-1834)
Rchb. – Heinrich Reichenbach (1793-1879)
A. Rich. – Achille Richard (1794-1852)
Robs. – Norman K.V. Robson (1928-   )
Roscoe – William Roscoe (1753-1831)
Rose – Joseph N. Rose (1862-1928)
Roth – Albrecht Wilhelm Roth (1757-1834)
Ruiz – Hipolito Ruiz Lopez (1754-1815)
Safford – William Edwin Safford (1859-1926)
St. Hill – Auguste de Saint Hilaire (1779-1853)
Sch. Bip. – Karl H. Schultz "Bipontinus"
(1805-1867)
Schott – Heinrich W. Schott (1794-1865)
Schum. – Karl M. Schumann (1851-1904)
Schumach. – H.C.F. Schumacher (1757-1830)
Scop. – G.A. Scopoli (1723-1788)
Seem. – Berthold C. Seeman (1825-1871)
Seib. – P.F. von Siebold (1796-1866)
Ser. – Nicolas C. Seringe (1776-1858)
Sm. – J.E. Smith (1759-1828)
H. Sm. – Henry G. Smith (1852-1924)
Soland – Daniel C. Solander (1733-1782)
Spach – Edouard Spach (1801-1879)
Spreng. – Kurt P.J. Sprengel (1766-1833)
Standl. – Paul Carpenter Standley (1884-1963)
Stapf – Otto Stapf (1857-1933)
Steud. – Ernst G. von Steudel (1783-1856)
Sw. – Olof Peter Swartz (1760-1818)
Taub – S. Taub (1965)
Thell. – A. Thellung (1881-1928)
Thonn. – H. Thonning
Thunb. – Carl P. Thunberg (1743-1828)
Trin. – K.B. von Trinius (1778-1844)
Trotter – Alesandro Trotter (1874-1967)
Ulbr. – Eberhard Ulbrich (1879-1952)
Urb. – Ignatz Urban (1848-1931)
Vahl – Martin H. Vahl (1749-1804)
Viv. – Domenico Viviani (1772-1840)
W. et A. –
Watson, S. – Sereno Watson (1826-1892)
Welw. – Friedrich Martin Welwitsch (1806-1872)
Willd. – Carl L. Willdenow (1765-1812)
Yates – B. Yates
Zucc. – J.G. – J.G. Zuccarini (1797-1848)

BIBLIOGRAPHY

Adams, C.D., *Caribbean Flora*, Thomas Nelson & Sons, Ltd., Nairobi, Kenya, 1967 (61 pp)

Adams, C.D., *Flowering Plants of Jamaica*, Robert MacLehose & Co., Ltd., Great Britain, 1972 (848 pp)

Ainslie, J.R., *A List of Plants Used in Native Medicine in Nigeria*, Forestry Inst., Oxford, 1937

Alan, Donald, *The Powerful Healing Magic of the Evening Primrose*, Reprint from Best Ways, Nevada, Sept., 1981

Allen, Grant, *The Story of the Plants*, D. Appleton & Co., New York, 1895 (218 pp)

Alston, A.H.G., *The Fern and Fern-Allies of West Tropical Africa*, Crown Agents for Overseas Governments, London, 1959 (89 pp)

Anderson, Frank J., *An Illustrated History of the Herbals*, Columbia Univ. Press, New York, 1977 (270 pp)

Ayensu, Edward S., *Medicinal Plants of the West Indies*, Reference Publications, Inc., Algonac, Mich., 1981 (282 pp)

Balls, Edward K., *Early Uses of California Plants*, University of California Press, Berkeley, 1962 (103 pp)

Bannerman, R.H., *Traditional Medicine in Modern Health Care Services*, W.H.O. Geneva Publication #TRM, Feb., 1980

Beebe, William, *The Book of Naturalists*, Alfred A. Knopf, Inc., New York, 1944 (499 pp)

Boedign, K.B. *Plants of the World: The Lower Plants*, W. Gaade Publisher, Netherlands, 1965 (312 pp)

Burtt-Davy, Joseph, & A.C. Hoyle, Ed.s, *Checklist of Forest Trees and Shrubs of Nayasaland*, Oxford, 1933 (111 pp)

Bramly, Serge, *Macumba*, St. Martin's Press, Inc., New York, 1977 (224 pp)

Brazilian Government Trade Bureau, *Medicinal and Useful Plants in Brazil*, 1946 (18 pp)

Bryant, A., C. Struik, *Zulu Medicine and Medicine Men*, Cape Town, 1970

Ciba Foundation Colloquia on Endocrinology, Vol. I *Steroid Hormones and Tumour Growth*, 1952 (315 pp)

Clarke, Charlotte Bringle, *Edible and Useful Plants of California*, University of California Press, Berkeley, 1977 (280 pp)

Cole, J.A. Abayomi, *Astrological Geomancy in Africa*, Women's Printing Society, London, 1898 (23 pp)

Compton, R.H., "An Annotated Check List of the Flora of Swaziland," Supplementary Vol. #6, *Journal of South African Botany*, 1966 (191 pp)

Conway, David, *The Magic of Herbs*, E.P. Dutton & Co., New York, 1973 (158 pp)

Cook, L. Russell, *Chocolate Production and Use*, Catalog & Book Division, Magazine of Industry, Inc., New York, 1963 (463 pp)

Craighead, Frank C., *The Trees of South Florida, Vol. I*, University of Miami Press, Coral Gables, Fl., 1971 (212 pp)

BIBLIOGRAPHY

Dalziel, J.M., *Hausa Botanical Vocabulary,* T. Fisher Unwin, Ltd., London, 1916 (119 pp)

Dalziel, J.M. *Useful Plants of West Africa,* Crown Agents for Overseas Gov., London, 1956

Dash, V.B. V.L. Kashyap, *Basic Principles of Ayurveda,* Concept Pub. Co., New Delhi, 1980

Dawodu, T.B., *A Provisional List of the Indigenous and Naturalised Flowering Plants of the Town and Island of Lagos and Etube Metta District,* Etube Metta, 1902, (22 pp)

Das, Sudhir Kumar, *Medicinal, Economic and Useful Plants of India,* Prachi Gobeson, Calcutta, India Undated (128 pp)

Dawson, A.G., *Health, Happiness and the Pursuit of Herbs,* The Stephen Green Press, Brattleboro, Vt., 1980 (278 pp)

Dayton, W.A., *Glossary of Botanical Terms Commonly Used in Range Research,* USDA # 110, 1931

DeWit, H.C.D., *Plants of the World, The Higher Plants I,* E.P. Dutton & Co., Inc., New York, 1966 (335 pp)

DeWit, H.C.D., *Plants of the World, The Higher Plants II,* E.P. Dutton & Co., Inc., New York, 1967 (340 pp)

Diguangco, Jose, *Philippine Medicinal Plants,* University of Santo Tomas Press, Manila 1950 (146 pp)

Dalziel, J.M., *Hausa Botanical Vocabulary,* T. Fisher Unwin, Ltd., London, 1916 (119 pp)

Dalziel, J.M. *Useful Plants of West Africa,* Crown Agents for Overseas Gov., London, 1956

Dash, V.B. V.L. Kashyap, *Basic Principles of Ayurveda,* Concept Pub. Co., New Delhi, 1980

Dawodu, T.B., *A Provisional List of the Indigenous and Naturalised Flowering Plants of the Town and Island of Lagos and Etube Metta District,* Etube Metta, 1902, (22 pp)

Das, Sudhir Kumar, *Medicinal, Economic and Useful Plants of India,* Prachi Gobeson, Calcutta, India Undated (128 pp)

Dawson, A.G., *Health, Happiness and the Pursuit of Herbs,* The Stephen Green Press, Brattleboro, Vt., 1980 (278 pp)

Dayton, W.A., *Glossary of Botanical Terms Commonly Used in Range Research,* USDA # 110, 1931

DeWit, H.C.D., *Plants of the World, The Higher Plants I,* E.P. Dutton & Co., Inc., New York, 1966 (335 pp)

DeWit, H.C.D., *Plants of the World, The Higher Plants II,* E.P. Dutton & Co., Inc., New York, 1967 (340 pp)

Diguangco, Jose, *Philippine Medicinal Plants,* University of Santo Tomas Press, Manila 1950 (146 pp)

Doane, Doris Chase and King Keyes, *How to Read Tarot Cards,* Funk & Wagnalls, A division of Readers Digest Books, Inc., New York, 1967 (207 pp)

Dorland's Medical Dictionary, Twenty Fifth Edition, W.B. Saunders Co., Philadelphia, London, Toronto, 1974

Espinal, Luis Sigifredo, *Plantas De La Medicina Popular En Cali,* Universidad Del Valle, Departmento De Biologia, 1968 (26 pp)

Esau, Katherine, *Plant Anatomy, Second Edit 'n,* John Wiley & Sons, Inc., New York, London, Sydney, 1953 (7676 pp)

Fairchild, David, *Exploring for Plants*, The MacMillan Company, New York, 1930 (591 pp)

Fernarld, Merritt Lyndon, & Alfred Charles Kinsey, *Edible Wild Plants of Eastern North America*, Idlewild Press, Cornwall-on-Hudson, N.Y. 1943 (452 pp)

Fielder, Mildred, *Plant Medicine and Folklore*, Winchester Press, New York, 1975 (268 pp)

Fisher, Helen Field and Gretchen Harshbarger, *The Flower Family Album*, University of Minnesota, 1941 (131 pp)

Florida Cooperative Extension Service, University of Florida, "Florida Weeds, Part I," a supplement to *Weeds of the Southern United States*, Circular 331, May, 1969 (10 pp)

Florida Cooperative Extension Service, University of Florida, "Florida Weeds, Part II," a supplement to *Weeds of the Southern United States*, Circular 419, (19 pp)

Florida Department of Education, Division of Vocational Education, *Plant Classification, Selection and Identification*, Tallahassee, Fl., 1977 (138 pp)

Florida Department of Education, Division of Vocational Educational, *A Guide to the Identification and Selection of Florida Ornamental Plants*, Tallahassee, 1977 (224 pp)

Ford, R.I., *The Nature and Status of Ethnobotany*, Edited with M.F. Brown, M. Hodge, & W.L. Merril, Ann Arbor, 1978

Foster, E.W., *Notes on Nigerian Trees and Plants*, Guildford, England, 1914 (69 pp)

Gamache, Henri, *The Magic of Herbs*, 6th Printing, Sheldon Publications, New York, Undated (96 pp)

Gilbert-Carter, H., *Glossary of the British Flora, 2nd Edition*, Cambridge, 1955 (88 pp)

Gottlieb, Karen, *Aloe Vera Heals—The Scientific Facts*, Royal Publications, Inc., Colorado, 1980 (31 pp)

Green, Aleph, "The Qabalistic Model of Wholeness," *Journal of Holistic Health*, Mandala Society, San Diego, CA 1975-76 (pg 96-101)

Greenway, P.J., *Swahili-Botanical-English Dictionary of Plant Names*, East African Agricultural Research Station, Amani, Tangayaki Territory, 1940 (308 pp)

Gonzales-Wippler, Migene, *Santeria: Caribbean Magic Cults*, Anchor Press, New York, 1976 (178 pp)

Gonzales-Wippler, Migene, *Santeria: Magia Africana en Latinoamerica*, The Julian Press, Inc., New York, 1976 (183 pp)

Hall, Manley P., *The Secret Teachings of All Ages*, The Philosophical Research Society, Inc., Los Angeles, CA, 1977 (245 pp)

Harris, Jessie Eubank, *Legend and Stories of Famous Trees*, Dorrance and Company, PA (77 pp)

Heath, A.E., *Scientific Thought in the Twentieth Century*, Watts & Co., London, 1951 (387 pp)

Hellyer,, A.G.L., *Sander's Encyclopaedia of Gardening*, The Hamlyn Publishing Group Ltd., London, New York, 1971, 1972

Hepper, F.N., and Fiona Neate, *Plant Collectors in West Africa*, A. Ooshoeks' Uitgeversmaatchappij N.V., International Bureau for Plant Taxonomy and Nomenclature, Netherlands, 1971

Herb Society of America, *The Herbalist*, #3%, Boston, MA, 1967

Herb Society of America, *Herbs for Use and Delight*, Boston, MA 1974 (323 pp)

Heslop-Harrison, J., *New Concepts in Flowering Plant Taxonomy*, Heinemann Ltd., London, 1953 (135 pp)

Higgins, Vera, *The Naming of Plants*, Longman, Green & Co., London, 1937 (103 pp)

Holland, J.H., *The Useful Plants of Nigeria*, Bulletin Misc. Info, Kew, 1908

Holt, Rachman, *George Washington Carver*, Doubleday, Doran & Co., Inc., New York, 1944 (342 pp)

Hooker, J.D. & George Bentham, *Flora Nigritiana*, London, 1849

Howes, F.N., *Vegetable Gums and Resins*, Chronica Botanica Co., Waltham, MA, 1949 (188 pp)

Hsu, Hon-Yen and William Peacher, *Chinese Herb Medicine and Therapy*, Oriental Healing Arts Institute, Hawaiian Gardens, CA & Aurora Publishers, Inc. Nashville, TN, 1976 (223 pp)

Humphreys, W.J., *Weather Proverbs and Paradoxes*, William & Wilkins Co., 1923 (125 pp)

Hutchinson, John, *A Contribution to the Flora of Northern Nigeria*, Bulletin Misc. Info., Kew, 1921

Hutchinson, J., *The Families of Flowering Plants*, The Clarendon Press, London, 1973 (968 pp)

Index Kewensis, *Plantarum Phanerogamarum Supplementum XVI*, Benthm-Moxon Trustees, Oxford University Press, New York, 1981 (309 pp)

Irvine, F.R., *Woody Plants of Ghana*, Oxford University Press, Amen House, London, 1961 (868 pp)

Jackson, B.D., *A Glossary of Botanic Terms*, Duckworth & Co., Philadelphia, J.B. Lippincott Co., London, 1916 (428 pp)

Jacobs, M.D. and H.M. Burlage, *Index of Plants of North Carolina With Reputed Medicinal Uses*, 1958 (322 pp)

Jain, S.K., *Medicinal Plants*, National Book Trust, India, 1968 (176 pp)

James, George G.M., *Stolen Legacy*, Richardson Associates, Publishers, San Francisco, 1976 (190 pp)

Jeffrey, C., *An Introduction to Plant Taxonomy*, J. & A. Churchill Ltd., London, 1968 (128 pp)

Jenkins, Glenn L., and Walter H. Hartung, *The Chemistry of Organic Medicinal Products*, Third Edition, John Wiley & Sons, Inc., New York, 1950 (745 pp)

Jimma Experimental Station, Bulletin No. 14, *Useful Plants of Ethiopia*, University of Addis Abba, 1960

Johnson, Arthur Monrad, *Taxonomy of the Flowering Plants*, The Century Co., New York & London, 1931 (864 pp)

Kaaiakamanu, D.M. and J.K. Akina, *Hawaiian Herbs of Medicinal Value*, Pacific Book House, Honolulu, Hawaii, 1922 (74 pp)

Kennedy, J.D., *Forest Flora of Southern Nigeria*, Lagos, 1936 (242 pp)

Kew, Royal Botanic Gardens, *Indigenous Plants of Yorubaland*, Bulletin Misc. Info., 1891 & 1908

Kew, Royal Botanic Gardens, *The Timbers of Southern Nigeria*, Bulletin Misc. Info, 1908

BIBLIOGRAPHY

Kellman, Martin C., *Plant Geography, Second Edition,* St. Martin's Press, Inc., New York, 1980 (181 pp)

Klein, Richard M., *The Green World: An Introduction to Plants and People,* Harper & Row, New York, 1979 (437 pp)

Kloss, Jethro, *Back to Eden,* Beneficial Books, New York, 1971 (671 pp)

Korach, Karen A., *Botanical Art & Illustration,* Pennsylvania, 1972 (187 pp)

Kunkel, Gunther, *The Vegetation of Hormoz, Qeshm and Neighbouring Islands (Southern Persia Gulf Area),* Strause and Cramer, Gmbh, Germany, 1977 (186 pp)

Lawson, G.W., *Plant Life in West Africa,* Oxford University Press, 1966 (150 pp)

Lely, H.V., *The Useful Trees of Northern Nigeria,* London, 1925 (128 pp)

Li, C.P., *Chinese Herbal Medicine,* U.S. Department of Health, Education and Welfare Publication No. (NIH) 75-732, 1974 (120 pp)

Li, Shih-chen, Porter F. Smith and G.A. Stuart, *Chinese Medicinal Herbs,* Georgetown Press, San Francisco, CA 1973

Linnean Society Symposium Series No. 10, *The Plant Cuticle,* U.S. Edition by Academic Press, Inc., 1982 (461 pp)

Leakey, Richard E., *The Illustrated Origins of Species by Charles Darwin,* The Rainbow Publishing Group, Ltd., 1979

Leyel, C.F., *Elixers of Life,* Edinburgh, Scotland, 1970 (220 pp)

Liogier, A.H., *Diccionario Botanico de Nombres Vulgares de la Española,* Santo Domingo, D.N. 1974 (813 pp)

Lundell, Cyrus, *Botany of the Maya,* Misc. Papers, Carnegie Institution of Washington, Publication #522, 1949

MacKnight, T.M., *Food for the Tropics,* W. Thacker & Co., 1904 (116 pp)

MacMillan, H.F., *Tropical Planting and Gardening,* MacMillan & Co., Ltd., London, 1956 (560 pp)

Mann, Felix, *Acupuncture: The Ancient Chinese Art of Healing and How it Works Scientifically,* Vintage Books, New YOrk, 1962

Mansfield, Louise, *An Artists's Herbal,* The MacMillan Company, New York, 1937 (77 pp)

Martin, Alexander C., *Weeds,* Western Publishing Company, Inc., 1972 (160 pp)

Martin, Keble W., *The Concise British Flora in Colour,* George Rainbird, Ltd., London, 1971, (254 pp)

Maxwell, Lewis S., *Florida Fruit,* Author/Publisher, Florida, 1967 (120 pp)

Mascarehnas, Ophelia, *A Preliminary Guide to Traditional Medicine in Tanzania,* Research Report No. 13 of the Bureau of Resource Assessment and Land Use Planning, University of Dar-Es-Ealaam, April, 1975

Mesmer, F.A., and George J. Bloch, Ph.D., editor, *Mesmerism: A Translation of the Original Medical and Scientific Writings of F.A. Mesmer, M.D.,* William Kaufmann, Inc., Los Altos, CA., 1981

Moore, David M., *Flora of Tierra del Fuego,* Anthony Nelson, England & Missouri Botanical Gardens, U.S.A., 1983 (396 pp)

Morton, Julia F., *Atlas of Medicinal Plants of Middle America, Bahamas to Yucatan*, Charles C. Thomas, Publisher, Springfield, Ill., 1981

Munz, Philip A., *California Mountain Wildflowers*, University of California Press, 1963 (122 pp)

Muhammed, Amir, Rustem Aksel and R.C. Borstel, *Genetic Diversity in Plants*, Plenum Press, New York, 1977 (506 pp)

Nelson, Alexander, *Medical Botany*, Edinburgh, Scotland, 1951 (544 pp)

North Carolina Flower Preservation Society, Inc., *North Carolina Native Plant Propagation Handbook*

Ossadcha-Janata, Natalia, *Herbs Used in Ukrainian Folk Medicine*, Research Program on the U.S.S.R. and the New York Botanical Garden, New York, 1952 (114 pp)

Parsons, Mary E., *The Wild Flowers of California*, Dover Publications, Inc., New York, 1966 (425 pp)

Pelaiseul, Jean, *The Green Guide to Health from Plants*, Redwood Burn, Ltd., 1977 (292 pp)

Perkins, K.D. and Willard W. Payne, *Guide to the Poisonous and Irritant Plants of Florida*, University of Florida Press, 1978 Circular 441

Perry, Mac, *Landscape Your Home*, E.A. Seeman Publishing, Inc., Miami, FL, 1972 (172 pp)

Phillips, Henry, *History of Cultivated Vegetables*, Henry Colburn & Co., London, Undated (432 pp)

Pursglove, John W., *Tropical Crops Dicotyledons I*, Longman, Green & Co., Great Britain, 1968, (332 pp)

Pursglove, John W., Tropical Crops Dicotyledons II, Longman, Green & Co., Great Britain, 1968 (719 pp)

Read, Bernard E., *Chinese Medicinal Plants from the Pen Ts'ao Kang Mu*, Peking Natural History Bulletin Publisher, Shanghai, China, 1936 (391 pp)

Rendel, A.B. E.G. Baker, H.F. Wernham, and L. LeM. Moore, *Catalogue of the Plants of the Oban District, South Nigeria*, London, 1913

Rennie, Professor, *Alphabet of Medical Botany*, Orr and Smith Publisher, London, 1833

Revolutionary Health Committee of Hunan Province, *A Barefoot Doctor's Manual, Revised and Enlarged Edition*, Madrona Publishers, Seattle, WA, 1977

Riva, Anna, *The Modern Herbal Spellbook*, International Imports, California, 1974 (74 pp)

Roberts, Daniel A., *Fundamentals of Plant Pest Control*, W.H. Freeman & Co., San Francisco, 1978

Robson, Vivian, *The Fixed Stars and Constellations in Astrology*, Samuel Weiser, Inc., New York, 1969

Rose, Donna, *Santeria: The Cuban-African Magical System*, Mi-World Publishing, Miami, 1980

Rose, Donna, *The Magic of Herbs*, Mi-World Publishing, Miami, 1978 (27 pp)

Sarton, George, *A Guide to the History of Science*, Chronica Botanica Co., Waltham, MA, 1952 (316 pp)

Schuman, Henry, *Main Currents of Scientific Thought: A History of Sciences*, New York, 1953 (520 pp)

BIBLIOGRAPHY

Sire, Marcel, *Secrets of Plant Life*, The Viking Press, New York, 1967 (140 pp)

Sofowora, Abayomi, *Medicinal Plants and Traditional Medicine in Africa*, John Wiley, New York, 1982 (234 pp)

Stearn, William T., *Botanical Latin*, Thomas Nelson Printers Ltd, London, 1966 (566 pp)

Stephenson, J., and H. Churchill, *Who's Who in Science International*, 1913 (572 pp)

Steyn, Douw G., *The Toxicology of Plants in South Africa*, Wm. Clowes & Sons, London, 1934 (631 pp)

Storer, John H., *The Web of Life*, New York, 1953 (142 pp)

Stott, Philip, *Historical Plant Geography: An Introduction*, Allen & Unwin, 1981 (151 pp)

Strybing Arboretum Society, San Francisco, *Garden Guide* 1977 (25 pp)

Sunset Magazine, *Sunset New Western Garden Book*, 4th Edition, 1979 (512 pp)

Swain, Tony, *Plants in the Development of Modern Medicine*, Harvard University Press, Cambridge, MA, and London, England, 1972 (367 pp)

Swift, Lloyd H., *Botanical Classifications: A Comparison of Eight Systems of Angiosperm Classification*, The Shoe-string Press, Inc., Hamden CN, 1974

Synge, Patrick M., *Plants with Personality*, E.P. Dutton & Co., Inc., New York (244 pp)

Symposium, *The HIstory of Science Origins and Results of the Scientific Revolution*, Cohen & West, Ltd., London,1951 (184 pp)

Symposium, *Tropical Botany*, University of Aarhus, Edited by Kai Larsen and Lauritz B. Holm-Nielsen, Academy Press Inc., Ltd., London, 1979 (453 pp)

Temple, Robert, *The Sirius Mystery*, St. Martin's Press, N2ew York, 1976 (290 pp)

Tetenyi, Peter, *Infra-specific Chemical Taxa of Medicinal Plants*, Akademiai Kiado, Budapest, Hungary, 1970 (225 pp)

Tompkins, Peter and Christopher Bird, *The Secret Life of Plants*, Harper & Row, Inc., New York, 1973 (402 pp)

UNESCO, *Medicinal Plants of the Arid Zones*, Paris, France, 1960

U.S. Department of Agriculture, Forest Service, Agricultural Handbook No. 41, *Check List of Native and Naturalized Trees of the United States Including Alaska*, 1953 (472 pp)

U.S. Department of Agriculture, Federal Extension Service, *Weeds of the Southern United States*, 1969 (42 pp)

Veith, Ilza, *The Yellow Emperor's Classic on Internal Medicine*, Translated, New Edition, University of California Press, Berkeley, 1966

Verdoorn, Frans. *Plants and Science in Latin America*, The Chronica Botanica Co., Waltham, MA 1945 (383 pp)

Verdcourt, Behard, and L.C. Trump, *Common Poisonous Plants of East Africa*, Collins, London, 1969

Verrill, A. Hyatt, *Wonder Plants and Plant Wonders*, Appleton-Century Co., Inc., 1939 (296 pp)

Watkins, John V., *Your Guide to Florida Landscape Plants*, University of Florida Press, 1961 (293 pp)